PSYCHOPATHOLOGY AND PHILOSOPHY OF MIND

This book explores how the human mind works through the lens of psychological disorders, challenging many existing theoretical constructs, especially in the fields of psychology, psychiatry, and philosophy of mind.

Drawing on the expertise of leading academics, the book discusses how psychopathology can be used to inform our understanding of the human mind. The book argues that studying mental disorders can deepen the understanding of psychological mechanisms such as reasoning, emotions, and beliefs alongside fundamental philosophical questions, including the nature of the self, the universal aspects of morality, and the role of rationality and normativity in human nature. By crossing different domains, this book offers a fresh perspective on the human mind based on the dialogue between philosophy, cognitive science, and clinical psychology. Mental disorders discussed include schizophrenia, anxiety disorders, major depression, obsessive-compulsive disorder, post-traumatic stress disorder, and paranoia.

This book caters to the increasing interest in interdisciplinary approach to solving some of the problems in psychopathology. Since this book treats psychological engagement with empirically informed philosophy of mind, it is essential reading for students and researchers of cognitive psychology, clinical psychology, and philosophy, as well as being of interest to clinicians and psychiatrists.

Valentina Cardella is Associate Professor of Philosophy of Language at the University of Messina, Italy. Her research interests encompass cognitive sciences, philosophy of language, and psychopathology. She is author of several books and papers on various topics of interest.

Amelia Gangemi is Full Professor of General Psychology at the University of Messina, Italy. Her research activity is in the area of thinking; she is, moreover, focused on examining the different ways in which emotional and motivational states affect intelligence and reasoning. She is author of several books and papers on various topics of interest.

PSYCHOPATHOLOGY AND PHILOSOPHY OF MIND

What Mental Disorders Can Tell Us About Our Minds

Edited by Valentina Cardella and Amelia Gangemi

Routledge
Taylor & Francis Group
LONDON AND NEW YORK

First published 2021
by Routledge
2 Park Square, Milton Park, Abingdon, Oxon OX14 4RN

and by Routledge
52 Vanderbilt Avenue, New York, NY 10017

Routledge is an imprint of the Taylor & Francis Group, an informa business

British Library Cataloguing-in-Publication Data
A catalogue record for this book is available from the British Library

Library of Congress Cataloging-in-Publication Data
A catalog record for this book has been requested

ISBN: 978-0-36744-457-0 (hbk)
ISBN: 978-0-36744-458-7 (pbk)
ISBN: 978-1-00300-985-6 (ebk)

Typeset in Bembo
by Apex CoVantage, LLC

This book is dedicated to our fathers, Antonio and Alfredo.
We miss you.

CONTENTS

CONTRIBUTORS

1 **Ines Adornetti,** University of Roma 3, Italy
2 **Isabelle Blanchette,** Université Laval, Canada
3 **Domenica Bruni,** University of Messina, Italy
4 **Alessandro Capodici,** University of Messina, Italy
5 **Valentina Cardella,** University of Messina, Italy
6 **Alessandra Falzone,** University of Messina, Italy
7 **Francesco Ferretti,** University of Roma 3, Italy
8 **Niall Galbraith,** University of Wolverhampton, UK
9 **Shaun Gallagher,** University of Memphis, TN, and University of Wollongong, United Arab Emirates
10 **Amelia Gangemi,** University of Messina, Italy
11 **Sara-Valérie Giroux,** Université du Québec à Trois-Rivières, Canada
12 **Philip N. Johnson-Laird,** Princeton University, NJ, and New York University, New York
13 **Francesco Mancini,** School of Cognitive Psychotherapy, Rome, Italy
14 **Antonino Pennisi,** University of Messina, Italy
15 **Giovanni Pennisi,** University of Messina, Italy
16 **Pietro Perconti,** University of Messina, Italy
17 **Guyonne Rogier,** School of Cognitive Psychotherapy, Roma, Italy
18 **Francesco Paolo Tocco,** University of Messina, Italy
19 **Leonarda Valana,** University of Messina, Italy

PREFACE

This book adopts a perspective which results from the interfaces between philosophy and cognitive psychology. The idea is that studying mental disorders can deepen our understanding of both psychological mechanisms, like reasoning, emotions, beliefs, and fundamental philosophical questions, like the nature of the self, the universal aspects of morality, the underpinnings of concepts like normality and normativity. Since mental disorders affect different, fundamental aspects of the human mind, they shed light on the mechanisms these aspects are grounded in, and, at the same time, they challenge many theoretical constructs, especially in the field of psychology, psychiatry, and philosophy of mind. Psychopathology is a challenging field, and this book aims to show how it can be used to inform our understanding of the human mind.

Part 1 of this book explores the way psychopathologies, from anxiety disorders and obsessive-compulsive disorder to schizophrenia and paranoia, offer a window into 'normal' cognition.

The opening chapter investigates the role of the mental in mental disorders. Cardella aims to show that the notion of mental disorders used by most psychiatrists is based on some philosophical assumptions, and that those assumptions are largely unwarranted. More precisely, the author focuses on realism and reductionism in psychiatry, that is, the idea that mental disorders are independent of the observer, and that they are essentially disturbances of the brain, showing that both of those assumptions are flawed. She argues then that a distinctive feature of psychiatric disorders is that they need the vocabulary concerning the mental, and she finally highlights the role of personal experience and ethics in psychiatry.

In Chapter 2, Johnson-Laird, one of the most influential psychologists of our times, presents his hyper-emotion theory of psychological disorders. His view is that mental illnesses are emotional disorders, in that their initial cause is a transition to an unusually intense emotion. Since individuals are aware of the emotion but don't know what caused its excessive intensity, they focus on it, and activate the deliberative system of thinking trying to understand it. But this kind of reasoning paradoxically amplify the emotion itself, and leads to a recursive loop between cognitions and emotions. Thus, mental illnesses can be defined as self-perpetuating hyper-emotions. The author highlights that the analysis of how patients reason and what they feel leads to a conclusion which is at odds with cognitive therapies. The latter rest on the assumption that patients make reasoning mistakes and hold irrational beliefs. But, in his chapter, Johnson-Laird shows not only that their reasoning is as good as that of control participants, but also that it is even better about the topics of their illnesses.

In Chapter 3, Gangemi and Mancini focus on the relationship between reasoning and goals. They claim that the analysis of the psychological illnesses' maintenance, one of the mysteries of psychopathology, indirectly shows something valid for pathological and healthy people, too, i.e., that reasoning is a tool at the service of our goals. More precisely, both normal and abnormal people choose the kind of reasoning that best helps them to achieve or protect their goals and reduce the costs of crucial errors. The authors show how this happens, in a context of danger, in the case of reasoning on danger hypothesis, where a confirmatory reasoning strategy is activated by both healthy and pathological people (i.e., in anxiety disorders), and in the case of safety hypothesis, where normal and abnormal individuals seek for falsifications. Finally, Gangemi and Mancini provide evidence that psychopathology would even improve reasoning, rather than worsening it, but only when topics are relevant to the disorder.

On the other hand, reasoning and emotions, and their interaction, are the topics of Chapter 4. Blanchette and Giroux focus on trauma because the interaction between emotion and cognition is involved in the very definition of it: trauma is an event that involves actual or threatened death or serious injury, and that evokes a specific emotional response of the victim (e.g., fear, helplessness, horror). Trauma studies provide important insights regarding the interaction between emotions and cognition, which can also have implications for ordinary emotional experiences. For example, although trauma usually decreases access to analytical reasoning, this effect can be mitigated by personal relevance. Another crucial insight is that higher level cognitive processes affect the encoding of emotional experiences. More precisely, symbolic processing, IQ, and education seem to have a protective influence. The authors also show the implications of these data in terms of psychological interventions.

In Chapter 5, Mancini, Rogier, and Gangemi focus on the feeling of guilt, or, better, the feelings of guilt. Psychopathology, and obsessive-compulsive disorder and major depression in particular, seem to show that there are admittedly two guilt experiences: deontological and altruistic. Their dualistic thesis affirms the non-reducibility of one guilt feeling to the other, contrasting the earlier monistic theses in which guilt feelings are described as the results of both the transgression of a moral norm, and harming a victim. In obsessive-compulsive disorder, different obsessions hide the same thing, the fear of being guilty, but this feeling is linked to the transgression of a moral norm. Even if there are no victims, even if no-one has been harmed, the feeling stays the same. In major depression, on the other hand, the presence of altruistic guilt is crucial; this can arise from the failure of one of two altruistic goals, closeness to the victim (not only physical closeness to the victim but also the sharing of the respective ill-luck or the participation in the suffering), or the sharing of one's joys with the other. All in all, this chapter shows how psychopathologies can enrich our psychological and philosophical view of morality.

In Chapter 6, Adornetti and Ferretti investigate the narrative self in one of the most severe mental disorders: schizophrenia. An increasing number of empirical findings have started to show that schizophrenic patients have an impaired dimension of the self, which involves both inability to temporally organize the events determining their personal identity and difficulty to extract meaning from these events. Narratives are generally considered a product of linguistic abilities, and thus the impairments showed by schizophrenics in the narrative self are usually ascribed to their alterations in language use. In contrast with this view, the authors claim that disorders of the self in schizophrenia are due to dysfunctions in cognitive processes that underlie both narrative and language, rather than reflecting a linguistic nature. To prove that, the authors focus on a specific mechanism, i.e., mental time travel, which governs the ability to project in time, and shows its independency from language and its role both in the construction of the self and in the processing of narrative discourse.

The last chapter of this part, by Galbraith, focuses on the pathologies of belief. The general idea of the author is that all psychotic disorders are related, and lie along an illness continuum (pace Kraepelin and the traditional psychiatry, which consider psychoses as discrete entities distinct from normal behaviour). Family studies, psychotic-like experiences in healthy individuals, and psychometric data all seem to provide evidence for this continuum model. Galbraith then considers the continuum of belief, i.e., how beliefs fit into the spectrum of psychosis, and, on the other side, how delusions are continuous with other beliefs. He shows evidence that paranormal beliefs feature in both psychotic delusions and subclinical delusional ideas, thus supporting the notion of a continuum of belief. Finally, he focuses on a specific kind of implausible belief: conspiracy theories. Conspiracy beliefs share many features with delusional ideas, like the presence of unwarranted claims and misinterpreted evidence, paranoid ideation, the need for cognitive closure, the preference to rely on intuitive judgements. This chapter concludes with a look at the role of social media, which easily propagate and reinforce conspiracy theories and other implausible beliefs, in a way that was inconceivable just a few decades ago.

Part 2 of this book collects contributions that lie at the intersection between psychopathology and philosophy, and that focus on the most specific features of human nature: language, normativity, morality, love, rationality, and identity.

Chapter 8 is dedicated to a preliminary, crucial concept for psychopathology, which is nevertheless very difficult to define: that of normality. Thanks to his historical background, Tocco offers a new way to look at this notion, through the analysis of the way insanity and madness were conceptualized throughout history, and focusing particularly on linguistic landmarks. In his survey, normality first appears in the Middle Ages, with a semantic field connected to 'rule', and to the Latin word 'norma', which originally indicated the carpenter's square. Until the medieval period, madness was a piece of the social world, but after that, we assist to both a linguistic process, in which the word 'normal' drifts from 'establishment of rules' to 'the usual and common functioning', and a social process, where 'abnormal' are marginalized, and finally hospitalized. The chapter concludes with the analysis of what is left of normality's conception today; Tocco claims that the apparent 'objectivity' of modern psychiatry, which speaks no more of 'abnormality', is another, new form of the psychiatric power, that, by its biological stance, tries to remove the social stigma, but yet offers pathological labels for every kind of oddity or distress, unreasonably increasing the number of mental illnesses.

Moral judgement and its relation with normativism are the topics of Chapter 9. After focusing on the way normality and normativity are conceived within the sciences of mental health, Vaiana investigates two approaches, legal practice and clinical practice, respectively, pointing out the necessary differences but also their interaction in the field of psychiatry. Then, to explore the way psychopathology can challenge the philosophical approach to ethical issues, she compares experimental psychology on moral reasoning and Kant's moral findings on mental disorders, finding unexpected consonances. Both seem to identify the distinctive features of mental disorder as the loss of common sense, which is replaced by a private sense, and a characteristic form of radical egoism.

Chapter 10 focuses on language through the lens of schizophrenia. Cardella and Falzone aim to show that language has some dark sides, and that schizophrenia reveals them. They start with the analysis of disorganized language, one of the most important features of schizophrenia, and focus then on the deep linguistic awareness showed by schizophrenic people. Furthermore, they describe how language is involved in the other typical symptoms of schizophrenia, hallucinations and delusions, showing that lives a life of its own, haunts the patients' heads with voices, and fills the world with meaning. In sum, the authors provide evidence of the fact that language is not just an aspect of schizophrenia, but something that has to do with the nature of this disorder.

In Chapter 11, Perconti focuses on the role of narratives in mental disorders. His claim, at odds with the recent growing popularity of narratives, is that the idea that most of the mental disorders involve the inability to manage personal stories in the right way is fundamentally wrong. Such view, according to which wrong stories are the mark of mental illness, while consistent narratives are the sign of a healthy inner life, essentially reflects an ethical stance. In other words, it is taken for granted that it is a value for individuals to always control their preferences and behaviour, and to create coherent stories through autobiography and public narratives. Perconti will show that personal identity is not only shaped by stories and storytelling, but also by psychological episodes and non-conceptual experiences.

In Chapter 12, Pennisi and Capodici analyse the phenomenology of a very peculiar syndrome, Body Integrity Dysphoria (BID), in which subjects aspire to the amputation or functional/sensory deprivation of a healthy body part. Focusing on this disorder that shows how the real body and the desired body can conflict, the authors aim to study the living body in a different, original way. Though a neurological origin is very likely, in BID other factors seem to play a crucial role, like a first phase of vulnerability in childhood, the neuroplastic retroaction related to simulation, and the influence of culture and sharing of experiences. The authors investigate the first-person perspective of those living with the BID also through a qualitative questionnaire, showing that the building up of the body image is a complex construct, made by neurological, cultural, social, and environmental factors.

In Chapter 13, Bruni shows us the dark side of love. Her claim is that love shapes the human nature in a unique, peculiar way, but, at the same time, it is a kind of addiction that can force people into pathological pathways. The perspective adopted by the author is the evolutionary one, which follows the traces of our biological history. According to this view, what we call 'romantic love' is a developed form of the mechanisms that have evolved in animals to attract conspecifics, and it is associated with the dopaminergic reward system, the circuit which controls motivation, associative learning, and emotions involving pleasure. For both evolutionary and neurobiological reasons, romantic love can be compared to a form of addiction, in that it shows all the typical symptoms of it: persistent desire, ecstasy, salience, mood swings, distortion of reality, anxiety, abstinence, and craving. This is also more evident when a love story ends, as Bruni shows in the last part of the chapter, dedicated to love rejection and its typical phases, protest and despair.

Finally, the last chapter is dedicated to one of the typical features attributed to human beings: rationality. Moving away from an intellectualist view of rationality, which conceives it as a series of syllogistic and inferential abilities relying entirely on the use of language, Pennisi and Gallagher develop the notion of embodied rationality, a kind of rationality which is deeply rooted on body-schematic processes and that involves performative awareness. The authors then show that in schizophrenia, there is a breakdown of this kind of rationality, which patients try to compensate through hyper-reflexivity and morbid rationalism, that is an exaggerated awareness of one's own body and a tendency to conceive all aspects of life under a set of schematic and often algorithmic rules. In the final part of the chapter, Pennisi and Gallagher investigate the consequences of this disembodied rationality in schizophrenia, i.e., the breakdown in body-schematic processes and the disruption of the protentional function of time consciousness.

PART 1

Cognition in the light of psychopathology

1

A PRELIMINARY STEP

Understanding the mental in mental disorders

Valentina Cardella

1 The challenge of psychopathology

A man is at his first meeting in acute inpatient care. He talks to the psychiatrist about his recent discovery: he is decomposing. During the session, he gives some evidence of this belief (e.g., the strong smell he can perceive, the worms he feels inside his body), and talks about the precautions he's taking (for example, he puts hydrochloric acid on his skin to kill the worms). Here's an excerpt of the interview with the psychiatrist:

Psychiatrist (PS): So . . . do these worms eat organs too?
Patient (PA): I think so.
PS: How do you survive then, when these worms eat your organs?
PA: Well, how do I know?
. . .
PS: Your parents, what do your parents for example say?
PA: They say that it is not true . . .
PS: Okay, they say that it is not true. And the fact that they say that it is not true, does not make you think that it is possible that it is not true, that it is perhaps rather your perception that you have worms in the body?
PA: I am decomposing (*Zangrilli et al.*, 2014: 3–6).

Another patient, with Parkinson's disease (Mr I.) is admitted to the department of neurology; during his meeting with the doctor, his wife is present. Suddenly, Mr I asks if it's alright if he blows in a bottle (something he usually does for his disease). His wife says he can, but adds that it would be better not to do it in public. Then Mr I says: "My wife usually says that too". Her wife's attempts to convince him that she is his wife are unsuccessful. Further during the conversation, while his wife is in a different room, he says that the person accompanying him is extremely like his wife and acts like her, but adds: "Even though she looks like her, it doesn't *feel* like it's her" (Alstadhaug, 2019: 85).

A 31-year-old woman starts seeking medical help for her obsessive-compulsive disorder. She is obsessed with cleaning, spends 12 hours a day cleaning her house and objects, washing clothes, and taking care of her personal hygiene. Every time she comes back home, she wipes down her shoes, bag, and cell phone and those of her husband. She would not dirty the kitchen, so she buys ready-to-eat meals. Her overuse of water and cleaning products has provoked physical injury on her skin, hands, and nails. Yet, she can't help but clean; she just can't stop (Justo et al., 2015).

Jaspers, the founder of modern psychopathology, cites one of his patients to illustrate thought insertion, one of the most bizarre symptoms of schizophrenia. The patient is perceiving an influence over him, and he's aware that the thoughts he's thinking are not his own.

> The thought arises and with it a direct awareness that it is not the patient but some external agent that thinks it. The patient does not know why he has this thought nor did he intend to have it. He does not feel master of his own thoughts and in addition he feels in the power of some incomprehensible external force.
>
> *(Jaspers, 1963: 122–123)*

What exactly happened to those people? We look at them, we listen to them, we read their stories, and we are under the impression that something terribly wrong occurred. How is it possible that they believe impossible things, like that they are decomposing or that their partners have been replaced by a double? How did they end up spending most of their time performing senseless rituals, and being totally absorbed by their obsessions? And, finally, how can they deny such a patent, evident, unmistakable true, as the authorship of their thoughts? To make people act this way, some mental mechanism should have broken down. And then, what happened to their *minds*? What went wrong with them?

Those questions seem absolutely appropriate. But even a trivial question, when including the word 'wrong', is not that trivial after all. 'Wrong' implies 'right', or also 'normal', 'correct', 'common', 'proper'. And those are value judgements. Now, common people, when facing mental illness, can sense that 'wrongness', in an instinctively, pre-theoretically, 'a-scientific' way. But psychiatry is a medical discipline. It has to endorse an objective, impersonal view of abnormal behaviour. It must be so, given that being diagnosed as mentally ill has serious consequences, at the personal, relational, and social levels. One has to be very cautious when a person's life is at stake.

However, what does it mean, for a discipline that deals with human fragility and suffering, to be 'objective'? Is a mental disorder something we can detect in an 'a-theoretic' way? Furthermore, is it possible, for any science, to be impartial, unbiased, absolutely neutral? Every scientific enterprise, every scientific paradigm (Kuhn, 1962) has its philosophical assumptions. The more implicit they are, the more important it is for a philosopher to detect them. Psychiatry makes no exception. In this chapter, I will first outline some of those assumptions which concern the nature of mental disorders. I will show that, despite the claim of being a practical discipline, which only aims to cure people, psychiatry starts from a series of postulations, i.e., notions and beliefs that are widely shared but largely unwarranted. I will criticize those assumptions, showing that most psychiatrists are committed to a notion of mental disorder that is flawed (or at least unjustified) and that neglects the very role of the mental. I will then show the importance, in defining mental disorders, of both a mentalist vocabulary and the reference to norms that are cultural, social, moral, and evaluative. At the end of the chapter, I will outline the importance of ethics in psychiatry.

2 The strange nature of mental disorders

> On the one hand our patients suffer greatly from psychiatric symptoms, and it seems wildly foolish to theorize away their suffering. On the other hand our efforts to organize and classify their suffering can seem arbitrary and confusing. We organize or categorize a symptom cluster and give it a diagnostic name, and it overlaps with another cluster. Or a patient simply has symptoms of both. We start off with the expectation that there will be a match-up between therapeutic agent and diagnostic cluster, and we discover that, at the extreme, most of our pharmacologic agents seem to treat most of our disorders. Finally, we somehow want to resolve this confusion by getting at the underpinnings of the identified disorders, and we discover that the genetics and neuroscience don't support our groupings.
>
> *(Phillips et al., 2012: 4)*

The practice of psychiatry, as described earlier, is very hard. But why is it so? Does it all come down to the mental disorder's label, which is still too elusive, as suggested by Philips and colleagues? Or does the reason lie in the confusion concerning the biological basis of mental disorder, as stated by the same authors at the end of this quote? In other words, is a complete neurobiological framework still to come, and do we only have to wait? I'll come back to these topics later. For the nonce, let's start with a simple question. What are mental disorders?

As strange as it may seem, psychiatry has always been more interested to identify the meaning of the word 'disorder', in the 'mental disorder' label, rather than the word 'mental'. Many authors (see Brulde and Radovis, 2006; Murphy, 2006; Graham, 2013) noted that what precisely is 'mental' in mental disorder remains unclear in the psychiatric literature. The philosopher George Graham, for example, remarks:

> The very idea of the mental deployed in psychiatry as well as in the theory of mental disorder typically is unexamined or at least under-examined by psychiatrists and other writing on mental disorder.
>
> *(Graham, 2013: 30)*

Murphy even claims that "psychiatry contains no principled understanding of the mental" (2006: 61). What does it mean? How is it possible that a medical discipline that has to do with disorders affecting the mind doesn't clarify properly the meaning of mental? I will elucidate this point later on, and, by now, I will come back to the initial question: what are mental disorders? To answer this question, let's start from another one, which looks quite trivial: are mental disorders real? That is, are mental disorders out there, existing independently of the observers, entities which psychiatric categories try to match with better and better? If this is the case, a correct nosography has to *correspond* to these entities, which in turn have to remain much or less the same independently from the historical and social contexts (Patil and Giordano, 2010; Kendler, 2016; Eronen, 2019). In other words, mental disorders should be what they are, regardless of our linguistic practices and social norms.

The claim that mental disorders are real phenomena is the ground for realism in psychiatry. And realism is one of the dominant conceptions of psychiatry; according to this perspective, mental disorders are discrete entities, existing independently of the way we study them, they are, in other words, natural kinds. The strong realist position is both ontological and epistemological (Pouncey, 2005): it has an ontological commitment about the existence of abstract entities called mental disorders, and an epistemological commitment about our possibility to genuinely know them. However, there is also a weaker realism, where the commitment is ontological only; in other words, one can believe that mental disorders exist in nature, but can doubt our capacity to know them as they are. This seems to be a more plausible position, because it is hard to deny that psychiatric categories are constructs, viz., the best attempts to describe mental disorders' abstract entities based on manifest symptoms alone. Thus, the vast majority of psychiatrists probably share this last position; maybe we aren't able to accurately characterize them, but mental disorders really exist out there. After all, does it make sense for a physician to doubt the reality of his patient's disease? The same should be valid for a psychiatrist.

But is this ontological commitment justified? For instance, is there, in nature, something like depression, a category with essential and specific features, that can be described with objectivity and is clearly distinct from other mental disorders? The answer is no, for several reasons. First of all, psychiatric disorders don't have sufficient and necessary conditions. To give an example, the DSM-5's criteria for major depression involve five or more symptoms among a list of nine; thus, no single symptom is sufficient, and, as strange as it may seem, the depressed mood is not even necessary (APA, 2013a). Secondly, the boundaries among psychiatric categories are fuzzy and blurred. For example, despite the claim, that dates back to Kraepelin (1883), that affective disorders and schizophrenia are two distinct categories, experience has shown that there are many hybrid cases (the schizo-affective disorder, see Jablensky, 2016), and the same can be said of affective disorder and personality disorders, or depression and anxiety disorders, or addiction and psychiatric disorders. In other words, comorbidity, that is, the presence of more mental disorders in a single person, is very common (Maj, 2005; Roca et al., 2009; Teesson et al., 2005). As pointed out by Jablensky "It is not surprising that disorders, as defined in the current versions of DSM and ICD, have a strong tendency to co-occur, which suggests that fundamental assumptions of the dominant diagnostic schemata may be incorrect" (2016: 28). It is not surprising, then, that the last edition of DSM shifted from a categorical to a dimensional approach, giving up the aim to identify distinct mental diseases, as one can read in the highlights of changes between DSM-IV and DSM-5:

> Because the previous DSM approach considered each diagnosis as categorically separate from health and from other diagnoses, it did not capture the widespread sharing of symptoms and risk factors across many disorders that is apparent in studies of comorbidity. . . . Indeed, the once plausible goal of identifying homogeneous populations for treatment and research resulted in narrow diagnostic categories that did not capture clinical reality, symptom heterogeneity within disorders, and significant sharing of symptoms across multiple disorders. The historical aspiration of achieving diagnostic homogeneity by progressive subtyping within disorder categories no longer is sensible.
>
> *(APA, 2013b: 12)*

However, it is worth noticing that, in DSM-5, this dimensional model often remains a declaration of intent, rather than being an actual paradigm shift, especially when the Manual has to deal with what makes a behaviour *abnormal*. A clear cut-off among the different mental disorders is often really hard to find, but, and this is also more striking, the same issue regards the boundary between clinical normality and abnormality, too. Evidence has started to show that the line between normality and insanity is not a sharp one, and that mental disorders are extreme variants of normal continua (Poulton et al., 2000; van Os et al., 2009; Freeman et al., 2005; see also Chapter 7 in this book). In the general population, psychotic-like experiences are more common than expected, and it is sometimes hard to divide 'normal' and pathological anxiety, or 'normal' grief and depression. But the DSM largely ignores those evidence supporting the dimensional approach. Actually, the last edition expands the concept of mental disorder, 'pathologizing' normal reactions to distress or loss, like normal grief (major depressive disorder can now include people who are grieving the loss of a loved one if a patient's distress and impairment last more than two months after the death), and including syndromes like premenstrual dysphoric disorder, caffeine withdrawal, disruptive mood dysregulation disorder, which many experts considered flawed and that, in some cases, even raised concerns of ethicality (see, for example, Frances, 2014; Browne, 2015; Parker and Tavella, 2018). Ironically, the dimensional approach led the DSM to enlarge the area of abnormality, contributing to overdiagnosis and overmedication. Given that normality and pathology are close, the DSM's response is to expand pathology.

Thus, it is hard to divide mental disorders into distinct categories, and, in many cases, it is also hard to identify a clear cut-off between normality and pathology. In other words, clinical reality is not the type of reality philosophers find in natural kinds: it is fuzzy, heterogeneous, with broad areas of ambiguity and uncertainty. And there's no need to say that, in the definition of mental illness, social and cultural norms play a role that is much more important than in medical diseases, as one can read even in the 'objective' and 'atheoretical' DSM-5: "an expectable or culturally approved response to a common stressor or loss, such as the death of a loved one, is not a mental disorder" (APA, 2013a: 20). Many criteria indicated in the DSM for different mental disorders have a culturally bound threshold; to give some examples, the definition of social phobia, as noted by Olbert and Gala, 2015, implies a fear which is out of proportion to the sociocultural context; the decision whether depression is present rather than being a 'normal' response "inevitably requires the exercise of clinical judgment based on what the clinician knows about the individual in question and the individual's cultural norms for the expression of distress in the context of loss". The concept of mental disorder is rooted in society and has a deep normative aspect, which is absent or much less essential in the other branches of medicine.

In sum, mental disorders are not discrete entities, they don't possess sufficient and necessary conditions for their diagnosis, there is often comorbidity within them, and, given their deep connection with cultural and social expectations, they are not independent of the observers. In other words, realism in psychiatry seems to be an assumption that lacks any evidence.

The other crucial assumption of modern psychiatry is reductionism. Reductionism is the claim that mental disorders have roots in biology, that is, they are disturbances in neural structures. The hope is that eventually, once the different mental disorders' biological underpinnings will be discovered, psychiatry will be reduced to neurobiology (White et al., 2012). This idea dates back to the very origins of psychiatry, in that Kraepelin (1883) endorsed it. According to him, mental disorders were somatic diseases, with causal roots in biology and physiology, and the lack of evidence for these roots was for him only a contingency, that the progress of medicine would overcome with time. After more than a century, the DSM-5 was released following this hope. The members of the Task Force who prepared this new edition had promised a 'paradigm shift' (another one, after that concerning the dimensional approach), since, thanks to the progress of neurosciences, it seems that the biological underpinnings of mental disorders have become much clearer. In the Preface of the Manual, the authors remark:

> The revised chapter structure was informed by recent research in neuroscience and by emerging genetic linkages between diagnostic groups. Genetic and physiological risk factors, prognostic indicators, and some putative diagnostic markers are highlighted in the text.
>
> *(APA, 2013a: xlii)*

The implied hope is that, eventually, in the DSM's next edition, psychiatric categories will be superseded by neurobiological categories, which in turn would have found the essence of the different mental disorders, in terms of the underlying biological mechanisms. As stated by Banner (who, as we will see later, is actually *against* this view):

> [D]isease and disorder should be understood in terms of morbid anatomy and physiology; eventually, it will be possible to generate causal hypotheses about psychiatric disorders in terms of neuropathology or dysregulation. Whether the key theoretical concepts come from cognitive neuroscience, molecular biology or some other basic brain science, the strong interpretation of the medical model assumes that explanations for mental disorders can be sought that cite pathogenic processes in brain systems, and that furthermore, future classifications should reflect this knowledge. Many different causal processes may operate, including social and psychological ones, but the strong interpretation relies on neurobiology and cognitive processes being fundamental.
>
> *(Banner, 2013: 510)*

Thus, Kraepelin's dream is finally beginning to come true. Mental disorders are brain disorders, and genetics and neurosciences have begun to show how. But, is it really so? It's time to ask another question that looks trivial: are mental disorders brain disorders? The reason why this question looks trivial is that there is a sense in which mental disorders are obviously in the brain: they are mental, so they are in the brain. In other words, the brain is the physical basis of the mind, so it is the physical basis of mental disorder, too. But does it follow that mental disorders are disorders of the brain, viz., that the brain itself is disordered?

Not necessarily. As claimed by Graham (2013), there could be a disturbance in the body without a malfunctioning of the body; for example, I can feel sick and vomit, but this doesn't imply that there is a damage in the body. On the contrary, this reaction is likely a body's defence mechanism (for instance, it is eliminating toxins), and therefore the body is functioning well, even if I feel sick. Coming back to mental disorders, these disorders may be *in* the brain, without being *of* the brain, or, in other words, mental disorders may be based in healthy brains (Graham, 2013; Poland, 2013; Nesse and Jackson, 2011).

Actually, despite the DSM's optimism about the discovery of neuroscientific underpinnings and genetics linkage between diagnostic groups, and despite initiatives like the Research Domain Criteria, aiming to detect biological factors in mental disorders (Insel et al., 2010), the neurobiological aetiology of mental disorders is still lacking evidence (Ghaemi, 2012; Lakhan and Kramer, 2009). No clear biomarkers have been found for schizophrenia or other mental disorders (Stein et al., 2010; Weickert et al., 2013; Prata et al., 2014; Venkatasubramanian and Keshavan, 2016), and no neuroscientific tests can diagnose mental illnesses (Kapur et al., 2012). As claimed by Olbert and Gala, "the thesis that mental disorders are brain disorders is best understood as an ontological hypothesis regarding the nature of mental disorders that awaits empirical validation" (2015: 204). In other words, and it comes as no surprise, reductionism is a philosophical assumption, rather than an empirical finding.

Furthermore, this philosophical assumption is controversial. Claiming that mental disorders are brain disorders implies, as remarked by the same authors,

> the perception that the physiological substrata of disorders are more important, basic, necessary, or causally relevant than social, psychological, or contextual aspects of disorders. Indeed, the clinical neuroscientist seems committed to the view that the psychological and social aspects of disorders possess only instrumental importance as signifiers of underlying dysfunction.
>
> *(ivi: 212)*

But the clinical experience shows that, in the vast majority of cases, the contextual aspects of disorders are extremely relevant for the very ascription of the disorder itself. I've already pointed out some of those aspects in depression and social phobia. But the same can be said for other psychopathologies. In specific phobias, fear must be "more intense than is deemed necessary", and "the individual's sociocultural context should also be taken in account", in that, for example "fear of insects may be more disproportionate in settings where insects are consumed in the diet" (APA, 2013a: 199). In generalized anxiety disorder, it is remarked the necessity to "consider the social and cultural context when evaluating whether worries about certain situations are excessive" (ivi: 224). In separation anxiety disorder, the anxiety "exceeds what may be expected" (ivi: 191). In personality disorders, the reference to community standards, social environment and others' judgement is quite impressive. For instance, the avoidant personality disorder is a "pervasive pattern of social inhibition, feelings of inadequacy and hypersensitivity to negative evaluation", and individuals with this disorder are "described by others as being 'shy', 'timid', 'lonely' and 'isolated'" (ivi: 672–3). The essential feature of histrionic personality disorder is "excessive emotionality and attention-seeking behaviour" (ivi: 667). The definition of obsessive-compulsive personality disorder is, if possible, even more normative: "a pervasive pattern of preoccupation with orderliness, perfectionism, and mental and interpersonal control, at the expense of flexibility, openness, and efficiency" (ivi: 678). It is clear that, in this definition, flexibility, openness, and efficiency are absolute values, and that being stubborn, rigid and "overconscientious about matters of morality, ethics, or values" (ibid.) is not merely a defect (thesis to be proved), but a pathology (Olbert and Gala, 2015).

Where has the brain gone? How can a brain disorder depend so much on a normative and social approach? Furthermore, is it *useful* to consider mental disorders as brain disorders? There is indeed a correlation between, for example, depression and low levels of serotonin. An individual with major depression usually presents this anomaly. However, one can find those depleted levels in a healthy individual in grief for the loss of her loved one, too. Is her brain malfunctioning, then? And why do we usually ascribe this malfunctioning to the first individual, and not to the second one? Where is the difference in their brains? Besides, the first subject can be a single parent with a low-paid job, who feels tired, isolated, and hopeless, and she can also feel guilty for losing her pleasure to play with her child. In saying that a course of selective serotonin reuptake inhibitors may help her, have we caught the essence of her disorder (Banner, 2013)? To be more direct: what's the point of reductionism in psychiatry?

My claim is that even if neural correlates will be found in the different mental disorders, describing mental illness as a kind of brain disorder completely misses the essence of mental disorder. In most mental disorders, like depression, anxiety disorders, and personality disorders, the normative criteria for dysfunctionality originate at the level of the mental. Thus, the concept of brain disorder is *inherited* from the mental dysfunction, rather than being the roots or the explanation of the mental disorder itself (Jefferson, 2020). This specific role of the mental in mental disorder, and its consequences, will be the focus of the next section.

3 What is mental in mental disorders?

> *Whatever* the aetiology of the condition or its causal pathways in the brain – whether it is genetic, the product of gene-environment interactions, psychological, social or spiritual causes – the attribution of 'disorder' applies to the thoughts, feelings and behaviours of the person. Mental disorders are not mental disorders because of an assumed mental cause, but rather because they identify problems in the *person's* mental life and relationships.
>
> (*Banner, 2013: 511*)

What is the correct level of analysis for understanding that something is wrong in one's mind? What does the attribution of disorder apply to? Does it apply to brain states or the individual? As observed by Fuchs (2010), it is hard to describe mental disorders in a detached way, using a third-person approach. But this is just what the DSM tries to do. It assumes a realist perspective, and endorses the idea that, for psychiatry to be a science, its object has to be exactly measurable; and only single symptoms and behaviours are so. It also assumes a reductionist perspective, and only very circumscribed and simplified behaviours can be reduced to brain dysfunctions. But the reality and the practice of psychiatry are totally different. Without a mentalist vocabulary, psychiatry would simply not exist. As remarked by Broome and Bortolotti (2009), a distinctive feature of psychiatric disorders is that they need the vocabulary concerning the mental. Someone has a mental disorder because she beliefs something, or she thinks something. In other words, what's wrong is the person, the way she feels, how she suffers, and her relationship with the environment and the others. We recognize that behaviour is pathological, only understanding deviations in the social, moral, and epistemic norms (that is, norms which govern the acquisition of beliefs, see Bortolotti, 2018). The patient we opened this chapter with is detected as 'abnormal' for the way he holds an impossible belief, that of being decomposing. We can scan its brain to find whether something is wrong in it, but this won't help us to understand the meaning of his delusion. Without reference to the reasons a person gives to her behaviour, without taking into account what she feels and thinks, it is impossible to detect any mental disorder. Brain abnormalities are indicative of a mental disorder only if they associate with deviations from cultural, social, moral, and evaluative norms.

Furthermore, the mentalist vocabulary is necessary not only for defining mental disorders but also for explaining the symptoms: the social isolation and the fear of going out of a paranoid subject are explained referring to his belief of being persecuted by the CIA, the compulsive cleaning of the girl I described in the first paragraph is justified by the fear to contaminate herself or her loved ones. How would we understand any symptom showed by a patient without referring to the meaning she ascribes to that symptom? As remarked by Banner (2013: 511), "in no other medical discipline is the subjective experience of the patient quite so crucial to diagnosis and the aims of treatment".

In 1992, Wakefield joined in the debate on the description of mental disorder with a definition that became quite prominent:

> I argue that a disorder is a harmful dysfunction, wherein harmful is a value term based on social norms, and dysfunction is a scientific term referring to the failure of a mental mechanism to perform a natural function for which it was designed by evolution. Thus, the concept of disorder combines value and scientific components.
>
> *(373)*

The success of this definition derives from the fact that it puts together the 'scientific' aspect of mental disorder ('dysfunction') with the social one ('harmful'). Given that some kind of dysfunction must be present, much importance should be ascribed to the social background, too. The role of the environment can hardly be overrated. It is society that decides whether some dysfunction is harmful or not. And, in many cases, it is society that *makes* this dysfunction harmful. This is one of the reasons why mental disorders are not brain disorders.

> [I]n championing the brain as the locus of disorder at the expense of the person-level, we are making a powerful, and in my view, mistaken, judgement about how the disorder is conceptualized and what kinds of approaches should be taken towards treatment. A recent controversial article in the New York Times sums up this problem well. Dr Michael Anderson, a child psychiatrist in Georgia, frequently prescribes medication such as Ritalin and Adderall to children from poor socio-economic backgrounds who are struggling academically in inadequate, underfunded schools. He argues 'we've decided as a society that it's too expensive to modify the kid's environment. So we have to modify the kid'.
>
> *(Banner, 2013: 511)*

As I tried to show in the previous paragraph, the DSM's last version didn't inherit Wakefield's view, in that the importance of the social aspect is almost entirely dismissed, except for the brief notes concerning the culture-related diagnostic issues of each mental disorder.

I'm in favour of Wakefield's definition, but in a stronger sense. In psychiatry, we can't divide the 'factual' component from the 'value' component. The two aspects are intertwined. There are no 'naked' facts, nor 'pure' abnormalities.

> The difference between fracture as a man made and a natural category is trivial, unless you're in a philosophical argument. But when it comes to psychiatry, something changes. To call a snapped femur an illness is to make only the broadest assumptions about human nature – that it is in our nature to walk and to be out of pain. To call fear generalized anxiety disorder or sadness accompanied by anhedonia, disturbances in sleep and appetite, and fatigue depression requires us to make much tighter, and more decisive, assumptions about who we are, about how we are supposed to feel, about what life is for. How much anxiety is a creature cognizant of its inevitable death supposed to feel? How sad should we be about the human condition? How do you know that? To create these categories is to take a position on the most basic, and unanswerable, questions we face: what is the good life, and what makes it good? It's the epitome of hubris to claim that you have determined scientifically how to answer those questions, and yet to insist that you have found mental illnesses in nature is to do exactly that.
>
> *(Greenberg, in Phillips et al., 2012: 11)*

Is there, in nature, the generalized anxiety disorder? The answer is no. As Greenberg suggests, this category is simply how we call something, something that depends on an evaluative stance. In this view, psychiatry is philosophical at its very core, in that being a psychiatrist means judging what a good life is, what amount of sadness is reasonable, what emotive reactions we are supposed to show, and so on.

> But that's not to say that you can't determine scientifically patterns of psychic suffering as they are discerned by people who spend a lot of time observing and interacting with sufferers. The people who detect and name those patterns cannot help but organize what they observe according to their lived experience. The categories they invent then allow them to call those diseases into being. They don't make the categories up out of thin air, but neither do they find them under microscopes, or under rocks for that matter. That's what it means to say that the diseases don't exist until the doctors say they do. Which doesn't mean the diseases don't exist at all, just that they are human creations, and, at their best, fashioned out of love.
>
> *(ivi: 12)*

In other words, does this unavoidable evaluative stance mean that mental disorders are not real? Not at all. Mental illness is real in that it changes a person's life, in that the individual must deal with it, in that, ultimately, she suffers because of it.

Suffering is real. We cannot deny what it feels to be a person with a mental disorder. Maybe, as claimed by Loughlin and Miles (2014), we need a less restrictive conception of reality. And, most of all, psychiatrists must be aware of the centrality of ethics in their discipline. It makes no sense to invoke an objective, scientific, atheoretical approach to mental illness. The difficulties of this approach are evident in the last version of DSM, with its increasing number of mental disorders and the mention of an underpinning biological cause which is still to be found. But what is problematic is this demand of scientificity:

> The problem is philosophical: the influence of scientism and the idea that 'objective reality' consists only of that which is detectable and measurable according to certain methods. Only when we make that idea explicit, identify it as the problem, and reject it, can we move forward and start to talk about the sort of value-judgments that unavoidably inform diagnosis, and discuss their rationale with reference to a defensible conception of the human good. That's the point to which we must return, before we can recommence our journey to validate our notions of mental health and illness. The debate we need to have is within the field of ethics. Ethics is not a side issue but conceptually central to psychiatry.
>
> *(Loughlin and Miles, 2014: 156)*

Psychiatry is not just a medical discipline among others. It has to do with ethics. Mental wellness is the aim of psychiatrists, that want people to feel better, but mental health is a practical concept, based on value judgements about what is good and what is not.

> It is not as though one can study the epistemology of psychiatry and then, as a separate task, discuss its ethics, as the latter forms an inseparable part of the former: taking up an evaluative stance toward the nature of psychiatric disorders is an essential component of understanding what a psychiatric disorder is.
>
> *(ivi: 161)*

What are the consequences of this ethical view of psychiatry? The first consequence concerns the very definition of mental disorder. The 'mental' in mental illness is not a 'temporary' label, intended to be replaced by the different brain anomalies that neuroscience or genetics will find someday. Even if those biological bedrocks will be found, the essence of mental disorder will still lie in the relationship with the others and the environment. A mental disorder is mental because it has to be described with a mentalist vocabulary, and because it needs the others' look at the patient's mind, be this look empathic, judgemental, scared, and so on.

The second consequence of this view is that the phenomenological approach, rather than being an alternative perspective on mental disorder, must be taken into account when trying to understand the nature of the mental disorder itself

(Fuchs, 2010). That is, symptoms can be described using an impersonal, third-person approach, but only when the psychiatrist becomes familiar with the way the patient experiences those symptoms, and the meanings she ascribes to them, a real comprehension (and a therapeutic path) is possible. Going back to the patient doubting the agency of his thoughts, only focusing on his self-experience, and understanding what this *passivity* phenomenon means for him, the psychiatrist can grasp the meaning of this symptom and what it is like to be schizophrenic for him. I'm not saying that the two approaches, the impersonal and the phenomenological one, are mutually exclusive, but on the contrary that the objectivity of the medical gaze must be combined, in psychiatry, with the phenomenological, empathic stance that recognizes the role of the mental in mental disorder.

A further implication of this view is the acknowledgement of psychiatry's subjective essence. Here, subjective doesn't mean that all considerations, opinion, and attitudes towards mental illness have the same value. For instance, a psychiatric diagnosis, even if it's value-laden, can be true or false. And incorrect diagnoses could be very harmful, as in all branches of medicine. However, psychiatry is subjective, in that it can't lose track of the subject. In psychiatry, it is not a matter of detecting symptoms, but of understanding the personal significance of those symptoms to the subject.

The last, but not least, implication is actually a lesson in humility. Uncertainty is at the core of psychiatry. It is hard to know someone else's mind for real. And when there is something fundamentally different in this mind, when the way this mind works challenges our intuitions and comprehension, the task gets harder. As Philips et al. rightly pointed out:

> [I]f psychiatry were to officially recognize this fundamental uncertainty, then it would become a much more honest profession – and, to my way of thinking, a more noble one. For it would not be able to lose sight of the basic mystery of who we are and how we are supposed to live.
>
> *(2012: 12)*

References

Alstadhaug, K. B. (2019). Misclassification and emotional logic: A case report and a narrative review of Capgras syndrome. *Current Neurobiology*, 10(2), 84–88.

American Psychiatric Association (APA). (2013a). *Diagnostic and statistical manual of mental disorders* (5th ed.). Arlington: American Psychiatric Publishing.

American Psychiatric Association (APA). (2013b). *Highlights of changes from DSM IV-TR to DSM 5*. Arlington: American Psychiatric Publishing.

Banner, N. (2013). Mental disorders are not brain disorders. *Journal of Evaluation in Clinical Practice*, 19(3), 509–513.

Bortolotti, L. (2018). *Delusions in context*. London: Palgrave Mcmillian.

Broome, M., and Bortolotti, L. (2009). Mental illness as mental: In defence of psychological realism. *Humana Mente*, 11, 25–43.

Browne, T. K. (2015). Is premenstrual dysphoric disorder really a disorder? *Journal of Bioethics Inquiry*, 12(2), 313–330.

Brulde, B., and Radovic, C. (2006). What is mental about mental disorder? *Philosophy, Psychiatry, and Psychology*, 13, 99–116.

Eronen, M. I. (2019). The levels problem in psychopathology. *Psychological Medicine*, 1–7. https://doi.org/10.1017/S0033291719002514

Frances, A. (2014). *Saving normal: An insider's revolt against out-of-control psychiatric diagnosis, DSM-5, big pharma, and the medicalization of ordinary life*. New York: William Morrow & Co.

Freeman, D., Garety, P. A., Bebbington, P. E., Smith, B., Rollinson, R., Fowler, D., . . . and Dunn, G. (2005). Psychological investigation of the structure of paranoia in a non-clinical population. *British Journal of Psychiatry*, 186, 427–435.

Fuchs, T. (2010). Subjectivity and intersubjectivity in psychiatric diagnosis. *Psychopathology*, 43(4), 268–274.

Ghaemi, N. (2012). Taking disease seriously: Beyond "pragmatic" nosology. In K. Kendler and J. Parnas (Eds.), *Philosophical issues in psychiatry. II: Nosology*. Oxford: Oxford University Press.

Graham, G. (2013). *The disordered mind: An introduction to philosophy of mind and mental illness*. London and New York: Routledge.

Insel, T., Cuthbert, B., Garvey., M, Heinssen, R., Pine, D. S., Quinn, K., . . . and Wang, P. (2010). Research domain criteria (RDoC): Toward a new classification framework for research on mental disorders. *American Journal of Psychiatry*, 167(7), 748–751.

Jablensky, A. (2016). Psychiatric classifications: Validity and utility. *World Psychiatry: Official Journal of the World Psychiatric Association (WPA)*, 15(1), 26–31.

Jaspers, K. (1963). *General psychopathology*. Manchester: Manchester University Press.

Jefferson, A. (2020). What does it take to be a brain disorder? *Synthese*, 197, 249–262.

Justo, A. P., Gomes de Matos, E., and Lipp, M. E. N. (2015). Cognitive-behavioral therapy of a case of obsessive-compulsive disorder. *Revista Brasileira de Terapias Cognitivas*, 11(1), 10–24.

Kapur, S., Phillips, A., and Insel, T. (2012). Why has it taken so long for biological psychiatry to develop clinical tests and what to do about it? *Molecular Psychiatry*, 17, 1174–1179.

Kendler, K. S. (2016). The nature of psychiatric disorders. *World Psychiatry*, 15, 5–12.

Kraepelin, E. (1883). *Compendium der Psychiatrie zum Gebrauche für Studirende und Aerzte*. Leipzig: Abel Verlag.

Kuhn, T. S. (1962). *The structure of scientific revolutions*. Chicago: The University of Chicago Press.

Lakhan, S. E., and Kramer, A. (2009). Schizophrenia genomics and proteomics: Are we any closer to biomarker discovery? *Behavioral and Brain Functions*, 5, 2. https://doi.org/10.1186/1744-9081-5-2

Loughlin, M., and Miles, A. (2014). Psychiatry, objectivity, and realism about value. In P. Zachar, Dr. St. Stoyanov, M. Aragona, and A. Jablensky (Eds.), *Alternative perspectives on psychiatric validation: DSM, IDC, RDoC, and beyond*. Oxford: Oxford University Press.

Maj, M. (2005). 'Psychiatric comorbidity': An artefact of current diagnostic systems? *British Journal of Psychiatry*, 186(3), 182–184.

Murphy, D. (2006). *Psychiatry in the scientific image*. Cambridge, MA: MIT Press.

Nesse, R. M., and Jackson, E. D. (2011). Evolutionary foundations for psychiatric diagnoses: Making DSM V valid. In P. Adriaens and A. DeBlock (Eds.), *Maladapting minds*. New York: Oxford University Press.

Olbert, C. M., and Gala, G. J. (2015). Supervenience and psychiatry: Are mental disorders brain disorders? *Journal of Theoretical and Philosophical Psychology*, 35(4), 203–219.

Parker, G., and Tavella, G. (2018). Disruptive mood dysregulation disorder: A critical perspective. *Canadian Journal of Psychiatry. Revue canadienne de psychiatrie*, 63(12), 813–815.

Patil, T., and Giordano, J. (2010). On the ontological assumptions of the medical model of psychiatry: Philosophical considerations and pragmatic tasks. *Philosophy, Ethics, and Humanities in Medicine*, 5, 3.

Phillips, J., Frances, A., Cerullo, M. A., Chardavoyne, J., Decker, H. S., First, M. B., . . . and Zachar, P. (2012). The six most essential questions in psychiatric diagnosis: A pluralogue part 1: Conceptual and definitional issues in psychiatric diagnosis. *Philosophy, Ethics, and Humanities in Medicine: PEHM*, 7, 3. https://doi.org/10.1186/1747-5341-7-3

Poland, J. (2013). Deeply rooted sources of error and bias in psychiatric classification. In J. Sullivan and H. Kincaid (Eds.), *Psychiatric classifications and natural kinds*. Cambridge: MIT Press.

Poulton, R., Caspi, A., Moffitt, T. E., Cannon, M., Murray, R., and Harrington, H. (2000). Children's self-reported psychotic symptoms and adult schizophreniform disorder: A 15-year longitudinal study. *Archives of General Psychiatry*, 57(11), 1053–1058.

Pouncey, C. L. (2005). Philosophy of psychopathology. *Current Opinion in Psychiatry*, 18, 659–663.

Prata, D., Mechelli, A., and Kapur, S. (2014). Clinically meaningful biomarkers for psychosis: A systematic and quantitative review. *Neuroscience and Biobehavioral Reviews*, 45, 134–141.

Roca, M., Gili, M., Garcia-Garcia, M., Salva, J., Vives, M., Garcia Campayo, J., and Comas, A. (2009). Prevalence and comorbidity of common mental disorders in primary care. *Journal of Affective Disorders*, 119(1–3), 52–58.

Stein, D. J., Phillips, K. A., Bolton, D., Fulford, K. W. M., Sadler, J. Z., and Kendler, K. S. (2010). What is a mental/psychiatric disorder? From DSM-IV to DSM-V. *Psychological Medicine*, 40(11), 1759–1765.

Teesson, M., Degenhardt, L., Proudfoot, H., Hall, W., and Lynskey, M. (2005). How common is comorbidity and why does it occur? *Australian Psychologist*, 40, 81–87.

van Os, J., Linscott, R. J., Myin-Germeys, I., Delespaul, P., and Krabbendam, L. J. P. M. (2009). A systematic review and meta-analysis of the psychosis continuum: Evidence for a psychosis proneness-persistence-impairment model of psychotic disorder. *Psychological Medicine*, 39(2), 179.

Venkatasubramanian, G., and Keshavan, M. (2016). Biomarkers in psychiatry: A critique. *Annals of Neuroscience*, 23, 3–5.

Wakefield, J. C. (1992). Disorder as harmful dysfunction: A conceptual critique of DSM-III-R's definition of mental disorder. *Psychological Review*, 2, 232–247.

Weickert, C. S., Weickert, T. W., Pillai, A., and Buckley, P. F. (2013). Biomarkers in schizophrenia: A brief conceptual consideration. *Disease Markers*, 35. https://doi.org/10.1155/2013/510402

White, P. D., Rickards, H., and Zeman, A. Z. (2012). Time to end the distinction between mental and neurological illnesses. *British Medical Journal*, 344: e3454.

Zangrilli, A., Ducci, G., Bandinelli, P. L., Dooley, J., McCabe, R., and Priebe, S. (2014). How do psychiatrists address delusions in first meetings in acute care? A qualitative study. *Biological and Medical Central Psychiatry*, 14, 178.

2

MENTAL ILLNESSES ARE EMOTIONAL DISORDERS

Philip N. Johnson-Laird

1 Introduction

Psychological illnesses are pandemic. Nearly half the population of the United States will succumb to such a disease, and suffer from anxiety, phobia, hypochondria, depression, explosive anger, or an obsessive compulsion (American Psychiatric Association, 2013). What is so odd is that their cause is psychological – a matter of thoughts and experiences rather than gross changes to the brain – yet their cure is so difficult. They are unlikely to strike a person at random: character and personality seem to make some people more vulnerable than others, and so too does a stressful situation. Scientists do not understand these illnesses. They know that the illnesses exist, that they are common, and that some treatments are helpful. But, the existence of hundreds of different sorts of psychotherapy (Herink, 1980) is a sign of ignorance.

Fifteen years ago, my colleagues and I published a theory of psychological illnesses – the hyper-emotion theory (Johnson-Laird et al., 2006; Mancini et al., 2007). This chapter aims to bring the account up to date, and it is designed for readers unfamiliar with the theory. It outlines what they need to know about emotions, how music arouses them (a useful analogy), and how humans reason. It then presents the theory and recent corroborations of its predictions about aetiology, prognosis, and treatment. Its range is wide but its focus is narrow: the hyper-emotion theory, and so it omits alternative points of view.

Human beings like all social mammals have to solve everyday problems that concern their bodily environment (sickness and pain), their physical environment (food, drink, and shelter), and their social environment (cooperation, mates, rearing offspring). They cope. But, they do sometimes make terrible errors – a fact impolitic to mention to theorists who believe that human thinking cannot err (e.g., Cohen, 1981; Henle, 1978). To borrow a remark from Ramsey (1929/1990), these theorists are like those bridge-players who argue that you cannot break its rules, because if you do, you are no longer playing bridge. One reason that social mammals cope is that evolution led to an efficient solution to their problems: emotions.

2 The communication of emotions

Emotions perplex philosophers. Plato regarded them as a force for irrationality (e.g., *Timaeus*, 86b). Many others have echoed him, and so a pure intellect unsullied by emotions is often treated as an ideal – from Sherlock Holmes to Mr. Spock of *Startrek* fame. Such characters are to be pitied, not emulated. In contrast, Aristotle grasped the cognitive roots of emotions (e.g., *Rhetoric*, Book II). He remarked that when someone insults you, it makes you angry (see *Politics*, line 1312b30), and he recognized that some emotions have characteristic facial expressions (*Physiognomics*, line 805b1).

His descendant in the study of facial expressions wrote:

> The power of communication between the members of the same tribe by means of language has been of paramount importance in the development of man; and the force of language is much aided by the expressive movements of the face and body. We perceive this at once when we converse on an important subject with any person whose face is concealed.
>
> *(Darwin, 1897: 354)*

What Darwin analysed are the causal roots of the ways in which individuals and animals express their emotions – from dogs wagging their tails to people weeping for joy. He noted that humans recognize emotions in others without knowing their exact cues. The emotions and their recognition are innate, and the same throughout the world (ibid: 359). He speculates that the free expression of an emotion intensifies it, whereas the suppression of these signs softens the emotion (ibid: 365).

2.1 The basis of emotions

The account that my colleagues and I adopted as basis for the hyper-emotion theory is Darwinian in essence. It is the "communicative" theory of emotions developed with Keith Oatley (Oatley and Johnson-Laird, 1987, 1996; Johnson-Laird and Oatley, 1992). It acknowledges that emotions are distinct, as Darwin did, and that they communicate themselves to others. They coordinate the collective lives of social mammals. But they are also internal communications in the brain. A rudimentary cognitive evaluation suffices to trigger such a signal. It is faster than deliberate thinking, and its consequences are general rather than particular. When, for instance, a stranger is rude to you, you understand the threat (a cognitive evaluation); various changes occur in your brain (neurophysiological processes); and, as a result, hormones are released into your bloodstream, your heart pumps faster (somatic changes), and so you are ready for action; you sense anger mounting within you (a subjective feeling); you frown (a facial expression); and you say something rude in reply (an intentional action).

From a simple cognitive evaluation of the situation, emotions prepare individuals for a general course of action. Hence, many different events in the world are mapped onto a small number of categories, each of which can elicit a distinct set of physiological, behavioural, and subjective consequences appropriate to the situation. If there were many such categories, then the problem of deciding amongst them could be as time-consuming as a deliberate choice. Likewise, the repertoire of physiological changes and behaviours that an emotion elicits must be useful preparations for the wide class of events that trigger the emotion. For human beings, this repertoire includes learned actions. Fire drills prepare them for practiced actions that can be carried out without much thought, e.g., what to do to leave the building.

Theorists squabble about which, if any, of the elements is the "emotion", about whether it is a separate entity or merely a cluster of values on multiple dimensions, and which element causes another. William James (1884) thought that your actions cause your feelings. You aren't rude because you're angry; you're angry because you're rude. This back-to-front view, however, is contrary to common sense and to the fact that total paralysis spares emotions.

Both the external and internal signals of basic emotions are innate. They are evolutionarily old and dependent on systems in the brain, such as the amygdala – two subcortical organs. Their interpretation differs from the interpretation of the cognition eliciting them. It can have propositional content, and it can be expressed in language, e.g., "His insult annoyed me". The meaning of such a proposition is composed from the meanings of its parts according to the grammatical relations amongst them. As semantic theorists say, it has a "compositional" meaning (Partee, 2014). In contrast, emotional signals have no such structure: they are more akin to one of a small set of alternative alarms. These signals propagate in the brain more rapidly than propositional messages. Their external propagation in facial and bodily expressions also has no compositional structure and is understood rapidly. You can tell a genuine smile from a posed one, but you cannot identify what cues the difference – unless you have studied the matter (Ekman and Friesen, 1982).

Emotional signals and their cognitive evaluations both can impinge on consciousness – in which case an individual is aware of a subjective feeling and of its cause. But each one may fail to impinge in this way. Individuals may be aware that they ought to feel an emotion, but experience nothing more than a sense of 'numbness'. Or, they may feel an emotion, but have no idea why they are experiencing it. And if they are unaware of the message and the signal, they can have an unconscious emotion manifest only in bodily changes and expressive behaviour. This claim sounds Freudian. But Freud (1915) went out of his way to deny this possibility: "It is surely of the essence of an emotion that we should be aware of it, i.e. that it should become known to consciousness".

The communicative theory identifies certain emotions as *basic*, such as happiness, sadness, anger, and fear, because they can be experienced without awareness

TABLE 2.1 Basic emotions that can be with or without a known object, and those that must have known objects, with their antecedents and the consequences

Emotion ± object	*Antecedent*	*Consequences in expressions and behaviours*
Happiness	Success, achievement of goals	Continue course of actions
Sadness	Loss, failure of goals	Withdraw, do nothing, cogitate
Irritation-anger	Obstruction to goals	Act aggressively
Anxiety-fear	Threat to preservation	Withdraw, protect, worry
Emotion + known object	**Object**	**Consequences in expressions and actions**
Parental love	Infant or child	Nurture
Sexual love	Partner	Court, be affectionate
Hatred	Rival, other	Act towards without care, ignore
Disgust	Noxious entity	Expel, reject, avoid

of any cognitive message. So, individuals may feel them for no reason of which they are aware, and they can underlie moods, that is, prolonged emotional states. Other basic emotions can be experienced only with an awareness of their objects, e.g., disgust or love. In sum, basic emotions are innate, they serve an adaptive function, and they prepare individuals for a general course of action or inaction.

Table 2.1 summarizes the principal basic emotions that can be experienced without a known object and those that have necessary objects.

Originally, the communicative theory postulated that lateral inhibition in the brain led a single basic emotion to be predominant at any one time (Oatley and Johnson-Laird, 1987). But, as a result of studies in which people kept diaries of their emotions (Oatley and Duncan, 1994), it became obvious that the assumption was false. People have mixed emotions. Before an examination of more complex emotions, it is sensible to consider emotional reactions to music, because they are analogous to those that occur in psychological illnesses.

2.2 *Music elicits basic emotions*

For an alien, music causes a universal psychological illness. In its pure form, it has no propositional content, yet it evokes emotions. And listeners can project all sorts of content onto it. But music itself conveys no propositions – entities that can be true or false, and whose meanings are compositional. Music is common to all cultures, and almost always social – the chief exception is Western music in the concert hall.

Music is popular, its listeners say, because it arouses their emotions. Its earliest psychological studies corroborated this claim (e.g., Gilman, 1891). It elicits basic emotions (e.g., Juslin et al., 2011). It can create a surprise, but surprise is nothing more than a sudden unexpected event eliciting a basic emotion. A piece of music that you have never heard before can make you happy, and so it contains cues that elicit the cognitive evaluations leading to a basic emotion. The process has innate roots: 2-day-old hearing infants of congenitally deaf parents prefer music intended for infants than music intended for adults (Masataka, 1999). And the process is rapid: in less than a second, you know whether an excerpt is happy or sad (Peretz et al., 1998). So, what is it that moves you? If you are not a musician, you cannot really say; and if you are a musician, you may say: it is up-tempo and in a major key. And why should these factors make you feel happy? You cannot say – or you make vague circular claims, such as "major scales signify happiness". The right answer is foreshadowed in Aristotle (*Politics*, 1340a11 et seq.) and in Helmholtz (1887/1912). Music is mimetic: it imitates the characteristic behaviours, tone of voice, and speed of thinking, which occur in different basic emotional states. When you are happy, you move and think quickly, and speak loudly with an intonation contour that leaps around for emphasis (unless you speak a 'tone' language). When you are sad, you move and think slowly, and speak softly with a low pitch, and not much change in your intonation contour. When you are angry, you are also quick but you shout at a high pitch. When you are fearful, you run and act in an agitated way. A bodily cause in all three of the negative basic emotions is pain.

Music imitates these characteristics. It has 'parameters' that can vary but that tend to remain constant for some time, such as tempo, volume, pitch, timbre, the range of pitches in a melody, key, and consonance or dissonance. In tonal music, the notes in melodies and chords tend to be from a major scale or a minor scale, which have a psychological reality (Krumhansl, 1990). Scales are subsets of notes that are possible to play, of which, ignoring octaves, there are 12 in conventional Western music. For example, the C major scale contains the seven notes, C D E F G A B – the white notes on the piano, and the C minor scale replaces the note E with E flat. And musical chords are the simultaneous playing of different notes from the scale.

What makes chords consonant or dissonant is the oldest puzzle in cognitive science. It goes back to Pythagoras, and Galileo, Euler, and many others who have proposed solutions. Helmholtz (1912) discovered an essential piece of the puzzle: when two overtones from notes are close together in frequency, they create an almost painful buzz. The reason is that they stimulate regions close together on the cochlear, which is the organ in the inner ear that converts auditory vibrations into nerve impulses. But Helmoltz realized that there was a cultural factor too, because chords once judged dissonant in Western music now seem consonant. He did not identify this cultural factor. But a recent theory locates it in major and minor keys, which are at the heart of tonal music – the genre that developed around 1600 and that persists to this day in some modern concert music, in jazz, and in rock (Johnson-Laird et al., 2012). Keys are matters of culture, not innate acoustics. Those chords with notes that only co-occur in a minor key are more dissonant than those that co-occur in a major key. The combination of the two factors, painful buzz and tonal keys, predicts listeners' ratings of dissonance for almost all the possible three-note chords and for a representative sample of four-note chords. These samples included tonal chords and those that are not. Likewise, a sequence of chords can follow tonal principles or not. Tonal chords are less dissonant in a tonal sequence than in a random sequence, whereas chords that are not tonal are highly dissonant in both contexts. In sum, consonance is pleasant, and dissonance is painful.

The communicative theory therefore postulates that music communicates cues analogous to those that humans communicate when they are in the grip of an emotion. Both sorts of cues elicit cognitive evaluations leading to basic emotions. For music, the cues are as follows (Johnson-Laird and Oatley, 2008):

Happiness: medium tempo, loud, wide range of pitches in melodies in a major scale, consonance.
Sadness: slow tempo, soft, low pitch, small range of pitches in a minor scale, mild dissonance.
Anger: rapid tempo, loud, high pitch, minor scale, large leaps in pitches in melodies, dissonance.
Anxiety: rapid tempo, moderate volume, low pitch, minor scale, dissonance.

Empirical studies show that settings of single parameters elicit appropriate emotions (for a review, see Johnson-Laird and Oatley, 2016). A major scale tends to elicit happiness, whereas minor and other scales tend to elicit negative emotions. Fast versus slow tempo has the same effect. When several parameters cue the same emotion, they increase the likelihood of its perception. A striking phenomenon occurs when music embodies conflicting cues to emotions, such as a major key but a slow tempo. Listeners experience mixed emotions. One study investigated happiness and sadness with recordings of real music (Hunter et al., 2008). And an unpublished study due to Olivia Kang exploited a computer program that creates music. The program builds up a matrix of transitions from one note to the next from a corpus of melodies. The transitions embody both pitch and rhythm. With an input of a chord sequence, the program uses the matrix to generate new melodies. With matrices based on corpora of music eliciting different basic emotions, and with appropriate settings of parameters, the resulting output is a novel piece of music expressing the relevant emotion. Kang's study confirmed the effect with music based on three corpora of melodies (happy, sad, and anxious). But, when the parameters were set to conflicting values, the listeners were less certain about what emotion the music conveyed, and their choice of terms to characterize it referred to mixed emotions.

In sum, the cues in music communicate emotions to listeners by mimicking behaviours of those in emotional states. The auditory system uses these cues to form a model of an emotional state, which in turn transmits a signal of a basic emotion in the brain. The underlying mechanisms are in large part innate. But no answer is available to the eternal question of what adaptive advantage music confers: the problem is the lack of pertinent evidence (Lewontin, 1998).

2.3 Complex emotions

Some emotions are complex in that they can be experienced only with knowledge of the circumstances initiating them. They depend on an awareness of the relevant situation and typically on conscious inferences concerning individuals' models of themselves. So, they can concern a comparison between actual events and alternative possibilities. These emotions therefore combine a signal of a basic emotion with a propositional message concerning the relation between a situation and a model of oneself. They include, for example, *guilt*, which is hatred of oneself for an action or inaction that was wrong – a deontic mistake; *remorse*, which is sadness in one's behaviour in the light of a model of one's ideal actions; and *embarrassment*, which is a self-conscious fear of looking bad, facing ridicule, and so on. Table 2.2 summarizes some complex emotions, their underlying basic emotions, and examples of their cognitive evaluations.

The transition from a cognitive evaluation to an emotion is itself unconscious and uncontrollable. You see something, and you have a rapid emotional reaction to it. You can control to some degree your behavioural expression of an emotion. You can use various other strategies such as trying to suppress the emotion itself. But evidence suggests the best strategy is to reappraise the situation creating the

TABLE 2.2 Some typical complex emotions, their underlying basic emotions, and examples of their typical cognitive evaluations

Complex emotion	*Underlying basic emotion*	*Typical cognitive evaluations in relation to models of the self*
Pride	Happiness	Action succeeds by one's own criteria
Hope	Happiness	Expectation of success in relation to one's goals
Despair	Sadness	No hope (ibid.) in relation to goals of one's life
Regret	Sadness	Action or inaction fails to achieve one's goal
Remorse	Sadness	Wrong action or inaction in relation to one's ideal
Pity	Sadness	Other's situation as one evaluates it
Grief	Sadness	Loss of loved one
Rage	Anger	Inability to control emotion against others
Panic	Fear	Inability to control emotion
Embarrassment	Fear	Awareness of one's situation as open to ridicule
Vanity	Self-love	Excessive pride (ibid.)
Bitterness	Hate	Others have wronged one
Envy	Hate	For another's desirable attributes or possessions
Jealousy	Hate	For another supplanting one in a person's love
Shame	Self-hate	Wrong action or inaction regarding collective ideal
Guilt	Self-hate	Deontically wrong action or inaction regarding one's own ideal

emotion if you are aware of it (Gross, 2002; McRae and Gross, 2020). What is indubitable is that a mere intention cannot stop the signal of a basic emotion and its outcomes. If you had such a control, then psychological illnesses would not exist to a degree that causes suffering.

The moral for psychological illnesses is that emotions can be evoked from rudimentary models outside awareness that embody nothing more than emotional characteristics of human behaviours. This primitive unconscious system creates basic emotions from music, but also from events in daily life. At the opposite extreme, if you read in an email that a dear friend has died, then this news triggers a feeling of grief – the propositional content of loss elicits a transition to an intense and uncontrollable feeling of sadness. The evaluative message is combined with the emotion it elicits and you are overcome by your awareness of the resulting grief at the feeling of loss. Figure 2.1 is a diagram representing the essentials of the communicative theory of emotions.

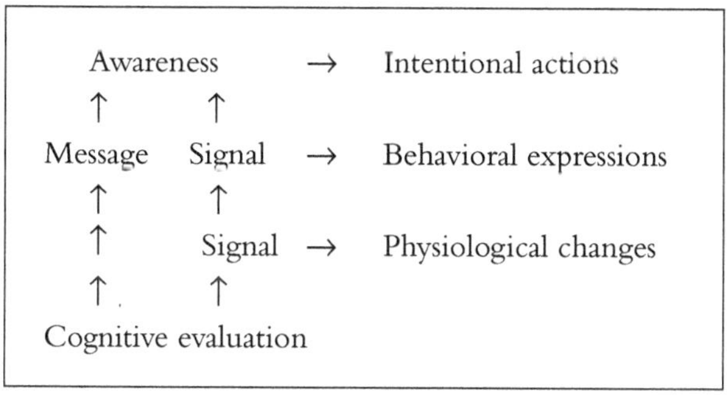

Figure 2.1 A schematic diagram of the communicative theory's account of emotional signals and propositional messages in the brain, from the initiating cognitive evaluation to its propositional message and emotional signal, and their respective outcomes. Message and signal may or may not impinge on the conscious system.

3 Thinking and reasoning

Thinking varies. It can have a goal or it can be goal-less. Without a goal, the mind wanders and one thought leads to another by association – a commonplace idea, but one for which no adequate theory exists. With a goal, thinking can be a sort of reasoning, deductive or inductive. But the goal can be too vague or too general so that it hardly constrains the process of achieving it – a person aims to compose a sonata, for instance, and so the constraints of creativity itself must take over. Psychologists divide thinking into these sorts of category in order to explain it, but its flow in daily life often moves so smoothly from one sort of process to another that you are not aware of the transitions. Indeed, you are more aware of the results of thinking than of how it proceeds from one thought to the next (Lashley, 1958).

Human reasoning is not all-powerful, despite leading to a deep understanding of mathematics and science and to sensible systems of law and governance. One source of difficulty is the human need to make sensible decisions when confronted with multiple and often incompatible goals, disparate beliefs, and the need to coordinate actions with other individuals. This social coordination of joint actions gets still worse when several people are trying to reach a decision, or when the number of beliefs to be taken into account is large. All reasoning is limited in power.

People with psychological illnesses think about them, and one influential view is that the origins of these illnesses are in faulty reasoning and irrational beliefs (Beck, 1976, 2019; Ellis, 1962). The idea is plausible, and the cognitive-behavioural therapy designed to correct these flaws is effective. So, the aim of this part of the chapter is to explain how individuals reason in daily life, and to do so it will rely on the theory of mental models (e.g., Johnson-Laird, 2006).

The basic idea is simple. People are not logicians. When they reason, they do not follow rules of inference such as those of a logic. Instead, they envisage the possibilities to which premises refer, and draw a conclusion from these mental models. A good way for you to envisage such models is to consider a building, such as a block of apartments or offices, with which you are familiar. Now, imagine that you are in, say, one such apartment or office, and have to get elsewhere on another floor in the building such as to its main entrance. Your task is to trace in the air with one finger the route that you take to get from your starting point to your destination. You can easily carry out this task. You trace the three-dimensional route with your finger. If you ask yourself how you were able to do so, the answer has to be that you had access to an internal representation of the three-dimensional layout of the building – a mental model – that enabled you to imagine the route. Some people report having visual images of the building, but many have no awareness of the model – it somehow guides their behaviour. In one experimental study, the participants likewise envisaged moving railway cars around a simple track, and in this case they constructed a kinematic model of a sequence of moves unfolding in time just as actual moves of the cars would do so (Khemlani et al., 2013). Even 10-year-old children could carry out this task, and they made many spontaneous gestures mimicking actual moves of cars. This outward sign of an inward mental simulation helped them to keep track of where the cars were, because when they were prevented from gesturing, their reasoning was worse (Bucciarelli et al., 2016).

When individuals reason from simple premises, the model theory postulates that they rely on intuitions; whereas in a task such as the rearrangement of cars on a railway, they rely on deliberations. This idea of two systems of reasoning is due to the late Peter Wason, who helped to explain performance in his well-known *selection* task (Wason, 1968). He invented the task to find out whether naive individuals – those with no training in science or logic – realized the importance of counterexamples to hypotheses. In the standard selection task, Wason put four cards down on the table in front of a participant as follows:

E F 3 4

and the participants knew that each card had a letter on one side and a number on the other side.

Their task was to select those cards that it was necessary to turn over to find out whether a hypothesis such as the following one was true or false:

> If a card has an E on one side, then it has a 3 on the other side.

They were told to be parsimonious in their selections. Most people selected E and 3, some selected only E, a few selected E, 3, and 4, but hardly anyone selected E and 4. Yet, it is the correct selection, because they are the only two cards that can yield counterexamples to the hypothesis. The almost universal failure to try to falsify the hypothesis shocked philosophers and psychologists. And over several decades it has led to more than 200 published experiments investigating the task.

The theory that Wason and the present author devised to explain performance in the task used his distinction between intuitive and deliberative sorts of reasoning, now often known as system 1 and system 2. The theory was formulated in an algorithm (Johnson-Laird and Wason, 1970). We recently implemented this algorithm in a computer program simulating mental models (Ragni et al., 2018). It makes a list of those items of evidence to be selected, i.e., cards in the selection task, and in intuitive mode it begins with those to which the hypothesis refers. So, for the hypothesis mentioned previously, the system 1 list is E and 3, but sometimes just E alone, depending on whether or not the hypothesis is taken to imply its converse. Intuitions therefore have no insight into counterexamples that could falsify the hypothesis: they select only evidence that matches the hypothesis. With a partial insight, system 2 adds any further item that could verify the hypothesis, or, failing that, any that could falsify the hypothesis. So, if 3 is not on the opening list, it is now selected. But if it is already on the opening list, deliberation now adds 4, yielding the selection of E, 3, and 4. With complete insight into falsification from the outset, the deliberations of system 2 select only items that could yield potential counterexamples to the hypothesis: E and 4. Although the selection of the three cards, E, 3, and 4 was rare in the initial studies, a procedure designed to elicit the selection of counterexamples led to it being the most frequent selection of all, followed by E and 4 (Wason, 1969).

The theory makes several predictions that a meta-analysis of the data corroborated, and its account of the selection task outperforms 15 alternative theories (Ragni et al., 2018). It also allows that people make sensible selections when they are tested in a repeated version of the task that gives them feedback on the status of each selection that they make, e.g., whether E occurs with 3 or 4 on its other side. The shocking neglect of falsifying selections in the original task therefore appears to be a consequence of participants having just one chance to make a correct selection for an abstract and arbitrary hypothesis. However, when the task is presented in a deontic framework, concerning acceptable and unacceptable actions, participants are also much more likely to deliberate and to select potential counterexamples.

The two systems of reasoning have continued to be part of the model theory (e.g., Johnson-Laird, 1983: Ch. 6, 2006), and other theorists have developed their own versions of "dual process" theories, e.g., Evans (2008); Sloman (1996); Kahneman (2011). In the recent model theory, intuitions rely on mental models, which represent what is true but not what is false, and focus on one model at a time. Consider, for instance, the following problem, in which both assertions refer to two alternative possibilities:

> Either the pie is on the table or else the cake is on the table.
> Either the pie isn't on the table or else the cake is on the table.
> Could both of these assertions be true at the same time?

Most people respond "yes" (Johnson-Laird et al., 2012). The model theory predicts this response, because intuition yields two mental models of what's on the table according to the first premise:

pie	
	cake

(Words here stand in for models of the items on the table.) And it yields two mental models of what's on the table according to the second premise:

not-pie	
	cake

Because the cake is on the table for both assertions, people think that they both could be true at the same time. They are wrong. Fully explicit models on which system 2 relies represent in addition what is false in each possibility, using negation to do so, and so for the two premises, they are

pie	not-cake
not-pie	cake

and

not-pie	not-cake
pie	cake

The cake occurs without the pie for the first assertion, but with the pie for the second assertion, and so the correct answer is that both the assertions cannot be true at the same time.

The model theory has led to many studies that have corroborated its account in comparison with alternatives based on logic or on the probability calculus (see, e.g., Johnson-Laird et al., 2015), and the computer programs that implement it are available online.[1]

3.1 *The interaction between emotions and reasoning*

If Plato and his ilk were right, then emotions, as a force for irrationality, should impede reasoning and even lead it astray. Suppose you're trying to carry out the selection task in a state of high dudgeon. Your feelings are likely to distract you – you pay attention to the emotion rather than to the task in hand, and so you fail to select falsifying cards in the selection task. An early study of the effects of emotion on reasoning corroborated this prediction using movies to induce emotions (Oaksford et al., 1996). This result is consistent with other studies, e.g., depression distracts its sufferers from thinking about other matters (Ellis and Ashbrook, 1987).

However, as Johnson-Laird and Oatley (2000: 464) suggested, a critical matter is the pertinence of an emotion to the task in hand. If it is irrelevant – as a movie-induced emotion is to the selection task – then it is likely to impede reasoning. But if it is relevant to your reasoning, then it should focus you to rely more on deliberation, and therefore to enhance your performance. Blanchette independently had the same idea, and has corroborated it in her ingenious studies (see, e.g., Blanchette and Richards, 2004, and Chapter 4 in this book).

Amelia Gangemi, Francesco Mancini, and the present author tested the effects of emotions on reasoning in an unpublished study. Their experiment manipulated whether or not psychologically healthy participants were feeling guilt, and whether or not the contents of a reasoning problem concerned guilt. The participants' task was to infer what was possible and what was impossible according to an assertion at the end of a brief description. One group of participants had to write down a vivid account of an autobiographical episode in which they had felt guilt. A control group wrote no such account. After the experiment, the experimental group felt more guilt than the control group did, so this manipulation worked. On each trial in the experiment proper, the participants read a brief description ending with a particular assertion, e.g., they read this description to elicit guilt:

> Suppose I am at my house with some friends. We decide to join some other friends in a bar. We leave the house joking amongst ourselves, but I forget to close the bathroom window. The burglar alarm rings or I feel guilt, or both.

They then had to list the possibilities and impossibilities for the final assertion. There are three main possibilities:

1 The burglar alarm rings and I feel guilt.
2 The burglar alarm rings (and I don't feel guilt).
3 (The burglar alarm does not ring and) I feel guilt.

And there is one impossibility:

4 The burglar alarm doesn't ring and I don't feel guilt.

Each of the groups of participants was further subdivided into two. In one case, the participants had to list possibilities for assertions in vignettes intended to induce guilt; and in the other case, the participants had to list possibilities for neutral assertions, which ended with an assertion: The burglar alarm rings or I feel tired, or both. Each participant carried out the task four times with different contents, and two of the vignettes had a test assertion based on "and" and two of the vignettes had a test assertion based on "or". The results showed that those participants who were feeling guilt performed more accurately with the contents concerning guilt than the control participants who were not feeling guilt, but no reliable difference occurred between the groups tested with the neutral vignettes.

A corollary in daily life is that individuals feeling guilt should tend to reason about matters relevant to the emotion in a more expert way, thinking of possibilities that might otherwise elude them. The emotion increases motivation and improves reasoning, perhaps because it pushes individuals to deliberate, that is, to use system 2.

4 The hyper-emotional theory of psychological illnesses

Given the preceding groundwork, the theory that psychological illnesses are emotional disorders is straightforward (Johnson-Laird et al., 2006). The initial cause of such an illness is a transition to an emotion appropriate to the situation but inappropriate in its intensity. A situation elicits a cognitive evaluation, perhaps an unconscious one, that leads to an emotional signal. This signal has a variable intensity, perhaps normally distributed, and so it can be more intense than the situation warrants. Both the constitution of individuals and their everyday circumstances should affect the mean and variance of this distribution. They are aware of the emotion and often of its object, but they are not aware of what caused its excessive intensity. Their intentional efforts to control or to dismiss it are useless, and so it becomes the focus of their thought. The problem leads to deliberation – an exercise of skill that otherwise would be lacking. One side effect of this reasoning is to elicit the emotion again and to amplify it. Another side effect is that it leads to complex emotions, such as embarrassment, guilt, shame, or despair. The unfortunate individual experiences a recursive loop of mental events: cognitions that lead to emotions, which lead to further cognitions, and so on and on. But an alternative possibility is that the initial overreaction wanes, and the individual returns to a customary state of mind. The episode is over with no long-lasting effects. The difference between the self-terminating episodes and those that lead to illness is not a matter of chance. Constitution and circumstances affect the susceptibility of individuals to succumb to recursive attacks.

4.1 Evidence for the hyper-emotion theory

The theory predicts that each basic emotion can give rise to a psychological illness, and that no psychological illness can occur without a concomitant basic emotion.

TABLE 2.3 The principal psychological illnesses in terms of their underlying basic emotions and origins in the ontogeny of daily life

Ontogeny in daily life	*Basic emotions*	*Psychological illnesses*
Bodily needs	Anxiety	Anorexia
Maintenance of health	Anxiety	Hypochondria
Avoidance of danger	Anxiety	Phobia
Avoidance of noxious things	Disgust	Obsessive-compulsive disorder
Socio-sexual relations and attachment	All basic emotions	Hypomania
		Depression
		Intermittent explosive disorder
		Agoraphobia
		Social anxiety
		Sexual disorders
		Attachment disorders

Table 2.3 presents the goals of daily life, the basic emotions they elicit, including those with known objects, and the corresponding psychological illness.

The theory predicts that psychological illnesses originate in the acquisition of an unconscious transition from a cognitive evaluation to a basic emotion. Evidence corroborating this claim comes from brain-imaging studies, which show that the amygdala is active whenever events elicit the signs and symptoms of a psychological illness, and these organs are known to mediate basic emotions (for a review, see Johnson-Laird et al., 2006). Such studies continue to proliferate for all the major psychological illnesses (e.g., Fullana et al., 2017; He et al., 2019; McCloskey et al., 2016; Shackman et al., 2017).

A different sort of corroboration is illustrated in a small scale epidemiological study (Johnson-Laird et al., 2006: Study 1). The participants were 24 Italian psychiatrists who had to consult their records for six or so of their most recent patients diagnosed as obsessive, agoraphobic, hypochondriac, or depressed. They then answered 15 questions about these patients, and the crucial ones, unbeknownst to the psychiatrists, were whether the patient remembered the onset of the illness and which of 11 words denoting emotions was the one that the patient had reported about this occasion. The psychiatrists could choose their own emotion word if it wasn't on the list, but they seldom had to. Only 5 patients could not recall the onset of their illness, and of the 101 who could, the overwhelming majority (83 of them) referred to basic emotions as occurring at the onset of their illness, namely, in rank-order of their frequencies: anxiety, fear, sadness, anger, and disgust. Of the remainder, the main exception was that 12 patients reported guilt, a complex emotion. The theory treats it as a complex emotion, because it depends on a self-conscious assessment, and because it does not have an innate facial expression (see, e.g., Ekman, 1993). In fact, some patients reported feeling guilty without knowing why, so perhaps the emotion is a borderline case. The most important datum, however, is that the vast majority of the patients recalled the onset of their illnesses, and those who did always reported the emotions that they experienced. People do not succumb to these illnesses without emotions.

The evidence that individuals differ in their susceptibility to psychological illness rests in part on studies of twins. Comparisons of monozygotic and dizygotic twins have shown that tendencies both to anxiety and to depression are heritable (e.g., Jang et al., 1998). More recent genetic studies have corroborated the interaction between such innate factors and the environment in which individuals live (e.g., Guintivano and Kaminsky, 2016; Lin and Tsai, 2020; Peña and Nestler, 2018).

The theory predicts that individuals with psychological illnesses should become skilled in reasoning about matters concerning their illnesses. The initial evidence corroborating this prediction was based on a study, akin to the one described previously, in which individuals enumerated what was possible and what was impossible given an assertion. It examined patients with obsessive compulsions and non-clinical controls. The patients were more accurate than the controls in enumerating the possibilities of an assertion referring to guilt, but there was no reliable difference between the groups who assessed the possibilities for a neutral assertion or for one about depression. A similar study with depressed patients and non-clinical controls also showed that the patients were better at reasoning than the controls but only when the possibilities concerned depression (see study 3, Johnson-Laird et al., 2006).

A more recent study examined the syllogistic reasoning of depressed patients and matched non-clinical controls (Gangemi et al., 2013). The patients drew more valid conclusions from premises about depression (77%) than from neutral premises (37%), and this difference was larger than the analogous difference for the control participants (33% depressing conclusions and 43% neutral conclusions). Likewise, for syllogisms with no valid conclusions, the patients responded correctly 'nothing follows' more often for neutral than for depressing conclusions (56% versus 8% correct rejections), and this difference was reliably larger than the analogous difference for the control participants (7% versus 28% correct rejections). A subsequent study showed the same two interactions in a comparison between a group of patients at high risk of panic attacks and a group of non-clinical controls.

The groups of participants in these studies were matched for age, gender, and level of education, which is a reasonable proxy for intelligence. Hence, overall, the evidence is that individuals suffering from psychological illnesses do not reason any worse than those who do not have such illnesses, and that the patients tend to cope better than the controls with inferences pertinent to their illnesses. This conclusion is contrary to the claim that faulty reasoning underlies psychological illnesses (pace Beck, 1976). Alas, the better reasoning of patients could lead to the persistence of their illness by way of the positive feedback loop described earlier.

A final strand of evidence concerns the typical strategies of reasoning that patients with different psychological illnesses adopt. These strategies relate to the different way in which healthy individuals select evidence to test hypotheses. As we described earlier, an intuitive approach (system 1) seeks evidence that matches the content of a hypothesis – its effect, which may not be an individual's conscious intention, is to seek its corroboration by selecting potential examples of it. For difficult tasks, such as a selection task with an abstract hypothesis, this approach is the most frequent. In contrast, a deliberative approach (system 2) seeks evidence that has the potential to falsify a hypothesis by selecting its potential counterexamples. Certain individuals tend to adopt this approach, and certain contents in the selection task, such as deontic ones, tend to elicit this search for counterexamples (see Ragni et al., 2018).

Initial studies of patients established different characteristic strategies in reasoning. Obsessive-compulsive patients tend to feel guilt: about a third of them reported the emotion at the onset of their illness, a greater proportion than for any other of the patients in the epidemiological study (see Johnson-Laird et al., 2006: Table 6). Indeed, those suffering from obsessive thoughts and compulsions tend to consider deontic matters, such as risk to others, and to reason in a deliberative way (system 2). They focus on an action that has a danger of contamination, and leads to feelings of anxiety, and thence to guilt because it could have harmed others. They deliberate about both examples of the risk and counterexamples to it, and they conclude that they have to act to minimize it.

In contrast, other sorts of psychological illness concern deontic matters much less often, and patients' characteristic strategies are intuitive (system 1). Hypochondriacs focus on a bodily sensation and infer that they are ill, which leads to an intense anxiety. They search for evidence matching this hypothesis, and they conclude that they have to go to a doctor. A diagnosis that nothing is wrong with them elicits a further search for evidence matching their hypothesis. And so they may make further visits to doctors. Phobic patients have an analogous intuitive strategy that leads them to evaluate a particular object or situation as a cause of fear. Safety dictates that they should avoid this potential cause. Likewise, depressed individuals infer that the initial loss that provoked their sadness can never be made good: they search for evidence that matches this hypothesis, and may idealize what was lost to make a substitute impossible.

Empirical studies showed that psychiatrists could identify these strategies even when they were described with different underlying contents (Johnson-Laird et al., 2006: Study 2). Their identifications were rapid, but they were unable to describe the cues on which they relied. Subsequent studies showed that patients themselves were able to identify their own characteristic strategies of reasoning (Gangemi et al., 2019). Obsessive patients identified protocols using their system 2 strategy of reasoning in protocols describing a different illness. They were more accurate than patients with anxiety disorders. And those suffering from various anxiety disorders were more accurate in identifying their system 1 strategy of reasoning than obsessive patients were. Independent evidence also corroborates these strategic differences (e.g., Vroling and de Jong, 2009).

4.2 Prognosis for psychological illnesses

Individuals suffering from psychological illnesses report recovering spontaneously (e.g., Sutherland, 2010). But what seems impossible is that they can do so as a result of a simple decision: emotions are not under intentional control. The hyper-emotion theory implies that gradual exposure to the object or situation causing excessive anxiety should be useful. Over time, individuals should habituate and the emotion should wane (see, e.g., Vinograd and Craske, 2020). The therapy works for phobias and obsessive compulsions, and it is effective for hypochondria when patients see images and documentaries about diseases (Weck et al., 2015).

Various sort of cognitive therapy are also helpful treatments for psychological illnesses (Cuijpers et al., 2016). No empirical studies have shown that other sorts of psychotherapy or psychoanalysis are more effective (David et al., 2018). But, as these authors point out, it does not follow that it is the best possible therapy. Music has been used in psychotherapy for many years (e.g., Capurso et al., 1952), and a meta-analysis of studies shows that it can alleviate depression (Aalbers et al., 2017). It is improbable that music alone can cure psychological illnesses. But one problem in assessing psychotherapies is that any sort of personal intervention may induce a Hawthorne effect: the mere fact that a therapist is trying to cure an individual may foster a beneficial 'transference' or a positive outcome.

To discover a better treatment for psychological illnesses, clinicians may need a better understanding of what has gone wrong in patients' mental life. Cognitive therapies rest on the assumption that patients make faulty inferences and hold irrational beliefs. As this chapter has laboured to show, their reasoning is as good as that of control participants, and better about the topics of their illnesses. Some patients do have false beliefs, but not all do. Consider the case of an electrician who came to work in the author's apartment. He arrived at the front door panting for breath, because he had walked up 12 flights of stairs. He couldn't use the elevator for fear of a panic. (His sympathetic boss excluded him from jobs on higher floors.) His problem had started when he got into an elevator and for no apparent reason felt very frightened. It is not an irrational emotion, because people do get stuck in elevators. But his fear was so strong that he'd had to get out of the elevator at once. He said: "I don't know why being in an elevator is so scary, other than the fear of losing control of myself". As far as one can tell, he holds no irrational beliefs about elevators or self-control, because he might panic in an elevator. His main inference was to avoid getting into them – a sensible precaution. Such a case illustrates a serious empirical problem: the lack of evidence about the cognitions of people at the onset of their illnesses. Our small-scale epidemiological study suggests that most patients recall the first episode of their illness and the emotion that they felt. They may know nothing else beyond the object or cause of their emotion. Suppose that a large-scale study corroborates these findings. It follows that psychological illnesses are self-perpetuating hyper-emotions. The illnesses *are* disorders of emotions. They should be the target of more effective therapies.

5 Conclusions

The hyper-emotion theory boils down to three principles.

1. *Hyper-emotions*: Psychological illnesses are emotional disorders in vulnerable individuals, and their origin is a basic emotion appropriate to the situation but aberrant in its intensity. These emotions continue to occur throughout the illness, and patients cannot control them.
2. *Basic emotions*: The taxonomy of psychological illnesses goes back to the situations that evoke basic emotions in everyday life – happiness, sadness, anger, anxiety. They can be triggered by rudimentary models of emotional behaviours as in the case of music. Other basic emotions with known objects also underlie illnesses, e.g., disgust and hatred, and patients' reasoning can elicit complex emotions such as guilt.
3. *Reasoning*: Uncontrollable emotions are the focus of patients' thoughts. They think about their causes, and, as a result, they become skilful in reasoning about their illness, adopting either the intuitive strategy of system 1 or the deliberative strategy of system 2 depending on its nature. Their reasoning maintains their illness.

The theme of the present book is what the reasoning of individuals suffering from a mental pathology teaches psychologists about human reasoning. It yields two principal lessons. First, psychological illnesses show that normal processes of reasoning still occur. It is business as usual. Second, they reinforce the point that emotions, which are endemic in psychological illnesses, can improve reasoning – they can lead people to deliberate, to think of possibilities that would not otherwise occur to them, and to reach valid conclusions that they would not otherwise infer.

Note

1 www.modeltheory.org/models/

References

Aalbers, S., Fusar-Poli, L., Freeman, R. E., Spreen, M., Ket, J. C., Vink, A. C., . . . and Gold, C. (2017). Music therapy for depression. *Cochrane Database of Systematic Reviews*, 11.

American Psychiatric Association. (2013). *Diagnostic and statistical manual of mental disorders (DSM-5)* (5th ed.). Washington, DC: American Psychiatric Association.

Beck, A. T. (1976). *Cognitive therapy and the emotional disorders*. New York: Meridian.

Beck, A. T. (2019). A 60-year evolution of cognitive theory and therapy. *Perspectives on Psychological Science*, 14, 16–20.

Blanchette, I., and Richards, A. (2004). Reasoning about emotional and neutral materials. Is logic affected by emotion? *Psychological Science*, 15, 745–752.

Bucciarelli, M., Mackiewicz, R., Khemlani, S. S., and Johnson-Laird, P. N. (2016). Children's creation of algorithms: Simulations and gestures. *Journal of Cognitive Psychology*, 28, 297–318.

Capurso, A., Fisichelli, V. R., Gilman, L., Gutheil, E. A., Wright, J. T., and Paperte, F. (1952). *Music and your emotions*. New York: Liveright.

Cohen, L. J. (1981). Can human irrationality be experimentally demonstrated? *Behavioral and Brain Sciences*, 4, 317–370.

Cuijpers, P., Cristea, I. A., Karyotaki, E., Reijnders, M., and Huibers, M. J. (2016). How effective are cognitive behavior therapies for major depression and anxiety disorders? A meta-analytic update of the evidence. *World Psychiatry*, 15, 245–258.

Darwin, C. (1897). *The expression of emotions in man and animals*. New York: Appleton. (Originally published 1872.)

David, D., Cristea, I., and Hofmann, S. G. (2018). Why cognitive behavioral therapy is the current gold standard of psychotherapy. *Frontiers in Psychiatry*, 9, Article 4.

Ekman, P. (1993). Facial expression and emotion. *American Psychologist*, 48, 384–392.

Ekman, P., and Friesen, W. V. (1982). Felt, false, and miserable smiles. *Journal of Nonverbal Behavior*, 6, 238–252.

Ellis, A. (1962). *Reason and emotion in psychotherapy*. Oxford, UK: Lyle Stuart.

Ellis, H. C., and Ashbrook, P. W. (1987). Resource allocation model of the effects of depressed mood states. In K. Fiedler and J. Forgas (Eds.), *Affect, cognition and social behaviour*. Toronto: Hogrefe.

Evans, J. S. B. (2008). Dual-processing accounts of reasoning, judgment, and social cognition. *Annual Review of Psychology*, 59, 255–278.

Freud, S. (1915). The unconscious. In J. Strachey (Ed. and Trans.), *The standard edition of the complete works of Sigmund Freud* (Vol. 14, pp. 161–214). London: Hogarth Press.

Fullana, M. A., Zhu, X., Alonso, P., Cardoner, N., Real, E., López-Solà, C., . . . and Simpson, H. B. (2017). Basolateral amygdala – Ventromedial prefrontal cortex connectivity predicts cognitive behavioural therapy outcome in adults with obsessive-compulsive disorder. *Journal of Psychiatry and Neuroscience, JPN*, 42, 378.

Gangemi, A., Mancini, F., and Johnson-Laird, P. N. (2013). Models and cognitive change in psychopathology. *Journal of Cognitive Psychology*, 25, 157–164.

Gangemi, A., Tentore, K., and Mancini, F. (2019). Two reasoning strategies in psychological illnesses. *Frontiers of Psychology*, 10, 2335.

Gilman, B. I. (1891). Report of an experimental test of musical expressiveness. *American Journal of Psychology*, 4, 558–576.

Gross, J. J. (2002). Emotion regulation: Affective, cognitive, and social consequences. *Psychophysiology*, 39, 281–291.

Guintivano, J., and Kaminsky, Z. A. (2016). Role of epigenetic factors in the development of mental illness throughout life. *Neuroscience Research*, 102, 56–66.

He, C., Gong, L., Yin, Y., Yuan, Y., Zhang, H., Lv, L., . . . and Zhang, Z. (2019). Amygdala connectivity mediates the association between anxiety and depression in patients with major depressive disorder. *Brain Imaging and Behavior*, 13, 1146–1159.

Helmholtz, H. (1912). *On the sensations of tone* (4th ed.). New York: Longmans, Green. (Original work published in German, 1877; 1st ed. in 1862.)

Henle, M. (1978). Foreword. In R. Revlin and R. E. Mayer (Eds.), *Human reasoning*. Washington, DC: Winston.

Herink, R. (Ed.). (1980). *The psychotherapy handbook: The A to Z guide to more than 250 different therapies in use today*. New York: New American Library.

Hunter, P. G., Schellenberg, E. G., and Schimmack, U. (2008). Mixed affective responses to music with conflicting cues. *Cognition and Emotion*, 22, 327–352.

James, W. (1884). What is an emotion? *Mind*, 9, 188–205.

Jang, K. L., McCrae, R. R., Angleitner, A., Riemann, R., and Livesley, W. J. (1998). Heritability of facet-level traits in a cross-cultural twin sample: Support for a hierarchical model of personality. *Journal of Personality and Social Psychology*, 74, 1556–1565.

Johnson-Laird, P. N. (1983). *Mental models: Towards a cognitive science of language, inference, and consciousness*. Cambridge: Cambridge University Press; Cambridge, MA: Harvard University Press.

Johnson-Laird, P. N. (2006). *How we reason*. Oxford: Oxford University Press.

Johnson-Laird, P. N., Kang, O. E., and Leong, Y. C. (2012). On musical dissonance. *Music Perception*, 30, 19–35.

Johnson-Laird, P. N., Khemlani, S. S., and Goodwin, G. P. (2015). Logic, probability, and human reasoning. *Trends in Cognitive Sciences*, 19, 201–214.

Johnson-Laird, P. N., Lotstein, M., and Byrne, R. M. J. (2012). The consistency of disjunctive assertions. *Memory and Cognition*, 40, 769–778.

Johnson-Laird, P. N., Mancini, F., and Gangemi, A. (2006). A hyper emotion theory of psychological illnesses. *Psychological Review*, 113, 822–841.

Johnson-Laird, P. N., and Oatley, K. J. (1992). Basic emotions, rationality, and folk theory. *Cognition and Emotion*, 6, 201–223.

Johnson-Laird, P. N., and Oatley, K. J. (2000). The cognitive and social construction of emotions. In M. Lewis and J. Haviland (Eds.), *Handbook of emotions* (2nd ed., pp. 458–475). New York: Guilford Press.

Johnson-Laird, P. N., and Oatley, K. J. (2008). Emotions, music, and literature. In M. Lewis, J. Haviland-Jones, and L. F. Feldman-Barrett (Eds.), *Handbook of emotions* (3rd ed., pp. 102–113). New York: Guilford Press.

Johnson-Laird, P. N., and Oatley, K. J. (2016). Emotions in music, literature, and film. In L. F. Barrett, M. Lewis, and J. M. Haviland-Jones (Eds.), *Handbook of emotions* (4th ed., pp. 82–97). New York: Guilford Press.

Johnson-Laird, P. N., and Wason, P. C. (1970). A theoretical analysis of insight into a reasoning task. *Cognitive Psychology*, 1, 134–148.

Juslin, P. N., Liljeström, S., Laukka, P., Västfjäll, D., and Lundqvist, L. O. (2011). Emotional reactions to music in a nationally representative sample of Swedish adults: Prevalence and causal influences. *Musicae Scientiae*, 15, 174–207.

Kahneman, D. (2011). *Thinking fast and slow*. New York: Farrar, Strauss, Giroux.

Khemlani, S. S., Mackiewicz, R., Bucciarelli, M., and Johnson-Laird, P. N. (2013). Kinematic mental simulations in abduction and deduction. *Proceedings of the National Academy of Sciences*, 110, 16766–16771.

Krumhansl, C. L. (1990). *Cognitive foundations of musical pitch*. New York: Oxford University Press.

Lashley, K. S. (1958). Cerebral organization and behavior. In H. C. Solomon, S. Cobb, and W. Penfield (Eds.), *The brain and human behavior* (pp. 1–18). Baltimore, MD: Williams and Wilkins.

Lewontin, R. (1998). The evolution of cognition: Questions we will never answer. In D. N. Osherson, D. Scarborough, and S. Sternberg (Eds.), *An invitation to cognitive science, Vol. 4: Methods, models, and conceptual issues* (pp. 107–132). Cambridge, MA: MIT Press.

Lin, E., and Tsai, S. J. (2020). Gene-Environment interactions and role of epigenetics in anxiety disorders. In *Anxiety disorders* (pp. 93–102). Singapore: Springer.

Mancini, F., Gangemi, A., and Johnson-Laird, P. N. (2007). Il ruolo del ragionamento nella psicopatologia secondo la Hyper Emotion Theory. *Giornale Italiano di Psicologia*, 4, 763–793.

Masataka, N. (1999). Preference for infant-directed singing in 2-day-old hearing infants of deaf parents. *Developmental Psychology*, 35, 1001–1005.

McCloskey, M. S., Phan, K. L., Angstadt, M., Fettich, K. C., Keedy, S., and Coccaro, E. F. (2016). Amygdala hyperactivation to angry faces in intermittent explosive disorder. *Journal of Psychiatric Research*, 79, 34–41.

McRae, K., and Gross, J. J. (2020). Emotion regulation. *Emotion*, 20, 1–9.

Oaksford, M., Morris, F., Grainger, B., and Williams, J. M. G. (1996). Mood, reasoning, and central executive processes. *Journal of Experimental Psychology: Learning Memory and Cognition*, 22, 476–492.

Oatley, K. J., and Duncan, E. (1994). The experience of emotions in everyday life. *Cognition and Emotion*, 8, 369–381.

Oatley, K. J., and Johnson-Laird, P. N. (1987). Towards a cognitive theory of emotions. *Emotion and Cognition*, 1, 29–50.

Oatley, K. J., and Johnson-Laird, P. N. (1996). The communicative theory of emotions: Empirical tests, mental models, and implications for social interaction. In L. L. Martin and A. Tesser (Eds.), *Striving and feeling: Interactions among goals, affect, and self-regulation.* Mahwah, NJ: Lawrence Erlbaum Associates.

Partee, B. H. (2014). A brief history of the syntax-semantics interface in western formal linguistics. *Semantics-Syntax Interface*, 1, 1–20.

Peña, C. J., and Nestler, E. J. (2018). Progress in epigenetics of depression. *Progress in Molecular Biology and Translational Science*, 157, 41–66.

Peretz, I., Gagnon, L., and Bouchard, B. (1998). Music and emotion: Perceptual determinants, immediacy, and isolation after brain damage. *Cognition*, 68, 111–141.

Ragni, M., Kola, I., and Johnson-Laird, P. N. (2018). On selecting evidence to test hypotheses. *Psychological Bulletin*, 144, 779–796.

Ramsey, F. R. (1990). Philosophy. In D. H. Mellor (Ed.), *F. R. Ramsey, philosophical papers* (pp. 1–7). Cambridge: Cambridge University Press. (Originally published posthumously, 1929).

Shackman, A. J., Fox, A. S., Oler, J. A., Shelton, S. E., Oakes, T. R., Davidson, R. J., and Kalin, N. H. (2017). Heightened extended amygdala metabolism following threat characterizes the early phenotypic risk to develop anxiety-related psychopathology. *Molecular Psychiatry*, 22, 724–732.

Sloman, S. A. (1996). The empirical case for two systems of reasoning. *Psychological Bulletin*, 119, 3–22.

Sutherland, S. (2010). *Breakdown: A personal crisis and a medical breakdown.* London: Pinter and Martin. (Originally published 1976.)

Vinograd, M., and Craske, M. G. (2020). History and theoretical underpinnings of exposure therapy. In T. S. Peris, E. A. Storch, and J. F. McGuire (Eds.), *Exposure therapy for children with anxiety and OCD: Clinician's guide to integrated treatment* (pp. 3–20). New York: Academic Press.

Vroling, M. S., and de Jong, P. J. (2009). Deductive reasoning and social anxiety: Evidence for a fear-confirming belief bias. *Cognitive Therapy and Research*, 33, 633–644.

Wason, P. C. (1968). Reasoning about a rule. *Quarterly Journal of Experimental Psychology*, 20, 273–281.

Wason, P. C. (1969). Regression in reasoning? *British Journal of Psychology*, 60, 471–480.

Weck, F., Neng, J., Richtberg, S., Jakob, M., and Stangier, U. (2015). Cognitive therapy versus exposure therapy for hypochondriasis (health anxiety): A randomized controlled trial. *Journal of Consulting and Clinical Psychology*, 83, 665.

3

REASONING AND GOALS

From psychopathological patients to healthy people

Amelia Gangemi and Francesco Mancini

1 Introduction

> *Laura is 55 years old, she's a doctor at the local hospital, her parents died two years ago and she's been living alone since then. She is not married, she has no children and since she was 30 she has had an affair with a married colleague, who is 25 years older. A few months ago she realized their relation has got no future and that not having children, she is going to live a solitary life. She's sad, she often bursts into tears, she lost interest in her work and friends. In addition, her sadness and apathy make her feel a complete failure.*
>
> *Giovanni thought he was dying when, while driving in a motorway, felt a sudden chest pain, his heart beating fast, he found it difficult to breathe and felt an annoying tingling in his arms. Convinced he was having a heart attack, he asked his fellow passenger to drive the car and take him to the nearest E.R., where the doctors, having done multiple tests, found nothing wrong with his heart.*
>
> *Sabrina is 15 years old, and since college she has had great difficulties in the oral tests, although she likes studying and she has no difficulties in learning. When under examinations, it often happens to her to be afraid of being unable to speak. She looks at her classmates and sees some of them giggling, some others minding their own business. She thinks she's going to make a fool of herself and that her classmates will laugh at her even more. Then she starts to stutter and she turns red*

Although apparently different, the stories of Laura, Giovanni, and Sabrina are likely: they concern someone who, starting from data that are far from remarkable, draws a negative conclusion which is exaggerated (*I'm a failed person, I'm having a heart attack, I'm making a fool of myself*).

Through these stories we can describe mood disorders, like depression (as in the case of Laura) which is characterized by sadness, pessimism, anhedonia, i.e., the inability to enjoy pleasures and interests, and reduced activity (American

Psychiatric Association, 2013), and anxiety disorders (as in the case of Giovanni and Sabrina), that is those pathologies which present symptoms as pounding heart, tachycardia, choking sensation, chest pain, and, in some cases, fainting. In the case of Giovanni, the disorder, called panic attack, involves feelings of overwhelming panic and, often, of an impending catastrophe. In the case of Sabrina, the disorder, called social phobia, leads to avoid social situations because of the fear of failure. The stories also show that these disorders can persist even when the sufferers have the available information to value the reality in a different way.

More generally, these stories point out to a crucial question in cognitivist clinical research. How can a wrong assessment of the social or body reality of one person lead to such consequences, and above all, why do these assessments persist even when facing with data which could easily change them? What maintains psychological disorders is indeed a topical question for clinical and cognitive scientists, including psychiatrists, psychologists, and neuroscientists.

In this chapter we want to show how, thanks to all the research aimed at trying to answer to this fundamental clinical question, the maintenance of psychological illnesses and their resistance to change, have deepened our understanding of a relevant general psychological process, such as reasoning, and how it is a tool at the service of our goals. According to a functional and pragmatic account of reasoning, we understood that the best kind of thinking is whatever kind of thinking that best helps people to achieve or protect their goals and reduce the costs of crucial errors. And surprisingly, we found out that this is valid for both normal and abnormal people.

2 Psychopathology and reasoning

Observations of behaviour show that all of us often fail to be rational. We make frequent errors, drawing fallacious inferences (e.g., Johnson-Laird, 2006; Gangemi et al., 2013). Yet, we usually function quite well and manage to survive, and so biases in reasoning are not always maladaptive and may even have real benefits (cf. Smeets et al., 2000). Cognitive theory of emotional disorders, however, commonly claims that biases in reasoning lead to dysfunctional behaviour and to psychological illnesses, including disorders in emotion, mood, and personality (e.g., Beck, 1976, 2019; Garety and Hemsley, 1997; Harvey et al., 2004), or to the interaction of patients' beliefs and concerns with normal processes of reasoning – an interaction that in turn leads to biased or irrational inferences (Beck, 1976, 2019). For this reason, cognitive biases have become an important part of cognitive models of psychopathology (e.g., Bögels and Mansell, 2004; Clark and McManus, 2002; Hirsch and Clark, 2004).

According to such accounts, we were in good company when we originally thought that patients were more irrational in reasoning about topics pertinent to their illnesses than healthy individuals were. According to Beck (1976), we were convinced that if patients made fewer logical mistakes, they would be able to counteract the effects of these biases on maintaining their illnesses. Logic should therefore help patients to recognize and to correct their flawed thinking (e.g., Leahy, 2004), and the identification of the inferential errors that lead to dysfunctional beliefs and psychopathology should contribute to cognitive therapies (Smeets and de Jong, 2005). In sum, psychotherapy should address errors in reasoning (Young and Beck, 1982). Here is an example of a man, under treatment (by F.M.) for paranoia, explaining why he thinks people are taking the mickey out of him (translated from Italian, Johnson-Laird et al., 2006):

> *As soon as I entered the lecture room I saw the students chatting together and among their almost imperceptible words I caught the word 'queer'. They were taking the mickey out of me. Did you see how they were sniggering yesterday at the lecture and in the corridors as I was going past? Then the other day one of them was sitting in the first row right in front of me; I was about to start the lecture and he addressed the student next to him in an effeminate tone of voice. He was clearly referring to me. It is a known fact that students are cruel to teachers and like to have fun at their expense. I remember that when I was in high school, there was a teacher, probably gay, and my friends and I had fun at his expense for years. And I remember how my friends made fun of him as soon as his back was turned. Of course they are taking the mickey out of me!*

This report is an example of the confirmatory pattern of inference: patient focuses only on the worst case (e.g., *students were taking the mickey out of me*), searching for confirmatory evidence (e.g., *a student addressed the student next to him in an effeminate tone of voice. He was clearly referring to me*, etc.) and ignoring disconfirming alternatives (e.g., *the student was not referring to me*). For this reason, this reasoning will likely end in the confirmation and strengthening of the worst initial hypothesis.

This form of reasoning seems to confirm the traditional thesis, supported originally by Beck: patients reason in a wrong way, since it involves the tendency to search only for confirmatory evidence, and it always leads to draw the same wrong conclusion and to hold the pathological conclusion or belief which creates, worsens, and maintains the pathology. However, thanks to a wide number of experiments, in the last years, it has been found out that:

1 It's not true that patients systematically confirm the worst hypothesis, but they can also falsify the safety hypothesis (i.e., reassurances), and this is a *very difficult cognitive process*!
2 It's not true that patients are not able to reason logically, they can even reason better than healthy people, but only when they reason on topics relevant to their disturbance.

Starting from these empirical observations, i.e., patients confirm the worst hypothesis and falsify the safety ones (i.e., reassurances), and their reasoning is not impaired, it has been argued that they are motivated to reason effortfully to pursue their goals, thus reducing the likelihood of crucial errors and thereby avoiding their costs (see Friedrich, 1993).

In what follows, we are going to examine the empirical evidence supporting these conclusions, and what this tells us about reasoning processes in normal people.

3 Patients can also falsify hypotheses

Starting from the end of the 1990s, a group of Dutch researchers examined the hypothesis-testing process in patients affected by anxiety disorders, such as specific phobia and hypochondria (de Jong et al., 1997; Smeets et al., 2000). And since the first experiments, they surprisingly demonstrated that patients' hypothesis-testing process is domain-specific and guided by the relevance of the hypothesis to their personal interests (Evans and Over, 1996; Kirby, 1994; Manktelow and Over, 1991; Smeets et al., 2000). In patients affected by anxiety disorders, a positive hypothesis-testing strategy (confirming information seeking) coexists with more normative test strategies (falsifying information seeking), and these variations in their testing strategy (confirmation vs. falsification) depend precisely on the perceived utility of the outcomes. In de Jong and colleagues' experiments, phobics, hypochondriacal patients, and healthy controls were presented with modified Wason Selection Tasks. The Wason Selection Task (WST, Wason, 1968) is a paradigm that is often used to investigate individuals reasoning strategy concerning conditional rules, and it indicates to what extent individuals tend to look for potentially confirmatory or for potentially disconfirmatory information concerning these rules (i.e., propositions). Using safety and danger rules, they found, for example, that in the context of health threats, individuals with hypochondriasis are not only more likely to selectively search for confirming information when asked to judge the validity of a danger conditional hypothesis (e.g., *if a person suffers from a headache, then that person has a brain tumour*), but that they can also search for falsifying information when asked to judge the validity of a safety conditional hypothesis (e.g., *if a person suffers from a headache, then that person has influenza*), that is they tend to look for falsifications in the case of safety rules (de Jong et al., 1998). Other research has demonstrated that similar reasoning processes are also involved in the context of phobic threat (e.g., de Jong et al., 1997). In two experiments, participants were presented with WST pertaining also to phobic threats. The WSTs contained safety rules (*if it is a new house, then there are only a few spiders*) and danger rules (*if it is a modern house, then there are a lot of spiders*). Both experiments showed that only clinically diagnosed phobics rely on corroborating information regarding danger rules and disconfirming information regarding safety rules. Thus, these results suggest that the perception of phobic threat is sufficient to activate a danger-confirming reasoning strategy, and such a reasoning pattern serves to maintain or even increase phobic fears.

The threat can also be related to guilt emotion and responsibility, which play a crucial role in the genesis and maintenance of obsessive-compulsive disorder (OCD, cf. Mancini and Gangemi, 2015). OCD is a mental disorder in which a person feels the need to perform certain routines repeatedly (*compulsions*), or has certain thoughts repeatedly (*obsessions*).

In their review, Shapiro and Stewart (2011) show that in healthy people, a mental state of guilt leads to obsessive-compulsive (OC)-like symptoms, including increased threat perception (see Gangemi et al., 2007), over-responsibility, and intrusive thoughts/impulses (Niler and Beck, 1989). Moreover, in healthy neuroimaging groups, the mental state of guilt is associated with brain activation in regions proximal to OCD-affected regions (Shin et al., 2000; Takahashi et al., 2004). In obsessive patients, reasoning processes should thus aim to reject the possibility of guilt in having done something wrong in creating, for example, a risk of contamination. If one wants to falsify a risk with certainty, s/he can only try to imagine all the possibilities in which it could be true, and falsify them one by one. This is an example of a real, typical protocol describing a problem relevant to an obsessive patients' illness, using the falsificatory strategy (translated from the Italian; comments in parentheses highlight the crucial cues to the strategy):

> *I get off the bus and I touch someone. I physically feel that my hand, or rather my fist, punched him. I think I hit him on the head. I think he could be dead (the patient focuses on his action, seeking to corroborate its negative consequences; he makes a transition to the emotion of guilt). I looked back, but the bus was already gone. I keep thinking about it. . . . If I had hit him he would have at least reacted, he would have called for help, he would have beaten me (he tries to infer counter-examples to the negative outcome of his having harmed the other person). Yes, but it all happened so fast. But people would have said something, they would have stopped me (he searches again for counter-examples to the negative outcome). What if no-one noticed it until it was too late? (He thinks again of a corroboration)*

Accordingly, in a recent research (Gangemi et al., 2019), we found that obsessive patients focus on all the possibilities that could put them at risk, and try to refute them beyond a reasonable doubt. This falsificationist strategy is chosen because there is no possibility of acting on the facts, for example, changing them (e.g., *I cannot go back, avoiding to touch someone*). In this case, not only the results obtained but also one's own efforts are evaluated against very high standards. The ultimate goal of this strategy is to prevent the self-accusation of having not been up to fulfilling one's duties. This goal has a paradoxical effect: it suggests possible mechanisms by which the risk could be real (see Johnson-Laird et al., 2006; Gangemi et al., 2019). The reasoning of obsessive compulsive patients should therefore be refutatory, searching for evidence falsifying the risk.

To examine this strategy in obsessive patients, in our experiment, we used vignettes in which the protagonist was guilty and responsible for the negative outcome. One vignette was as follows:

> *Imagine that it's Sunday afternoon and I'm with my niece. I'm playing with her on the sofa, when my nose starts itching and I sneeze. I don't care and keep on playing with her. Later, it strikes me that my niece might be sick because of my sneeze. It would because of my carelessness. I should have been more careful.*

After reading the story, all participants were asked to try to reassure themselves about this possibility, beyond any reasonable doubt. According to the idea that obsessive symptomatology is based on the threat of being guilty, assessed as being imminent and the goal being to prevent it, we found that obsessive patients used the falsificationist strategy in this kind of scenario. For example, in the attempt to reassure himself, a patient wrote:

- *Surely it doesn't depend on that, but if I was cold it is. The mere fact that I sneezed made the air full of germs* (the participant corroborates the negative outcome).
- *Maybe the window was open. Therefore, the germs could have gone out* (to refute the negative outcome).
- *Nevertheless, they could have contaminated the kid; they could have been everywhere in the air* (to corroborate the negative outcome).
- *Surely it was a coincidence. Maybe she already had a cold* (a refutation).
- *But what if this is not the case* (a corroboration).

Our findings appear to add to the growing list of studies showing that the effects of reasoning in psychological disorders run counter to the real intentions of patients. For example, the falsificationist strategies used by obsessive patients are counterproductive and lead to an increase, instead of a decrease, in confidence that there will be a negative outcome, and this in turn leads to the maintenance of the dysfunctional beliefs.

In general, thanks to all these studies with clinical populations, we concluded that a context of threat mental state attracts all patients' attention to the importance of more effectively avoiding the harm. Thus, participants take account of their beliefs (e.g., they have a very serious illness, or they are going to cause harm due to their irresponsibility) and their goals (e.g., to avoid a late diagnosis, or to avoid guilt due to irresponsibility), and manage hypotheses (safety versus danger) following the kind of strategy that helps them to achieve the goals (Baron, 2008). In all the research reviewed, patients tended to consider only the hypothesis that best served their goal (e.g., to prevent feeling guilty due to irresponsibility, or to avoid a late diagnosis) or that best fitted their beliefs (e.g., they were going to cause harm; the harm was imminent and probable); moreover, they tended to seek evidence and draw inferences in a way that favoured the hypothesis that already appealed to them, and thus the one they focused on (Baron, 2008). In this way, patients put themselves in a position that makes it harder to revise a hypothesis.

4 Hypothesis-testing process: from psychopathology to normal reasoning

But what do we learn from these findings on the hypothesis-testing process as regard to reasoning processes in normal people? The answers come again from de Jong and colleagues' studies (e.g., de Jong et al., 1998). They started from the question whether it was the threat mental state that leads anxious patients to test their hypotheses to prevent the crucial error of underestimating a danger, thus confirming the danger hypothesis and disconfirming the safety hypothesis. To answer, the authors decided to induce a threat mental state in healthy individuals to check whether they used the same reasoning strategy observed in patients. In a further experiment (Smeets et al., 2000) with hypochondriacs and normal controls, after having given the same conditional rules (danger versus safety) used in the previous studies (e.g., de Jong et al., 1998), they demonstrated that the threat mental state induction in normal controls leads to testing information *as if* they were worried. Healthy controls showed indeed the same threat-confirming or safety-disconfirming strategy in the domain of health threats that was, for example, the characteristic strategy for hypochondriacal individuals in the context of health threats. In other words, the addition of the sentence "*After hearing this you get worried*", changed the sensitivity of normal controls to the WST's conditionals, leading them to change their usual hypothesis-testing strategies.

In line with this procedure, we decided to examine whether the induction of the mental state of responsibility and fear of guilt in healthy people resulted in the same reasoning strategy observed in obsessive patients. Using the WST, we thus investigated the influence of the induction of this mental state on the hypothesis-testing strategies (confirmation vs. falsification) adopted by participants in the case of both the danger (e.g., *if my patient's symptoms, then Ebola virus*) and the safety (e.g., *if my patient's symptoms, then influenza*) hypotheses. The task instructions to activate responsibility and guilt in the participants were as follows:

> *You are the only doctor in your ward, and are solely responsible for several patients. In the few last months, although you had everything necessary, i.e., diagnostic equipment, time and medical know-how, you made several mistaken diagnoses due to superficiality, inattention and lack of commitment that led to serious consequences for your patients. You feel guilty about this and are fearful of making new serious mistakes.*

And in line with de Jong and colleagues' results, we found that in the responsibility and fear of guilt mental state, control participants became interested in seeking examples confirming the worst hypothesis (danger rule). By contrast, responsible and guilt-fearing individuals faced with a positive hypothesis (safety rule) prudentially tended to search for falsifying information about it. Thus, in a prudential way, responsible and guilty participants tended to select potentially confirming information in the case of the danger rule, and potentially disconfirming information in the case of the safety rule.

All these results are consistent with research results on reasoning, and show that both the mental state (i.e., mental state of threat) and the kind of conditional rule (safety vs. danger) have a strong impact on the reasoning strategy that participants tend to use when asked to check its validity (e.g., Cheng and Holyoak, 1985; Cosmides, 1989; Smeets et al., 2000). Indeed, in the domain of threats, it is adaptive to rely on confirming information concerning danger rules. For example, given the rule "If the alarm bell rings, then there is a fire", one is well advised to check whether *the bell rings* is indeed followed by *the fire* and whether *the fire* is indeed preceded by *the bell rings*. The logical possibility of false alarm (the bell rings in the absence of fire) is less relevant for survival. In other words, although it is very uncomfortable to escape for nothing on some circumstances, only one time ignoring the bell may be fatal. Thus, individuals' interests are better served knowing whether the bell rings when there is a fire than whether the bell sometimes rings in the absence of a fire. The opposite is true for safety rules such as "If the dog barks, then it will not bite". In this example, it is adaptive to test whether it is, indeed, safe when the signal is present. That is, maybe there are barking dogs that bite. Thus, in the case of safety rules, individuals' interests are best served by searching for potentially disconfirming information. In line with the idea that individuals reasoning in the context of threat is guided by perceived utilities, it has been thus demonstrated that healthy people, indeed, rely on a confirmatory reasoning strategy when reasoning about danger rules, whereas individuals actively seek for falsifications in case of safety rules. To sum up, all people adopt a *better-safe-than-sorry reasoning strategy* (e.g., Smeets et al., 2000; Gangemi et al., 2015). People tend to adopt this strategy in the face of exposure to a threat. It focuses them on the danger and leads them to search for examples confirming it. Such a reasoning pattern is functional and adaptive when faced with threats. However, if the perceived threats are related to the disorders, and thus exaggerated (e.g., dysfunctional beliefs, as in case of hypochondriacal concerns), actively searching for danger confirming information in combination with ignoring disconfirming evidence logically serves to maintain dysfunctional beliefs.

5 Patients can even reason better

In the previous section, we demonstrated that reasoning in psychological disorders works in the same way as it does in normals, and that it departs from normative rules no more so than usual, and, above all, that it is goal-directed just like in healthy people (cf. Harvey et al., 2004). In what follows, we will not only see that faulty reasoning does not characterize psychopathology, but that, on the contrary, psychopathology would improve reasoning, but only when topics are relevant to the disorder. In other words, patients can even be better reasoners than normal, when they are in their pathological domain. This means again that their reasoning is goal-directed and directed in a specific way, that is, as a way to minimize and contain the risk of catastrophic errors! (cf. the principle of *Primary Error Detection and Minimization*, Friedrich, 1993, and Trope and Lieberman, 1996).

Our clinical observations suggest indeed that patients are highly competent reasoners, at least about matters related to their psychological illnesses. For example, Francesco Mancini treated a patient suffering from obsessive-compulsive disorder. She was worried that she might have contracted the HIV after having touched a magazine photograph of Rock Hudson, who had died from AIDS. To justify her worries, she said as follows (translated from the Italian):

> *The photographer must have been near to Hudson because the photograph was a close-up. So, he might have been contaminated. So, when he developed the negative, he*

could have contaminated it. The photographic negative was in contact with the print and so could have contaminated it. The man in charge of printing the newspaper used the print, and so, he could have passed its contamination on to the newspaper's printer. The printing press could have passed the contamination on to the picture in every newspaper. So, when I touched the newspaper, I too might have been contaminated.

Like expert reasoners, the patient constructed a long chain of interconnected inferences, and she envisaged more than just obvious possibilities. She recognized that her conclusion was questionable, yet, typically for this kind of patients, she could not reject it, and so she obsessed about that possibility. Clinical observations of this kind led us to doubt whether faulty reasoning is the cause of psychological illnesses.

Also in research, the assumption that patients and non-patients with propensities towards psychological illness are more irrational than normals has not found robust support. In that regard, again the studies conducted by the Dutch group of researchers seem rather interesting. For example, Smeets and de Jong (2005) found that in solving linear syllogisms, patients are not poorer reasoners than normal controls. Other studies have even shown that patients reason better than normal controls, but only when the contents of the task are relevant for their pathology (Jonson-Laird et al., 2006; Johnson-Laird, 2006; Mancini et al., 2007). For example, in two initial experiments, we examined the reasoning of participants with obsessive-compulsive tendencies and those with depressive tendencies (Johnson-Laird et al., 2006). The first experiment compared individuals with obsessive-compulsive tendencies and normal controls. All participants read a short scenario that ended with a specific proposition: *The alarm rings or I feel guilty, or both.* They were then asked to list what was possible and what was impossible according to this sentence. With this proposition, there are three different possibilities: (a) the alarm rings, (b) I feel guilty, and (c) the alarm rings and I feel guilty. There is only one impossibility instead: the alarm doesn't ring and I don't feel guilty. Each group of participants was further subdivided into two. In one group, the participants had to list possibilities for assertions in scenarios aimed at eliciting guilt, such as:

Suppose I am at my house with some friends. We decide to join some other friends in a bar. We leave the house joking amongst ourselves, but I forget to close the bathroom window. The burglar alarm rings or I feel guilty, or both.

They listed possibilities for the final sentence. In the other group, the participants listed possibilities for neutral scenarios, which ended with a sentence: *The burglar alarm rings or I feel tired, or both*, for which they listed possibilities. All the participants carried out the task four times with different contents, and two of the scenarios had a test proposition based on "and", while the other two vignettes had a test proposition based on "or". The obsessive individuals listed many more correct possibilities for sentences about guilt than the control participants did, but no reliable difference occurred between the two groups for neutral or depressing propositions.

The second experiment was the same, but the participants were at risk for depression. Again, depressed individuals listed many more correct possibilities for propositions about being depressed than the normal controls did, but no reliable difference occurred between the two groups for neutral propositions or those about guilt.

What both studies showed is that participants with tendencies towards mental illness reason about topics relevant to their illness better than about other topics, and better than control participants do.

In two further studies we examined participants who drew their own conclusions from syllogistic premises (Gangemi et al., 2013). In a first experiment we compared depressed patients and control participants. All the participants stated in their own words what followed, if anything, from several pairs of syllogistic premises. One set had premises (e.g., *Sometimes when I think of my future, I feel sad. Every time I feel sad, I'm very pessimistic*) and conclusions (e.g., *Therefore, sometimes when I think of my future, I'm very pessimistic*) that were depressing, and the other set had premises (e.g., *Sometimes when I look back at my life, I find myself smiling. Every time I find myself smiling, I feel very satisfied with myself*), and conclusions (e.g., *Sometimes when I look back at my life, I feel very satisfied with myself*) that were neutral. Overall, the depressed patients were more correct in their reasoning when they drew conclusions from premises about depression than the control participants. A second study compared the reasoning of students who were at high risk of panic attacks with controls who were not. The experiment was identical to the previous study apart from the different participants and contents. As in the previous experiment, anxious participants outperformed control participants when the premises and the conclusions (e.g., *Sometimes when I am in an elevator I find it difficult to breathe*) were relevant to their disturbance.

Overall, all the previous studies falsify the hypothesis that psychological illnesses impair reasoning: both the obsessive, depressed, and anxious participants outperformed control participants, but tended to draw conclusions relevant to their illnesses (e.g., Goel and Vartanian, 2011).

These findings suggest that psychological disorders help patients to explore more possibilities in reasoning about their symptoms, and this is because they are more motivated to draw conclusions about these symptoms. This could mean that individuals feeling anxious, depressed, or guilty should tend to reason about this kind of topic more expertly, thinking of possibilities that might otherwise escape them. The effect is to increase motivation and to improve reasoning, perhaps because emotions enable individuals, whether they are psychologically ill, to think of possibilities that they would otherwise not imagine.

The crucial question is now, why do clinical people reason better than non-clinical individuals when topics are pertinent to their illnesses?

According to the hyper-emotion theory (Johnson-Laird et al., 2006, see also Johnson-Laird in this book), psychological illnesses are disorders in which individuals have emotions that are appropriate to the situation but inappropriate in their intensity. This theory combines a theory of emotions and a theory of reasoning.

The theory of emotions is based on a cognitive view of emotions in which they dispose individuals to some thought and action, and can be caused by both unconscious and conscious evaluations of situations (see, e.g., Oatley and Johnson-Laird, 1987). An individual suffering from panic attack says, for example, "I don't know why I am so frightened in highway, other than that I feel that I might lose control of myself". Thus, although individuals may be aware of the cause of an emotion, they cannot be aware of the process that makes the transition to the emotion itself, which is exaggerated in its intensity. Individuals have no voluntary control over them. The best they can do is to adopt some method to decrease the emotion, such as avoiding its object.

The theory about reasoning assumes that it depends on envisaging the possibilities to which propositions refer, and on drawing conclusions that hold in those possibilities (Johnson-Laird, 2006). A common error in reasoning is to overlook a possibility (Barres and Johnson-Laird, 2003), and so any factor that can diminish such mistake should improve reasoning. One such factor is an emotion concerning the topic of inference. When these individuals experience this emotion, they are bound to reason about its cause. This focus, in turn, leads to the maintenance of the emotion and its concomitant pathology, which are beyond the reach of reason. But what this theory tells us about reasoning in healthy people?

6 Reasoning and emotion: from psychopathology to normal people

Before answering this question, we want to focus on what is the relation between rational thinking and emotion. A wide literature tends to see this relationship as a simple contrast between the two. Indeed, many scholars tend to use the term "emotion" as a substitute for the word "irrationality". They say that rational thinking needs to be always cold. We cannot thus reason well, reaching our goals, if we are influenced by our emotions. In this perspective, emotions should always worse our reasoning, making us irrational. Yet, this is not the position of the Appraisal Theories of reasoning. In general, these theories assume that an individual's goals (i.e., desires, needs, values) and beliefs (i.e., cognitions, representations, assumptions) are proximal determinants of our behaviour (cf. Castelfranchi and Paglieri, 2007). In particular, the appraisal-based theories claim that all emotional states and behaviours are based on "*a person's subjective evaluation or appraisal of the personal significance of a situation, object, or event on a number of dimensions or criteria*" (Scherer, 1999: 637). Among these dimensions or criteria, our own goals or interests are the most important. When we believe that they could be compromised, then our reasoning becomes a tool to make them safe. Accordingly, these theories claim that our emotions can even improve our capacity to protect our goals driven by our reasoning processes. And emotions can improve our reasoning in some contexts, as demonstrated by several studies (e.g., Blanchette and Richards, 2010, see also Chapter 4 in this book). Let's see what are these contexts. Some research shows that when emotions are incidental, and they are, for example, induced by music, they actually burden the system and lead to bad performance in a reasoning task (e.g., Blanchette, 2006; Blanchette and Richards, 2004). But, when emotions are integral, and so they are induced by the topic of reasoning, they improve it (e.g., Johnson-Laird et al., 2006; Gangemi et al., 2013). For example, Blanchette and her colleagues have shown these effects in a study with war veterans suffering from post-traumatic stress disorder. In this experiment, war veterans solved syllogisms better when the conclusions referred to a topic relevant for them, i.e., war, than to neutral topics (Blanchette and Campbell, 2005). Similar effects were found in the evaluation of syllogisms after the terrorist attacks in London, UK, in July 2005 (Blanchette et al., 2007). Participants who lived in London, UK, were more correct in drawing conclusions from syllogisms concerning terrorism than those living in Manchester, UK, who in turn were more accurate than those living in another country (e.g., Canada). In other words, the closer the geographical proximity of the participants was to the attacks, the greater was the proportion of them who correctly evaluated syllogisms. The difference between the Londoners and Canadians disappeared six months later, even though the Londoners still reasoned more accurately about terrorism than the other two groups. These results were due to the emotion related to the terrorist attack. The three groups differed indeed in the reported intensity of their basic emotions.

So, how do emotions explain an improvement in reasoning? The mental model theory of reasoning offers a hypothesis (e.g., Johnson-Laird, 2006; Johnson-Laird et al., 2015). The theory postulates that reasoning depends on imagining possibilities, and so emotions induced by the topic lead individuals to make a more exhaustive search for possibilities relevant to their cause than the search they make in other cases (e.g., Bucciarelli and Johnson-Laird, 1999; Johnson-Laird et al., 2006; Gangemi et al., 2013; Gangemi et al., 2015; Gangemi et al., 2019). In this way, our emotions may help people to achieve or protect their goals, orienting their reasoning processes. Reasoning thus becomes a tool to make them safe. This means that rational reasoning does not need to be cold. In many contexts, such as in a danger one, emotion can even improve our capacity to reason on the threat. An example of a functional reasoning strategy activated by our emotions is the previously mentioned Better Safe than Sorry strategy. In a context of danger, we focus on the threat and this leads us to feel a congruent emotion, such as anxiety. This emotion leads us to prudentially seek for evidence confirming the danger hypothesis. The confirmation of the threat protects us from crucial errors, i.e., undervalue a danger, when it is true. For example, if we are worried because of a persistent symptom, such as stomach pain, we could make a transition to great anxiety, focusing on the worst case as a result of our own anxiety: we could have a serious illness. This danger hypothesis is likely to start a confirmatory pattern of inferences, rather than a falsification process. We thus search for evidence confirming this hypothesis from an available source of information, such as an analogy with a friend, a relative, or a case in a newspaper, and this strengthens our belief in the worst-case scenario (see, e.g., Gangemi et al., 2019). We then infer that we should consult a doctor. If we are mistaken about our illness, no harm is done, but if we fail to consult a doctor and we have the illness, the consequences will be disastrous. We are adopting the better-safe-than-sorry reasoning strategy (de Jong et al., 1998) that helps us to focus on the danger and leads us to search for examples confirming it.

In summary, the relationship between rational thinking and emotion is more complex than a simple contrast between the two, if we avoid using the term "emotion" as a substitute for the word "irrationality". Emotions can make our reasoning rational, when they orient it to help our relevant goals, for example, by achieving or protecting them. This interpretation accords with the general principle that individuals think more carefully about what is important to them than about what is unimportant (Blanchette and Richards, 2010; Tanner and Medin, 2004).

7 Conclusions

Thanks to a wide number of experiments, we know now that patients' reasoning is not impaired, and that the source and the maintenance of their illnesses are not in faulty inferences. We argued that they are motivated to reason effortfully to pursue their goals, thus reducing the likelihood of crucial errors, and thereby to avoid their costs (see Friedrich, 1993). And this makes their reasoning rational. The same is for normal people. All of us are rational every time we think to achieve a relevant goal or to avoid compromising it. Our thinking depends on the relevance of the hypothesis we have to test and on the context in which we test it. In other words, what makes our reasoning process rational or irrational is not, for example, the systematic use of a falsification strategy, but choosing the strategy (confirmatory vs. falsificatory) that could avoid us to commit crucial errors, from the point of view of our goals. Our hypothesis testing is indeed a pragmatic directed process, mainly motivated by the costs of our inferential errors. Several studies demonstrated that people's hypothesis-testing process is indeed domain-specific and guided by their relevant goals: individuals' reasoning performances depend on the perceived relevance of the hypothesis to one's personal interests. (Baron, 2008; Evans and Over, 1996; Kirby, 1994; Manktelow and Over, 1991; Smeets et al., 2000).

Moreover, we now know that individuals suffering from mental illness experience intense emotions, and that, thanks to these emotions, can even reason better than those who are mentally healthy (e.g., Johnson-Laird et al., 2006; Owen et al., 2007; Vroling and de Jong, 2009). Yet, cognitive therapists keep on suggesting that the source of illnesses is in faulty inferences. The correction of these inferential errors would contribute to preventing their aberrant emotions. The hyper emotion theory postulates instead that the emotion directs attention, interpretation, and reasoning to its potential cause (Johnson-Laird et al., 2006). And again, this is valid for every one of us. The emotions, whether they are induced by the task or are a result of a psychological disorder, lead individuals to be more likely to construct models of possibilities pertinent to their source than to do so for other contents. It postulates indeed that reasoning depends on imagining possibilities – the key assumption in the model-based account of reasoning (see, e.g., Bucciarelli and Johnson-Laird, 1999; Johnson-Laird, 2006; Johnson-Laird and Byrne, 1991). It follows that all human beings will be more likely to envisage the possibilities needed to infer conclusions about the source of an emotion than about other matters. Several experiments (cf. Johnson-Laird et al., 2006; Gangemi et al., 2019) corroborated this prediction, and are consistent with a growing body of evidence suggesting that individuals showed increased normatively correct thinking when reasoning about "protected value", that is, issues they felt very strongly about, relative to other more neutral issues (Blanchette and Richards, 2010; Tanner and Medin, 2004).

References

American Psychiatric Association. (2013). *Diagnostic and statistical manual of mental disorders (DSM-5)* (5th ed.). Washington, DC: American Psychiatric Association.

Baron, J. (2008). *Thinking and deciding*. Cambridge: Cambridge University Press.

Barres, P., and Johnson-Laird, P. N. (2003). On imagining what is true (and what is false). *Thinking and Reasoning*, 9, 1–42.

Beck, A. T. (1976). *Cognitive therapy and the emotional disorders*. New York: Meridian.

Beck, A. T. (2019). A 60-year evolution of cognitive theory and therapy. *Perspectives on Psychological Science*, 14, 16–20.

Blanchette, I. (2006). The effect of emotion on interpretation and logic in a conditional reasoning task. *Memory and Cognition*, 34, 1112–1125.

Blanchette, I., and Campbell, M. (2005). The effect of emotion on syllogistic reasoning in a group of war veterans. In *Proceedings of the XXVIIth annual conference of the Cognitive Science Society* (p. 1401). Mahwah, NJ: Erlbaum.

Blanchette, I., and Richards, A. (2004). Reasoning about emotional and neutral materials. Is logic affected by emotion? *Psychological Science*, 15, 745–752.

Blanchette, I., and Richards, A. (2010). The influence of affect on higher level cognition: A review of research on interpretation, judgement, decision-making and reasoning. *Cognition and Emotion*, 15, 561–595.

Blanchette, I., Richards, A., Melnyk, L., and Lavda, A. (2007). Reasoning about emotional contents following shocking terrorist attacks: A tale of three cities. *Journal of Experimental Psychology. Applied*, 13, 47–56.

Bögels, S. M., and Mansell, W. (2004). Attention processes in the maintenance and treatment of social phobia: Hypervigilance, avoidance and self-focused attention. *Clinical Psychology Review*, 24, 827–856.

Bucciarelli, M., and Johnson-Laird, P. N. (1999). Strategies in syllogistic reasoning. *Cognitive Science*, 23, 247–303.

Castelfranchi, C., and Paglieri, F. (2007). The role of beliefs in goal dynamics: Prolegomena to a constructive theory of intentions. *Synthese*, 155, 237–263.

Cheng, P. W., and Holyoak, K. J. (1985). Pragmatic reasoning schemas. *Cognitive Psychology*, 17, 391–416.

Clark, D. M., and McManus, F. (2002). Information processing in social phobia. *Biological Psychiatry*, 51, 92–100.

Cosmides, L. (1989). The logic of social exchange: Has natural selection shaped how humans reason? Studies with the Wason Selection Task. *Cognition*, 31, 187–276.

de Jong, P. J., Haenen, M.-A., Schmidt, A., and Mayer, B. (1998). Hypochondriasis: The role of fear-confirming reasoning. *Behaviour Research and Therapy*,36, 65–74.

de Jong, P. J., Mayer, B., and van den Hout, M. (1997). Conditional reasoning and phobic fear: Evidence for a fear-confirming pattern. *Behaviour Research and Therapy*, 35, 507–516.

Evans, J. St. B. T., and Over, D. E. (1996). Rationality in the selection task: Epistemic utility versus uncertainty reduction. *Psychological Review*, 103, 356–363.

Friedrich, J. (1993). Primary Error Detection and Minimization (PEDMIN) strategies in social cognition: A reinterpretation of confirmation bias phenomena. *Psycological Review*, 100, 298–319.

Gangemi, A., Mancini, F., and Dar, R. (2015). An experimental re-examination of the inferential confusion hypothesis of obsessive-compulsive doubt. *Journal of Behavior Therapy and Experimental Psychiatry*, 48, 90–97.

Gangemi, A., Mancini, F., and Johnson-Laird, P. N. (2013). Models and cognitive change in psychopathology. *Journal of Cognitive Psychology*, 25, 157–164.

Gangemi, A., Mancini, F., and van den Hout, M. (2007). Feeling guilty as a source of information about threat and performance. *Behaviour Research and Therapy*, 45, 2387–2396.

Gangemi, A., Tenore, K., and Mancini, F. (2019). Two reasoning strategies in psychological illnesses. *Frontiers of Psychology*, 10, 2335.

Garety, P. A., and Hemsley, D. R. (1997). *Delusions: Investigations in the psychology of delusional reasoning*. Hove: Psychology Press Ltd.

Goel, V., and Vartanian, O. (2011). Negative emotions can attenuate the influence of beliefs on logical reasoning. *Cognition and Emotion*, 25, 121–131.

Harvey, A., Watkins, E., Mansell, W., and Shafran, R. (2004). *Cognitive behavioural processes across psychological disorders: A transdiagnostic approach to research and treatment*. Oxford: Oxford University Press.

Hirsch, C. R., and Clark, D. M. (2004). Information-processing bias in social phobia. *Clinical Psychology Review*, 24, 799–825.

Johnson-Laird, P. N. (2006). *How we reason*. Oxford: Oxford University Press.

Johnson-Laird, P. N., and Byrne, R. M. J. (1991). *Deduction*. Hillsdale, NJ: Erlbaum.

Johnson-Laird, P. N., Khemlani, S. S., and Goodwin, G. P. (2015). Logic, probability, and human reasoning. *Trends in Cognitive Sciences*, 19, 201–214.

Johnson-Laird, P. N., Mancini, F., and Gangemi, A. (2006). A hyper-emotion theory of psychological illnesses. *Psychological Review*, 113, 822–842.

Kirby, K. N. (1994). Probabilities and utilities of fictional outcomes in Wason's four card selection task. *Cognition*, 51, 1–28.

Leahy, R. L. (2004). *Contemporary cognitive therapy: Theory, research, and practice*. London: Guilford Press.

Mancini, F., and Gangemi, A. (2015). Deontological guilt and obsessive compulsive disorder. *Journal of Behavior Therapy and Experimental Psychiatry*, 49, 157–163.

Mancini, F., Gangemi, A., and Johnson-Laird, P. N. (2007). Il ruolo del ragionamento nella psicopatologia secondo la Hyper Emotion Theory. *Giornale Italiano di Psicologia*, 4, 763–793.

Manktelow, K. I., and Over, D. E. (1991). Social roles and utilities in reasoning with deontic conditionals. *Cognition*, 39, 85–105.

Niler, E. R., and Beck, S. J. (1989). The relationship among guilt, disphoria, anxiety and obsessions in a normal population. *Behaviour Research and Therapy*, 27, 213–220.

Oatley, K. J., and Johnson-Laird, P. N. (1987). Towards a cognitive theory of emotions. *Emotion and Cognition*, 1, 29–50.

Owen, G. S., Cutting, J., and David, A. S. (2007). Are people with schizophrenia more logical than healthy volunteers? *British Journal of Psychiatry*, 191, 453–454.

Scherer, K. R. (1999). Appraisal theory. In T. Dalgleish and M. J. Power (Eds.), *Handbook of cognition and emotion* (pp. 637–663). Chichester, UK/New York: John Wiley and Sons Ltd.

Shapiro, L. J., and Stewart, E. S. (2011). Pathological guilt: A persistent yet overlooked treatment factor in obsessive-compulsive disorder. *Annual Clinical Psychiatry*, 23, 63–70.

Shin, L. M., Dougherty, D. D., Orr, S. P., Pitman, R. K., Lasko, M., Macklin, M. L., et al. (2000). Activation of anterior paralimbic structures during guilt-related script-driven imagery. *Biological Psychiatry*, 48, 43–50.

Smeets, G., and de Jong, P. J. (2005). Belief bias and symptoms of psychopathology in a non-clinical sample. *Cognitive Therapy and Research*, 29, 377–386.

Smeets, G., de Jong, P. J., and Mayer, B. (2000). If you suffer from a headache, then you have a brain tumour: Domain specific reasoning "bias" and hypochondriasis. *Behaviour Research and Therapy*, 38, 763–776.

Takahashi, H., Yahata, N., Koeda, M., Matsuda, T., Asai, K., and Okubo, Y. (2004). Brain activation associated with evaluative processes of guilt and embarrassment: An fMRI study. *Neuroimage*, 23, 967–974.

Tanner, C., and Medin, D. L. (2004). Protected values: No omission bias and no framing effects. *Psychonomic Bulletin and Review*, 11, 185–191.

Trope, Y., and Lieberman, A. (1996). Social hypothesis testing: Cognitive and motivational mechanism. In E. Higgins and A. Kruglanski (Eds.), *Social psychology: Handbook of basic principles* (pp. 239–270). New York: Guilford.

Vroling, M. S., and de Jong, P. J. (2009). Deductive reasoning and social anxiety: Evidence for a fear-confirming belief bias. *Cognitive Therapy and Research*, 33, 633–644.

Wason, P. C. (1968). Reasoning about a rule. *Quarterly Journal of Experimental Psychology*, 20, 273–281.

Young, J. E., and Beck, A. T. (1982). Cognitive therapy: Clinical application. In A. J. Rush (Ed.), *Short-term psychotherapies for depression*. London: Guilford Press.

4

REASONING, TRAUMA, AND PTSD

Insights into emotion–cognition interactions

Isabelle Blanchette and Sara-Valérie Giroux

1 Introduction

Certain experiences in life are extremely distinctive. Situations where an individual's safety or integrity is compromised can generate extreme levels of emotion: fear, horror, and anguish. These experiences mark significant moments in life and lay down long-lasting and vivid memory traces. What is their impact on other cognitive processes such as reasoning? Emotions are typically thought of as antithetic to rational thought, but research in the past 40 years has provided a much richer portrait of the complex interactions between emotion and cognition. In this chapter, we examine how the experience of highly emotional events is associated with higher level cognitive function, and what this may tell us about the interaction between emotion and cognition.

We focus on reasoning as one example of a higher level cognitive process. Higher level cognitive function requires complex operations, often voluntary control and awareness. Reasoning is the process through which inferences are drawn. The ability to reason analytically is commonly held as one of the hallmarks of the rational mind. In this chapter, we ask how reasoning is affected by trauma, but also how analytic thinking can shape the experience of trauma.

Before diving into the cognitive aspects, we explore how prevalent the experience of trauma is. To determine implications for the normal mind, we need to know what normal is. While traumatic events are exceptional, in the sense that they occur rarely and that they generate incomparable levels of emotion, they are nevertheless normal, in the sense that they are experienced by a majority of the population. Following this global portrait of trauma, we examine how trauma exposure and post-traumatic stress disorder (PTSD) negatively impact analytic reasoning. We then explore how trauma affects precursor mechanisms, specifically working memory and attention, and how this may have cascade effects on reasoning. We review studies showing that higher level cognitive abilities, indexed by IQ or developed through education, can influence the experience of trauma. We draw on all this research to present novel insights into the emotion–cognition interactions and integrate these in a preliminary theoretical model.

2 Prevalence of trauma exposure

About 69–89% of individuals will experience a traumatic event at one point in their life (Breslau, 2009; Resnick et al., 1993; Van Ameringen et al., 2008). A traumatic event is defined in the DSM-V (American Psychiatric Association, 2013) as an event that involves actual or threatened death or serious injury, or a threat to the physical integrity of self or others. Such events evoke feelings of intense fear, helplessness, or horror. Hence, a traumatic event is defined by the person's emotional reaction, not solely by the characteristics of the event itself. Trauma, therefore, necessarily involves the interaction between emotion and cognition as it rests on the person's representation of the event as being life-threatening and the associated emotional reactions. Strictly speaking, certain events such as car accidents, physical assaults, or natural disasters are 'potentially traumatic'; whether they are traumatic varies across individuals. For short, we will use the term 'trauma exposure' to refer to exposure to a potentially traumatic event.

Epidemiological studies assessing the prevalence of trauma typically present a list of potentially traumatic events. Participants must indicate whether they have experienced each event. There is usually an 'all other traumas' category, where participants can report any other event that has evoked these feelings of fear, helplessness, or horror, or when they have felt that their safety or integrity was threatened.

In high-income countries (where the majority of studies have been conducted), the most common traumas reported are the unexpected death of a loved one, sexual assault, and seeing someone badly injured or killed (see Breslau, 2009; Van Ameringen et al., 2008). Exposure to at least one potentially traumatic event is very high even in relatively young individuals; for instance, up to 85% of college students report experiencing at least one potentially traumatic event (Frazier et al., 2009).

Recent worldwide surveys confirm similar levels of exposure globally. The World Health Organisation Mental Health Survey combines epidemiological surveys with nationally representative samples from 26 countries, ranging from lower income countries such as Nigeria and the Ukraine to higher income countries such Italy and New-Zealand (Kessler et al., 2017). More than 70,000 respondents were asked about 29 types of events, including war, accidents, and interpersonal violence. Global exposure rate was 70.4%. The most frequently reported traumas were the unexpected death of a loved one and witnessing death or serious injury.

In specific areas of the globe, where political and economic instability are high, or where there is war or armed conflicts, exposure to trauma can be even more prevalent and more severe. We have worked with participants in Rwanda and the Democratic Republic of Congo (DRC). During the 1994 genocide against the Tutsis in Rwanda, and over the period of chronic armed conflicts in the North-East of the DRC since 1994, individuals have been exposed to a range of traumatic events. In one of our studies in Rwanda, more than 90% of participants (from an *n* > 700) experienced the death of a loved one during the genocide, more than 80% had to flee their home, and more than 10% reported being raped. In the DRC, over 70% of the 220 participants in one of our studies directly witnessed armed combat. Over half were physically assaulted, threatened with a machete, or tortured. Kidnapping of a loved one was reported by half of participants. One out of two women experienced rape or sexual assault. Again, trauma exposure is not restricted to adults. One study conducted in Butembo, in the DRC, found that close to 75% of children had lost a family member and over 95% had experienced shooting (Masinda and Muhesi, 2004). These data illustrate the cumulation of potentially traumatic events faced by individuals living in parts of the globe afflicted by armed conflicts.

While trauma exposure is prevalent, only a minority of individuals will develop a post-traumatic stress disorder following such events. PTSD is a psychological disorder characterized by the persistent re-experiencing of a traumatic event, as well as alterations in mood, cognition, arousal, and reactivity (American Psychiatric Association, 2013). Intrusions are a cardinal feature of PTSD. These are unsolicited memories of negative past events, often in the form of images or sensory impressions, that are experienced as if occurring in the present. Breslau (2009) estimates that 6.8% of participants exposed to trauma will develop PTSD, based on the combined prevalence across nine studies. In the World Health Organisation (WHO) surveys conducted with representative community samples, lifetime prevalence of PTSD was estimated at 3.9% in the total sample, and 5.6% among trauma-exposed participants (Koenen et al., 2017). Certain types of traumas, notably sexual violence, intimate partner violence, and physical assault are more likely to lead to the development of PTSD, compared to others such as natural disasters (Breslau, 2009; Kessler et al., 2017). The cumulation of trauma also increases the likelihood of developing PTSD. Nevertheless, while a large majority of the population will be exposed to at least one form of trauma during their lifetime, only a minority of participants will suffer from PTSD.

The rates of PTSD may however be much higher in geographic areas such as Rwanda or the DRC where people experience a multitude of potentially traumatic events. In Rwanda, one study with a nationally representative sample estimated the prevalence of PTSD to be 26%, 14 years after the end of the 1994 genocide (Munyandamutsa et al., 2012). In our own sample of over 700 participants (not intended to be representative), tested between 2014 and 2018, the estimated rate of PTSD was 21%. The rate is higher when focusing on genocide survivors. In 2018 and 2019, 181 mothers who were genocide survivors participated in one of our studies; 61 of them (34%) met the criterion for probable PTSD. In North Kivu (DRC), we conducted a study in a period of ongoing armed conflicts; one out of three participants met the criteria for probable PTSD.

The rates observed in our studies generally concur with a recent meta-analysis of 33 studies of mental health in civilians exposed to war that estimated PTSD rates of 26% (Morina et al., 2018). A different recent study quantified the global prevalence of war exposure and PTSD by combining geolocated data on armed conflicts (from the Uppsala Conflict Data Program) and epidemiological surveys of mental health (Hoppen and Morina, 2019). Between 1989 and 2015, 1.45 billion people were exposed to war, of which 452 million likely suffered from PTSD. Most war survivors live in low-income countries like Uganda, Liberia, Sudan, and Palestine.

Altogether trauma exposure is highly prevalent, across the globe. In high-income and relatively safe countries, only a minority of participants exposed to trauma will suffer from PTSD. In areas exposed to armed conflicts, individuals are more likely to be exposed to a cumulation of events that threaten their safety and integrity. In such circumstances, rates of PTSD in the population are much higher, and may remain high for very long periods. Traumatic events are associated with intense feelings of fear, helplessness, or horror. They are exceptional in the sense that they evoke a level of emotional intensity that is rarely experienced in a lifetime. Investigating how these experiences, with or without PTSD, may be related to cognitive function offers a window into the interaction between emotion and cognition.

3 Reasoning and other cognitive correlates of trauma

In this section, we examine how trauma is related to reasoning. We will use the term trauma to refer to trauma exposure and PTSD indistinctly and use the specific terms when an effect is uniquely related to either PTSD or trauma exposure. We will present how trauma is negatively related to analytic reasoning. To explain this deleterious effect, we will draw upon the effect of trauma on two antecedent processes: working memory (WM) and attention. This will lead us to the hypothesis that attentional prioritizing of trauma-related information may start a cascade of cognitive operations resulting in reduced availability of cognitive resources, which negatively impacts analytic reasoning.

Reasoning and higher level cognitive processes

Reasoning is a complex process that can be accomplished through explicit, systematic processing of the structural features of arguments, for instance, through logic or statistical reasoning (Ball and Thompson, 2018). This type of process can be labelled analytic thinking. It can be contrasted with heuristic processing, which subsumes the reasoning processes that are less systematic, more likely to be based on intuition, influenced by semantic content, beliefs, and context. Analytic reasoning exemplifies the human capacity for abstract thinking. It can be influenced by a number of things, including emotion (Blanchette and Richards, 2004, 2010).

Trauma-related contents can decrease analytic thinking. In one study (Eliades et al., 2012), women survivors of sexual violence and controls reasoned about logical problems with neutral, emotional, or sexual abuse-related contents. Responses could be based on logic or belief. When participants reasoned about sexual abuse contents, they were more likely to display heuristic thinking and less likely to display analytic thinking. This was the case for both victims and non-victims. The sexual abuse–related contents were judged to be highly emotional, and personally relevant, by both groups of women, whether they reported personal experiences of sexual violence or not (we come back to the role of personal relevance later in the chapter).

We observed analogous results in a study examining statistical reasoning emotion (Eliades et al., 2013). We used the base rate task which indexes the extent to which participants rely on statistical vs. anecdotal information in drawing inferences. We compared problems with neutral contents to problems related to sexual abuse, using stimuli such as: *In a sample of 1000 persons, 5 are rapists. Mike is 30 years old. He enjoys watching child pornography, has few friends, and is generally a mysterious person. . . .* Participants were more likely to rely on heuristic processing, in this case anecdotal information, as opposed to statistical information when the contents were trauma related. In this study, the difference between trauma and neutral problems was greater for survivors of sexual violence than controls; they also judged these contents to be more emotional.

These two studies illustrate how reasoning about trauma-related contents can be associated with decrements in analytic thinking. Other studies have documented generic deficits in analytic thinking as a function of PTSD. For instance, in a group of UK veterans, logical reasoning was reduced for participants suffering from PTSD, compared to non-PTSD veterans (Blanchette et al., 2014). In our studies in Rwanda, trauma exposure and PTSD symptoms are negatively correlated with analytic reasoning (Caparos et al., 2018). In addition to the reasoning tasks, we also measured symbolic thinking using the matrices subtest of the Weschler Adult Intelligence Subscale, and this was also negatively related to both trauma exposure and PTSD symptoms.

PTSD may also be associated with more encompassing deficits in higher order cognitive function, notably in so-called executive functions (Polak et al., 2012; Scott et al., 2015). While this is a very broad category, some studies of executive function have included tasks measuring analytic or symbolic thinking, often taken from intelligence tests (Scott et al., 2015). Most findings confirm a negative correlation between PTSD and performance on these tests of analytic thinking.

Altogether studies suggest that trauma-related contents and the experience of trauma or PTSD are associated with decreased analytic reasoning or symbolic thinking. Analytic reasoning has been measured using syllogisms, conditional reasoning, or base rate tasks, taken from the psychology of reasoning literature. Symbolic or abstract thinking has often been measured using neuropsychological tests, for instance, subscales from IQ tests. The two cognitive abilities are highly related, though not entirely overlapping (Stanovich, 2009). Both, however, rely heavily on WM, which is also related to trauma. In the next section, we examine the link between trauma and WM as a potential precursor of its effect on reasoning.

Working memory

The experience of trauma is associated with working memory deficits. In one study with patients suffering from psychiatric disorders, a history of trauma was associated with lower performance on three different working memory tasks (alphabetic span, OSpan, and running span; El-Hage et al., 2006). In non-psychiatric samples, the number of stressful life events reported negatively correlates with working memory performance, measured with the OSpan task (Klein and Boals, 2001). Similarly, in four studies, we found that women who experienced sexual abuse, on average, showed lower WM performance (measured using the Reading Span task) than non-victims matched for age and education (Blanchette and Caparos, 2016). Women who suffered experiences of sexual abuse also reported a greater number of stressful life events generally; the number of life events reported was negatively correlated with WM performance. A failure to replicate the link between stressful life events and WM performance has recently been reported (Goller et al., 2020), so the link be restricted to potentially traumatic events, and not negative, or stressful life events generally.

Our studies in Rwanda further document the link between trauma exposure, PTSD, and WM (Blanchette et al., 2019). Participants completed a measure of verbal storage (a forward digit span task). They also answered questions about the severity of their experiences during the 1994 genocide. Participants who reported a greater number of potentially traumatic experiences showed poorer performance on the digit span task. This was more than 20 years after the events occurred. We more recently observed the same negative correlation between trauma exposure and performance on the digit span (both forwards and backwards) in the DRC, during a time of ongoing violence (Kankunda, Balumé, Caparos and Blanchette, in preparation).

The relationship between trauma and WM has also been observed in children, in this case using both visual and verbal WM tasks. Children exposed to family violence (DePrince et al., 2009) or chronic stress (Masson et al., 2016) show poorer WM performance, even when controlling for anxiety, socioeconomic status, and potential brain trauma. Effects of early childhood adversity on WM can persist into adulthood (see Goodman et al., 2019, for a meta-analysis).

In addition to trauma exposure, psychopathological symptoms are also related to WM function. Patients suffering from PTSD show poorer WM performance compared to healthy controls exposed to the same events. For instance, Iraqi, American and Bosnian veterans suffering from PTSD presented lower WM performance than healthy veterans exposed to similar combat experiences (Honzel et al., 2014; Koso & Hansen, 2006). Different meta-analyses and narrative reviews confirm that participants suffering from PTSD generally show poorer WM performance than age- and education-matched controls (Aupperle et al., 2012; Buckley et al., 2000; Polak et al., 2012; Scott et al., 2015).

One hypothesis suggests that thoughts related to negative events compete for working memory resources (Klein and Boals, 2001). One feature of emotional memories, particularly of highly emotional events, is that they are more likely to be activated, spontaneously or as a result of retrieval cues, in memory networks. The activation of trauma-related thoughts may capture WM resources, leaving less resources available to process task-related stimuli, especially in cognitively demanding tasks. This hypothesis has yet to be tested directly.

One important methodological issue needs to be considered: in most studies of trauma and WM, participants answer questions about their difficult past experiences and their psychological symptoms in the same session as they complete the cognitive assessments. Trauma-related thoughts have thus typically been primed through answering the questionnaires. This may increase the strength of the link between WM and trauma. The correlation between trauma and WM may be weaker when trauma-related thoughts have not been primed. Studies examining the impact of task order (WM first vs. questionnaires first) or using separate sessions to assess trauma experiences and cognitive function are required to explore this further.

Nevertheless, the negative link between trauma and WM appears to be robust. It is also consistent with the effects observed for analytic reasoning and symbolic thinking, which heavily rely on WM (Süß et al., 2002). If intrusive thoughts related to trauma weigh on WM, especially in individuals suffering from PSTD, this would decrease the likelihood of conjuring analytic processes when reasoning.

Most WM and trauma studies have examined performance with neutral (or trauma-unrelated) contents. Some studies have compared WM for emotional and neutral information. One recent meta-analysis suggests that in healthy populations, the affective nature of the information does not have an important impact on WM processing, but that it does in patients suffering from mental health problems (Schweizer et al., 2019). This meta-analysis did not break down results by type of psychopathology but it did include studies with patients suffering from PTSD. In patients, WM accuracy was negatively impacted by the presence of emotional contents. This points to a possible link between attention, WM, and trauma, this is what we explore next.

Attention

At least two dimensions of attention are impacted by trauma: attentional control and attentional bias. Attentional control refers to the ability to focus on relevant stimuli and ignore irrelevant stimuli. It is closely related to WM capacity (Oberauer, 2019). Attentional bias describes the extent to which the processing of specific types of contents, for example, trauma-related information, is prioritized over other information.

Attentional control can be examined using tasks such as the go-no-go, the Stroop task, and the Attentional Network Task. Meta-analyses confirm that attentional control is generally impaired in individuals suffering from PTSD, relative to non-exposed controls, and compared to exposed participants who do not suffer from PTSD (Aupperle et al., 2012; Polak et al., 2012). One meta-analysis estimates that the difference in executive function, including attentional control, is of moderate amplitude, between $d = -.45$ and -0.5. Thus, individuals suffering from PTSD have more difficulty focusing on task goals and/or inhibiting the processing of distracters.

An attentional bias towards trauma-related contents has been documented in many studies. One popular paradigm is the emotional Stroop task, where words are presented in different colours that participants must identify. Longer reaction times to name the colour of trauma-related contents is taken as an indication of increased attentional allocation to these semantic contents. The experience of trauma is closely related to this interference. For instance, in one study, sexual abuse victims and non-exposed controls named the colour of trauma-related, generally emotional and neutral words (Caparos and Blanchette, 2014). Trauma-related contents led to longer reactions times, compared to the emotional and neutral contents. The level of interference from trauma-related contents was linearly related to the severity of the abuse reported (r = 0.27) and to participants' subjective emotional evaluation of the contents. This type of attentional bias has been confirmed in a number of reviews of the literature on sexual abuse (Latack et al., 2017) as well as other types of traumas (Buckley et al., 2000; McNally, 2006).[1]

Trauma-related stimuli are thus prioritized. Further, it may be more difficult for individuals suffering from PTSD to inhibit distracters, including task-irrelevant thoughts related to trauma, to effectively allocate attentional resources towards task-relevant stimuli. This has implications for analytic thinking, which relies heavily on working memory and effective attentional control.

Personally relevant semantic contents

The evidence reviewed so far establishes that PTSD and trauma exposure have a deleterious impact on reasoning, and this impact is coherent with the effect of trauma on working memory and attention. Most studies of trauma and reasoning have evaluated cognitive function using generic, neutral contents. Analytic reasoning is impaired when reasoning about neutral contents; similarly, working memory is depleted when evaluated with digits, letters, or abstract shapes.

Research shows that semantic content can have a formidable impact on reasoning and other higher level cognitive processes. Thus, it may be important to consider what happens when trauma victims are processing information semantically related to trauma, which is personally relevant.

Personal relevance can indeed modulate the impact of emotion on analytical reasoning. For instance, we studied reasoning following coordinated terrorist attacks that occurred in London in 2004 (Blanchette et al., 2007). In one of these attacks, a bomb exploded on a bus. This occurred close to a university where we were able to interview people in the following week. We presented reasoning problems with neutral, emotional, or terrorism-related contents. We expected that participants would report higher levels of emotion and be more likely to reason based on beliefs (and stereotypes) when they were closer to the events. We used syllogisms such as the following: *Some Muslims are terrorists; Some terrorists are suicide bombers; Therefore, some suicide bombings are done by Muslims*, where logical and belief-based answers conflict. We compared the answers of participants in London to those of participants in Manchester, in the North of England, London, Ontario, and Canada. As predicted, participants in London reported higher levels of emotion. Contrary to expectation, they provided more logical answers to conflict problems related to terrorism.

Participants were thus more likely to reason analytically, and less likely to reason heuristically, when reasoning about emotional personally relevant topics.

We observed similar mitigation of the effect of emotion by personal relevance in another study with victims of severe car accidents or sexual abuse (Caparos and Blanchette, 2017). Participants reasoned about neutral contents, car accidents, or sexual abuse. Personal relevance systematically mitigated the effect of emotion on reasoning: victims of car accidents made more errors of logic on the sexual abuse than the neutral problems, but not on the car accident problems. Inversely, sexual abuse victims made more errors of logic on accident-related contents, but not sexual-abuse related contents, compared to neutral problems. Thus, emotional contents decreased analytic reasoning, except when these contents were personally relevant.

Studies exploring the role of personal relevance in emotional reasoning are still scarce. One other program of research confirms similar emotion-enhancing effects of emotion in psychopathology (Gangemi et al., 2014; Johnson-Laird et al., 2006). Participants suffering from varied psychopathologies, including depression and obsessive-compulsive disorder, displayed more logical reasoning when reasoning about contents related to their condition.

Nevertheless, emotion-enhancing effects on reasoning can be small and inconsistent. For example, in the study of belief bias and base rate neglect reported at the beginning of this chapter, sexual abuse victims did not exhibit more analytic reasoning than non-exposed women even though problems concerned sexual abuse. This may be because of the unfortunately high prevalence of sexual abuse; all women may process these contents as personally relevant. More research is needed to confirm that personal relevance mitigates the impact of trauma on reasoning.

There are however parallel findings concerning episodic memory illustrating that relevance can moderate the impact of trauma on cognitive function. The experience of trauma negatively impacts generic episodic memory. Individuals who have experienced trauma and/or suffer from PTSD show deficits in verbal episodic memory compared to non-exposed controls (Brewin et al., 2007). For example, victims of sexual abuse show poorer free recall and recognition of neutral and generally emotional short stories narrated to them, compared to non-exposed controls matched for age and education (Grégoire et al., 2020). There is a negative association between PTSD and verbal episodic memory, estimated to be of small to moderate size (Brewin et al., 2007; Buckley et al., 2000).

Trauma-related contents however mitigate these observed deficits in episodic memory (Grégoire et al., 2020). In our studies, victims did not differ from controls in their memory for short stories related to sexual abuse (a date rape scenario). Analogous findings were observed in a study of Holocaust survivors who showed no deficit in remembering paired-associates when the contents were related to the Holocaust (Golier et al., 2003).

Results from studies of episodic memory are consistent with those observed in reasoning studies. Both could be explained by the attentional prioritizing of personally relevant, trauma-related contents. This would counteract the depletion of attentional or working memory resources. The increased motivation to accurately process and represent these contents in working memory may also play a role (Blanchette and Caparos, 2013).

Altogether these studies highlight the important point that trauma does not necessarily have a universally negative impact on cognitive function. Trauma does not necessarily impair episodic memory or analytic reasoning. Before exploring the mechanisms responsible for the impact of trauma on cognition further, we examine the reverse relation: the impact of higher level cognition on the experience of trauma.

4 Impact of cognitive function on trauma

Experiencing highly emotional events can influence cognitive function, for participants who develop PTSD as well as those who do not. There is also evidence for the reverse relation: that higher level cognitive function can impact the experience of trauma. In this section, we present studies showing that IQ and education protect against the development of PTSD. We also describe the role granted to symbolic processing in PTSD models. These two lines of research suggest that symbolic thinking may be intrinsically related to the encoding (and subsequent regulation) of emotional experiences.

Intelligence, education, and PTSD

IQ is correlated with PTSD symptoms. Across studies of adults and children, individuals with lower IQ on average experience more severe PTSD symptoms (Buckley et al., 2000; Malarbi et al., 2017).

The relationship between IQ and PTSD may run in both directions. Trauma and PTSD could reduce global cognitive functioning; however, increased cognitive ability may also protect against the development of PTSD symptoms. Most studies are correlational and do not make it possible to differentiate between these two options. But there are a few studies using prospective and other designs showing that IQ represents a pre-existing vulnerability for the development of PTSD.

In one such study, Gilbertson and colleagues (Gilbertson et al., 2006) tested the IQ of 49 Vietnam veterans and that of their identical twin brothers. About half of the veterans had developed PTSD following combat exposure. These veterans suffering from PTSD had lower IQs than the non-PTSD veterans (the average difference was of 14 IQ points). However, the same difference existed for the brothers who had not been exposed to combat. This strongly suggests that the lower IQ of the veterans who developed PTSD existed prior to combat exposure rather than result from PTSD.

Similar conclusions were reached in a prospective study of 4000 young adults in Australia (Parslow and Jorm, 2007). The sample had been constituted to examine the factors that affect cognitive functioning over the years. Participants were tested for a wide range of cognitive functions, including verbal intelligence, episodic memory, and working memory. Three years after the initial test, a severe bushfire occurred in the area, resulting in over 5000 evacuations, 400 injuries, and 5 deaths.

Of the original participants, 1500 experienced a form of trauma related to this event. They were tested again, 36 weeks after the events, and their PTSD symptoms were evaluated. Participants with lower performance on all initial neurocognitive measures showed higher levels of PTSD symptoms. This evidence also supports the conclusion that lower IQ represents a risk factor for the development of PTSD.

Education also seems to protect against the development of PTSD symptoms. One study examined the PTSD symptom trajectory of over 10,000 responders (police officers and others) involved in rescue, recovery, and clean-up after the attacks on the World Trade Centre in 2001 (Pietrzak et al., 2014). Higher education attainment protected against the more negative trajectories (severe chronic, delayed onset, etc.). Another prospective study confirms this in the Israel military (Kaplan et al., 2002). Intellectual functioning and educational attainment were measured before exposure to operations, as part of the screening process. Participants who later suffered from PTSD (n = 901) had lower IQ and educational attainment compared to their age-matched healthy controls, who were adolescents attending the same high schools. In another study in Armenia, researchers interviewed the survivors of a major earthquake (that caused 25,000 deaths) 23 years after the event (Goenjian et al., 2018). Those with higher levels of education were less likely to suffer from chronic PTSD.

Education and IQ are highly correlated. In high-income countries, where general levels of educational attainment are quite high, IQ (or general cognitive ability) is an important determinant of educational success (Strenze, 2007). Most studies on trauma, IQ, and education have been conducted in high-income. In lower-income countries, the number of years in formal schooling is more variable across the population and depends on a wide range of factors unrelated to cognitive ability. Conducting studies in such countries should provide important insights concerning the potential protective role of formal education and may allow us to tease apart the influence of education and cognitive ability. Preliminary evidence suggests that in the DRC, for children exposed to high levels of violence and interpersonal trauma, a secondary education reduces the level of PTSD symptoms, relative to a primary education, particularly for girls (Duagani Masika et al., 2019).

Altogether these results strongly support the conclusion that IQ and education affect the encoding or subsequent regulation of highly emotional events. Both IQ and education are critically related to the capacity for symbolic thinking, abstract reasoning, and decontextualized processing (Stanovich and West, 2000). The impact of trauma exposure may be more pronounced for individuals who have lower levels of cognitive abilities or limited access to the thinking tools developed through education. Several theoretical models of PTSD grant a central place to symbolic processing in the encoding of emotional experiences. This is what we review next.

PTSD models: cognitive function and PTSD

According to theoretical models of PTSD, higher level cognitive processes determine the nature of trauma memories. For example, Brewin's (2014) and Dalgleish's

(1999) theories of PTSD rest on the distinction between two modes of cognitive processing: a more abstract, symbolic, verbal, or propositional mode and a more perceptual, sensory, and associative mode. Intrusive memories are thought to result from an imbalance favouring the latter, leading to a more perceptual encoding of the traumatic event. Conversely, a more abstract encoding would result in less intrusive memories and less PTSD symptoms. Ehlers and Clark (2000) also base their analysis of PTSD on a dual pathways model of autobiographical memories. One path to encode memories relies on propositional knowledge and uses language or symbolic representations. This allows integration with other knowledge stored in semantic or autobiographical memory. The other path is based on associative memory and encodes more data-driven and implicit memory representations. Traumatic events may shift processing towards associative encoding. This can result in more intrusions, which are often evoked by non-semantic cues (temporal or perceptual) and generate disorganized sensory impressions, without explicit recollections or integration with other knowledge.

Thus, models suggest that symbolic processing has a strong impact on the encoding of the event and the integration of the memory trace in existing knowledge structures. Most models do not explicitly specify what will affect the extent of propositional vs. perceptual encoding. It could be hypothesized that situational factors (for instance, the current availability of cognitive resources) may play a role. Dispositional factors such as individual differences in symbolic cognitive ability, resulting from IQ or educational history, may also have an impact. Although the models do not explicitly draw this connection, the propositions are compatible with the empirical link between IQ, education and PTSD symptoms. However, IQ and education are not the unique determinants of symbolic processing. Experimental studies will be necessary to examine the causal role of symbolic processing in the encoding of emotional events.

5 Implications for understanding the 'normal' mind

We started this chapter by providing an overview of the prevalence of potentially traumatic events, events that pose a significant threat to a person's safety and integrity and bring about intense feelings of fear, hopelessness, and terror. Statistically, the experience of trauma is quite common, hence completely in the realm of 'normal' experiences. PTSD is much less frequent and only a minority of individuals exposed to trauma will develop PTSD.

In our review, we did not draw a sharp distinction between the effects of trauma exposure and those of PTSD. While it was not our goals to examine this systematically, our overview suggests that the effect of the two can often be similar in nature. Researchers oriented towards understanding individual differences will focus specifically on discerning the effects specifically related to PTSD. This requires experimental designs with three groups of participants: suffering from PTSD, exposed non-PTSD, and non-exposed healthy controls. While this is often difficult to achieve, an increasing number of studies present such a design. For some cognitive processes (attentional bias), these studies have provided evidence that effects of PTSD are stronger than those of trauma exposure (see, for example, Latack et al., 2017). The evidence is currently lacking for other processes such as reasoning and working memory. More studies are needed to provide an exhaustive portrait and to be able to determine where differences are merely quantitative and where there are qualitative differences. For our purpose, we conclude that both trauma exposure and PTSD are related to reasoning, working memory, and attention in important ways.

While trauma is ordinary in the statistical sense, it is extraordinary in the intensity of emotions associated. We can ask whether insights from the trauma studies help understand more 'normal' emotion–cognition interactions, those involving the milder, more mundane emotions ubiquitous in everyday life. We focus on three insights from trauma research that might have implications for ordinary emotional experiences: the role of relevance in emotional reasoning, the impact of symbolic reasoning on emotion encoding, and the mechanisms linking attention, working memory, and emotional reasoning.

Studies of reasoning and trauma have provided two important insights: trauma can decrease access to analytical reasoning, and the effect of emotion can be mitigated by personal relevance. The first point has been extensively supported in laboratory studies. Inducing mild levels of emotion either through mood inductions (Oaksford et al., 2004) or by manipulating the emotional content (Blanchette, 2006) reduces analytic responses on a range of reasoning problems. This effect is linked to working memory load. In one study (Trémolière et al., 2016), participants were given the dual task of maintaining visual matrices in working memory while they reasoned about emotional and neutral logical problems. Participants were slower on the working memory task when the reasoning contents were emotional, suggesting these problems had taken up a greater portion of available cognitive resources.

The second important insight is that relevance may modulate the effect of emotion on reasoning. We examined this experimentally in a study of deductive reasoning where we manipulated the emotional value and relevance of photographs presented along the reasoning problems (Blanchette et al., 2014). Drawing on the trauma studies, we hypothesized that emotional images might hinder analytic reasoning when they were irrelevant for the task, but not when they were relevant for the task. We reasoned that irrelevant emotional images would distract resources away from the inference-making process, but relevant images might help focus attentional resources on the task and support inference making. When the images were emotional but irrelevant, participants made more logical errors, compared to when the images were neutral. However, when the images were semantically related to the reasoning statements, emotional images did not lead to more errors. Response times were generally consistent with the hypothesized mechanism: emotional-unrelated images led to longer response times, but emotional-related images did not. This confirms that relevance may moderate the impact of milder emotional experiences on reasoning, similar to trauma.

Another important insight from trauma studies is that higher level cognitive processes affect the encoding of emotional experiences. This stems from research on the link between IQ, education, and PTSD symptoms, but also from the theoretical models of PTSD. To our knowledge, this has not been explored very much in experimental studies. We have started to do this in "trauma analogue" studies, in which participants view a video presenting shocking images that can lead to intrusions. We examine how the encoding of the emotional event is affected by (a) individual differences in cognitive ability, including WM and symbolic reasoning, and (b) experimental inductions of symbolic processing. In one study, we found that higher verbal abilities and WM capacities measured a priori were related to less intrusions and a reduced attentional bias following the trauma-analog video (Grégoire, Gagnon and Blanchette, in preparation). In an experimental study, we induced more symbolic processing in one group of participants using semantically distant, abstract analogies. Another group of participants processed more concrete analogies, which induced less symbolic processing. The abstract group showed reduced sensory encoding of the emotional video, as measured by evoked potentials (Leblanc-Sirois, Chouinard and Blanchette, submitted). This suggests that symbolic processing can have a causal impact on the way emotional events are encoded. This line of research is still in its infancy but exemplifies another insight from trauma studies that offers parallels to more 'normal' emotion–cognition interactions.

One final important insight concerns the consistency of the effect of trauma across functionally related cognitive processes. Trauma exposure and PTSD are negatively related to analytic or symbolic reasoning, working memory, and attentional control. There is a functional link between these three processes. Individual differences in WM and attentional control are highly correlated (Robison et al., 2018). Analytic reasoning processes heavily draw on WM resources. The causal link between these three functions is easy to imagine: depleted attentional control (particularly in conjunction with an attentional bias) leads to a loading of WM by irrelevant trauma-related stimuli which hinders analytic processing. This relationship would be moderated by the status of the distracters; when processing the trauma-related contents is relevant for the task, it would not have a deleterious effect. As far as we know, no experimental studies have yet examined this causal chain. This could be done using different methodologies acting on cognitive load and attentional control. The consistency of individual differences effects identified in the trauma studies suggests that this is a fruitful avenue to explore. It informs the initial sketch of a theoretical model we present shortly.

The trauma studies have thus generated interesting hypotheses to be explored in experimental studies. The correlational nature of the trauma and PTSD studies, bar a few exceptional prospective studies, makes it difficult to identify causal mechanisms. On the cognitive side, IQ is related to much more than symbolic processing abilities (speed of processing, confidence, occupational 'success', income, etc.). On the trauma side, exposure to potentially traumatic events is correlated with many other personal and socio-demographic variables (income, education, health, personality, etc.) that may all impact cognitive function. Experimental studies are necessary to disentangle these complex arrays of influence. Laboratory studies are useful both for drawing implications for normal experience and for understanding the causal mechanisms at play in trauma.

Such studies can also help understand the mechanisms responsible for the effect of different psychological interventions. These most often necessitate symbolic processing. Clients need to put their experiences into words, which represents a first level of abstraction. With the help of their therapist, they will try to extract meaning from their experiences and reactions. Parts of this process can occur in expressive writing, where writing about negative painful experiences can have a positive impact on mental and physical health (Pennebaker, 1997). Using experimental studies, it will be possible to understand more precisely the mechanisms through which these interventions operate and maybe identify cognitive interventions that can increase symbolic processing and facilitate this process.

Beyond psychotherapeutic interventions, our work introduces the idea that cognitive interventions could help mitigate the affective impact of traumatic experiences. If symbolic thinking can be increased through education, then investing in education could act upon mental health following trauma exposure. This is an important idea to explore in post-conflict, often in low-income countries faced with challenges of reconstruction. In these situations, very high levels of PTSD are often documented and resources are scarce. Individual mental health services are often impossible, and it can be a challenge to develop a culturally appropriate model of intervention. Our work suggests that investing in education, apart from its numerous other positive effects, may also decrease psychopathological symptoms. Experimental studies are needed to establish the causal protective influence of education, and to identify the active cognitive ingredient, but this is a promising avenue for investigation.

A word of caution is needed when drawing parallels between studies conducted in high-income, often Western cultures, and those conducted in varied other cultures, often in low-income countries. This requires careful consideration of certain unquestioned methodological and theoretical assumptions. To highlight a few examples, there are immense challenges in determining the appropriate way to measure cognitive function and psychopathological symptoms. In our own work, for example, the ubiquitous use of computers and reaction times does not transfer easily to samples in Rwanda or the DRC, where many of our participants have never used a computer. Reading is not universal, especially in areas afflicted by violence, poverty, and instability, where access to education is difficult. Challenges with translation are abundant. More fundamentally, there are questions about the theoretical cross-cultural validity of constructs such as PTSD or intelligence. This points to the complexities of conducting such research in intercultural contexts; however, we believe this should not deter us from undertaking that challenge. If we want to understand the "normal" mind, our studies need to include the diversity of human contexts, cultures, and experiences. This is especially important in relation to trauma, as traumatic events disproportionately afflict individuals underrepresented in psychological research.

Altogether trauma studies can make an important contribution to understanding how higher level cognitive processes interact with emotion, both in high-intensity traumatic situations and in milder everyday emotional experiences, in both psychological disorder and healthy populations. We are still far from a comprehensive account of such interactions. Nevertheless, we draw together some elements to sketch a model that integrates these insights and provides a road map for our future work.

6 Sketching a theoretical model

Existing models of PTSD provide detailed accounts of the ways in which higher level cognitive processing can influence the experience of trauma. To our knowledge, no model has yet been proposed to account for the reverse relation, between trauma and higher level cognition.

We suggest that exposure to highly emotional events generally leads to an attentional prioritization of threatening stimuli (attentional bias) (Buckley et al., 2000) coupled with facilitated memory activation for concepts related to these events, both in working memory, semantic memory, and episodic memory (Falsetti et al., 2002). In the short term, this would result in intrusions (Verwoerd and Wessel, 2010) or ruminations. Ruminations are verbal thoughts about emotional events. This is likely to lead to a reduction in working memory capacity, as cognitive resources are partially allocated to the processing of trauma-related contents. This has immediate effects on all processes that require WM. Hence, trauma exposure and PTSD symptoms are likely to decrease the extent of symbolic or analytic reasoning, especially in contexts where the semantic contents of the task are irrelevant.

Individual differences can modulate this in important ways, notably differences in attentional control and WM capacity. Individuals who have a greater ability to inhibit the processing of task-irrelevant distracters, including intrusive trauma-related thoughts, would be less affected by trauma exposure. Furthermore, individuals with a greater propensity or capacity for symbolic encoding may also be less likely to experience intrusions in the first place. A more abstract encoding of the traumatic events should allow more contextualization of the memory trace in existing memory networks and mitigate the spontaneous activation of trauma-related thoughts (Sheppes et al., 2009). While individual differences in symbolic reasoning abilities may play an important role, situational factors may also promote a more abstract encoding or re-encoding of traumatic experiences (for instance, psychotherapy, expressive writing, etc.). Education, which develops abstract thinking and reasoning, could facilitate this process.

7 Conclusions

Human experience includes situations that evoke incomparable levels of emotions, emotions that signal a threat to the most basic human need to preserve safety and integrity. These situations occur in most people lives', even is safe and prosperous countries. There are areas where these threats are numerous and recurrent. Some individuals will experience more chronic distress following such experiences, but everybody's cognitive processes are likely to be altered by such experiences. Studying how these experiences shape higher level cognition provides a window into the mechanisms that link emotions and cognitive processes.

Note

1 One recent meta-analysis has provided different conclusions, suggesting that the attentional bias towards threatening information in anxiety and PTSD is not significantly different from zero (Kruijt, Parsons & Fox, 2019). This meta-analysis however focused on the baseline data from RCT trials of a cognitive intervention aimed at modifying attentional bias in anxiety and PTSD. Of the 18 studies included, only 4 focused on PTSD. Furthermore, the analysis only included studies using the dot-probe task, ignoring the vast literature using the Emotional Stroop paradigm.

References

American Psychiatric Association. (2013). *Diagnostic and statistical manual of mental disorders* (5th ed.). Washington, DC: American Psychiatric Association.

Aupperle, R. L., Melrose, A. J., Stein, M. B., and Paulus, M. P. (2012). Executive function and PTSD: Disengaging from trauma. *Neuropharmacology*, 62(2), 686–694.

Ball, L. J., and Thompson, V. A. (2018). *The Routledge international handbook of thinking and reasoning*. New York: Routledge/Taylor Francis Group.

Blanchette, I. (2006). The effect of emotion on interpretation and logic in a conditional reasoning task. *Memory and Cognition*, 34(5), 1112–1125.

Blanchette, I., and Caparos, S. (2013). When emotions improve reasoning: The possible roles of relevance and utility. *Thinking and Reasoning*, 19(3–4), 399–413.

Blanchette, I., and Caparos, S. (2016). Working memory function is linked to trauma exposure, independently of post-traumatic stress disorder symptoms. *Cognitive Neuropsychiatry*, 21(6), 494–509.

Blanchette, I., Lindsay, P., and Davies, S. (2014). Intense emotional experiences and logicality: an exploration of deductive reasoning in survivors of sexual abuse. *Psychological Record*, 64(4), 859–867.

Blanchette, I., and Richards, A. (2004). Reasoning about emotional and neutral materials: Is logic affected by emotion? *Psychological Science*, 15(11), 745–752.

Blanchette, I., and Richards, A. (2010). The influence of affect on higher level cognition: A review of research on interpretation, judgement, decision making and reasoning. *Cognition and Emotion*, 24(4), 561–595.

Blanchette, I., Richards, A., Melnyk, L., and Lavda, A. (2007). Reasoning about emotional contents following shocking terrorist attacks: A tale of three cities. *Journal of Experimental Psychology: Applied*, 13(1), 47–56.

Blanchette, I., Rutembesa, E., Habimana, E., and Caparos, S. (2019). Long-term cognitive correlates of exposure to trauma: Evidence from Rwanda. *Psychological Trauma: Theory, Research, Practice, and Policy*, 11(2), 147–155.

Breslau, N. (2009). The epidemiology of trauma, PTSD, and other posttrauma disorders. *Trauma, Violence, and Abuse*, 10(3), 198–210.

Brewin, C. R. (2014). Episodic memory, perceptual memory, and their interaction: Foundations for a theory of posttraumatic stress disorder. *Psychological Bulletin*, 140(1), 69–97.

Brewin, C. R., Kleiner, J. S., Vasterling, J. J., and Field, A. P. (2007). Memory for emotionally neutral information in posttraumatic stress disorder: A meta-analytic investigation. *Journal of Abnormal Psychology*, 116(3), 448–463.

Buckley, T. C., Blanchard, E. B., and Neill, T. M. (2000). Information processing and PTSD: A review of the empirical literature. *Clinical Psychology Review*, 28(8), 1041–1065.

Caparos, S., and Blanchette, I. (2014). Emotional stroop interference in trauma-exposed individuals: A contrast between two accounts. *Consciousness and Cognition*, 28, 104–112.

Caparos, S., and Blanchette, I. (2017). Independent effects of relevance and arousal on deductive reasoning. *Cognition and Emotion*, 31(5).

Caparos, S., Giroux, S. V., Rutembesa, E., Habimana, E., and Blanchette, I. (2018). Twenty years later, the cognitive portrait of openness to reconciliation in Rwanda. *British Journal of Psychology*, 109(2), 362–385.

Dalgleish, T. (1999). Cognitive theories of post-traumatic stress disorder. In W. Yule and W. Yule (Eds.), *Post-traumatic stress disorders: Concepts and therapy* (pp. 193–220). New York: John Wiley and Sons Ltd.

DePrince, A. P., Weinzierl, K. M., and Combs, M. D. (2009). Executive function performance and trauma exposure in a community sample of children. *Child Abuse and Neglect*, 33(6), 353–361.

Duagani Masika, Y., Leys, C., Matonda-Ma-Nzuzi, T., Blanchette, I., Mampunza Ma Miezi, S., and Kornreich, C. (2019). Peritraumatic dissociation and post-traumatic stress disorder in individuals exposed to armed conflict in the Democratic Republic of Congo. *Journal of Trauma and Dissociation*, 20(5), 582–593.

Ehlers, A., and Clark, D. M. (2000). A cognitive model of posttraumatic stress disorder. *Behavior Research and Therapy*, 38, 319–345. https://doi.org/10.1016/S0005-7967(99)00123-0

El-Hage, W., Gaillard, P., Isingrini, M., and Belzung, C. (2006). Trauma-related deficits in working memory. *Cognitive Neuropsychiatry*, 11(1), 33–46.

Eliades, M., Mansell, W., and Blanchette, I. (2013). The effect of emotion on statistical reasoning: Findings from a base rates task. *Journal of Cognitive Psychology*, 25(3), 277–282.

Eliades, M., Mansell, W., Stewart, A. J., and Blanchette, I. (2012). An investigation of belief-bias and logicality in reasoning with emotional contents. *Thinking and Reasoning*, 18(4), 461–479.

Falsetti, S. A., Monnier, J., Davis, J. L., and Resnick, H. S. (2002). Intrusive thoughts in posttraumatic stress disorder. *Journal of Cognitive Psychotherapy*, 16(2), 127–143.

Frazier, P., Anders, S., Perera, S., Tomich, P., Tennen, H., Park, C., and Tashiro, T. (2009). Traumatic events among undergraduate students: Prevalence and associated symptoms. *Journal of Counseling Psychology*, 56(3), 450–460.

Gangemi, A., Mancini, F., and Johnson-Laird, P. N. (2014). Emotion, reasoning, and psychopathology. In I. Blanchette (Ed.), *Emotion and reasoning* (pp. 44–83). Hove, Sussex: Psychology Press.

Gilbertson, M. W., Paulus, L. A., Williston, S. K., Gurvits, T. V, Lasko, N. B., Pitman, R. K., and Orr, S. P. (2006). Neurocognitive function in monozygotic twins discordant for combat exposure: Relationship to posttraumatic stress disorder. *Journal of Abnormal Psychology*, 115(3), 484–495.

Goenjian, A. K., Khachadourian, V., Armenian, H., Demirchyan, A., and Steinberg, A. M. (2018). Posttraumatic stress disorder 23 years after the 1988 Spitak earthquake in Armenia. *Journal of Traumatic Stress*, 31(1), 47–56.

Golier, J. A., Yehuda, R., Lupien, S. J., and Harvey, P. D. (2003). Memory for trauma-related information in Holocaust survivors with PTSD. *Psychiatry Research*, 121(2), 133–143.

Goller, H., Banks, J. B., and Meier, M. E. (2020). An individual differences investigation of the relations among life event stress, working memory capacity, and mind wandering: A preregistered replication-extension study. *Memory and Cognition*, 48(5), 759–771.

Goodman, J. B., Freeman, E. E., and Chalmers, K. A. (2019). The relationship between early life stress and working memory in adulthood: A systematic review and meta analysis. *Memory*, 27(6), 868–880.

Grégoire, L., Gosselin, I., and Blanchette, I. (2020). The impact of trauma exposure on explicit and implicit memory. *Anxiety, Stress and Coping*, 33(1), 1–18.

Honzel, N., Justus, T., and Swick, D. (2014). Posttraumatic stress disorder is associated with limited executive resources in a working memory task. *Cognitive, Affective and Behavioral Neuroscience*, 14(2), 792–804.

Hoppen, T. H., and Morina, N. (2019). The prevalence of PTSD and major depression in the global population of adult war survivors: A meta-analytically informed estimate in absolute numbers. *European Journal of Psychotraumatology*, 10(1).

Johnson-Laird, P. N., Mancini, F., and Gangemi, A. (2006). A hyper-emotion theory of psychological illnesses. *Psychological Review*, 113(4), 822–841.

Kaplan, Z., Weiser, M., Reichenberg, A., Rabinowitz, J., Caspi, A., Bodner, E., and Zohar, J. (2002). Motivation to serve in the military influences vulnerability to future posttraumatic stress disorder. *Psychiatry Research*, 109(1), 45–49.

Kessler, R. C., Aguilar-Gaxiola, S., Alonso, J., Benjet, C., Bromet, E. J., Cardoso, G., . . . and Koenen, K. C. (2017). Trauma and PTSD in the WHO World Mental Health Surveys. *European Journal of Psychotraumatology*, 8. https://doi.org/10.1080/20008198.2017.1353383

Klein, K., and Boals, A. (2001). The relationship of life event stress and working memory capacity. *Applied Cognitive Psychology*, 15(5), 565–579.

Koenen, K. C., Ratanatharathorn, A., Ng, L., McLaughlin, K. A., Bromet, E. J., Stein, D. J., . . . and Kessler, R. C. (2017). Posttraumatic stress disorder in the World Mental Health Surveys. *Psychological Medicine*, 47(13), 2260–2274.

Koso, M., and Hansen, S. (2006). Executive function and memory in posttraumatic stress disorder: A study of Bosnian war veterans. *European Psychiatry*, 21(3), 167–173.

Kruijt, A.-W., Parsons, S., and Fox, E. (2019). A meta-analysis of bias at baseline in RCTs of attention bias modification: No evidence for dot-probe bias towards threat in clinical anxiety and PTSD. *Journal of Abnormal Psychology*, 128(6), 563–573.

Latack, J. A., Moyer, A., Simon, V. A., and Davila, J. (2017). Attentional bias for sexual threat among sexual victimization survivors: A meta-analytic review. *Trauma, Violence, and Abuse*, 18(2), 172–184.

Malarbi, S., Abu-Rayya, H. M., Muscara, F., and Stargatt, R. (2017). Neuropsychological functioning of childhood trauma and post-traumatic stress disorder: A meta-analysis. *Neuroscience and Biobehavioral Reviews*, 72, 68–86.

Masinda, M. T., and Muhesi, M. (2004). Children and adolescents' exposure to traumatic war stressors in the Democratic Republic of Congo. *Journal of Child and Adolescent Mental Health*, 16(1), 25–30.

Masson, M., East-Richard, C., and Cellard, C. (2016). A meta-analysis on the impact of psychiatric disorders and maltreatment on cognition. *Neuropsychology*, 30(2), 143–156.

McNally, R. J. (2006). Cognitive abnormalities in post-traumatic stress disorder. *Trends in Cognitive Sciences*, 10(6), 271–277.

Morina, N., Stam, K., Pollet, T. V., and Priebe, S. (2018). Prevalence of depression and posttraumatic stress disorder in adult civilian survivors of war who stay in war-afflicted regions. A systematic review and meta-analysis of epidemiological studies. *Journal of Affective Disorders*, 239(May), 328–338.

Munyandamutsa, N., Nkubamugisha, P. M., Gex Fabry, M., and Eytan, A. (2012). Mental and physical health in Rwanda 14 years after the genocide. *Social Psychiatry and Psychiatric Epidemiology*, 47(11), 1753–1761.

Oaksford, M., Carlile, J., and Moore, S. C. (2004). The effects of reasoning, prior mood, and personality on emotion. *Psychologia: An International Journal of Psychology in the Orient*, 47(4), 250–263.

Oberauer, K. (2019). Working memory and attention: A conceptual analysis and review. *Journal of Cognition*, 2(1), 1–23.

Parslow, R. A., and Jorm, A. F. (2007). PTSD symptoms in a community sample of young adults. *American Journal of Psychiatry*, 164(3), 509–515.

Pennebaker, J. W. (1997). *Opening up: The healing power of expressing emotions* (Rev. ed.). New York: Guilford Press.

Pietrzak, R. H., Feder, A., Singh, R., Schechter, C. B., Bromet, E. J., Katz, C. L., . . . and Southwick, S. M. (2014). Trajectories of PTSD risk and resilience in World Trade Center responders: An 8-year prospective cohort study. *Psychological Medicine*, 44(1), 205–219.

Polak, A. R., Witteveen, A. B., Reitsma, J. B., and Olff, M. (2012). The role of executive function in posttraumatic stress disorder: A systematic review. *Journal of Affective Disorders*, 141(1), 11–21.

Resnick, H. S., Kilpatrick, D. G., Dansky, B. S., Saunders, B. E., and Best, C. L. (1993). Prevalence of civilian trauma and posttraumatic stress disorder in a representative national sample of women. *Journal of Consulting and Clinical Psychology*, 61(6), 984–991.

Robison, M. K., Miller, A. L., and Unsworth, N. (2018). Individual differences in working memory capacity and filtering. *Journal of Experimental Psychology: Human Perception and Performance*, 44(7), 1038–1053.

Schweizer, S., Satpute, A. B., Atzil, S., Field, A. P., Hitchcock, C., Black, M., . . . and Dalgleish, T. (2019). The impact of affective information on working memory: A pair of meta-analytic reviews of behavioral and neuroimaging evidence. *Psychological Bulletin*, 145(6), 566–609.

Scott, J. C., Matt, G. E., Wrocklage, K. M., Crnich, C., Jordan, J., Southwick, S. M., . . . and Schweinsburg, B. C. (2015). A quantitative meta-analysis of neurocognitive functioning in posttraumatic stress disorder. *Psychological Bulletin*, 114(1), 105–140.

Sheppes, G., Catran, E., and Meiran, N. (2009). Reappraisal (but not distraction) is going to make you sweat: Physiological evidence for self-control effort. International Journal of. *Psychophysiology*, 71(2), 91–96.

Stanovich, K. E. (2009). Rational and irrational thought: The thinking that IQ tests miss. *Scientific American Mind*, 20(6), 34–39.

Stanovich, K. E., and West, R. F. (2000). Individual differences in reasoning: Implications for the rationality debate? *Behavioral and Brain Sciences*, 23(5), 645–726.

Strenze, T. (2007). Intelligence and socioeconomic success: A meta-analytic review of longitudinal research. *Intelligence*, 35(5), 401–426.

Süß, H. M., Oberauer, K., Wittmann, W. W., Wilhelm, O., and Schulze, R. (2002). Working-memory capacity explains reasoning ability: And a little bit more. *Intelligence*, 30(3), 261–288.

Trémolière, B., Gagnon, M.-È., and Blanchette, I. (2016). Cognitive load mediates the effect of emotion on analytical thinking. *Experimental Psychology*, 63(6).

Van Ameringen, M., Mancini, C., Patterson, B., and Boyle, M. H. (2008). Post-traumatic stress disorder in Canada. *CNS Neuroscience and Therapeutics*, 14(3), 171–181.

Verwoerd, J., and Wessel, I. (2010). Unwanted traumatic intrusions: The role of pre-trauma individual differences in executive control. In J. Mace (Ed.), *The act of remembering: Toward an understanding of how we recall the past* (pp. 337–360). Hoboken, NJ: Wiley Blackwell.

5

THE DISTINCTION BETWEEN ALTRUISTIC AND DEONTOLOGICAL GUILT FEELINGS: INSIGHTS FROM PSYCHOPATHOLOGY

Francesco Mancini, Guyonne Rogier, and Amelia Gangemi[1]

1 Introduction

In a review of the literature about feelings of guilt, Carnì et al. (2013) distinguish three main approaches: intrapsychic, interpersonal, and integrated.

The intrapsychic approach is well expressed by Freud, who assumes that guilt is the manifestation of the intervention of the Superego, which sanctions impulses, desires, and actions that violate internalized norms. Hence, guilt would express an intrapsychic conflict. In line with Kugler and Jones, "Guilt can be defined as the dysphoric feeling associated with the recognition of having violated a moral or social standard of personal relevance (1992: 218)".

Fromm (1985) claimed that the fear of being guilty is the fear of having outraged an authority, albeit an unreal, internalized one, and that guilt is a kind of power that authority wields over people. To alleviate their guilt, individuals who feel guilty are particularly disposed to do everything they can to get the authority's approval (Carnì et al., 2013).

> The psychoanalytic approach describes guilt, and the psychological distress that characterizes it, as not necessarily related to others. From this theoretical perspective, all the actions of people who experience guilt are aimed at diminishing their own discomfort, regardless of whether there is any actual damage repair. Thus, we can feel guilty and act to alleviate our guilt but not necessarily another's suffering.
>
> *(Carnì et al., 2013: 6)*

Consequently, all feelings of guilt, even the survivor's guilt, would translate into internal conflict, where transgression of a moral norm is not at all evident.

On the other hand, the interpersonal approach (Baumeister et al., 1994; Hoffman, 1982, 1998) shifted the attention from people's internal states to the relational effects of their actions/omissions. This approach attributes feelings of guilt to the assumption of having harmed or failed to help another person, with the feeling of guilt being crucially affected by the affection and empathy that unite the 'guilty' to the 'victim' (Kubany and Watson, 2003). Individuals feel guilty not towards an internalized authority but another person, particularly if they are tied to the other by affection or, at least, by a common belonging. It is worth noting that the interpersonal approach also suggests a monistic conception of feelings of guilt, including those guilt feelings in which it seems that the good of another person is not involved (Carnì et al., 2013).

Prinz and Nichols (2010) argued for an integrated approach, which describes the psychological guilt-related state as follows: "Someone I am concerned about has been harmed and I have responsibility for what I have done or failed to do". This schema includes two components: the perceived transgression of an internalized moral norm that defines responsibility and the idea of not having preserved the other's well-being. According to the monistic thesis of Prinz and Nichols (2010), any kind of guilt would therefore derive from these two ingredients, often mixed: having transgressed an internalized moral norm and having caused damage to a victim.

These three approaches share the idea that guilt is a single emotional state. However, two psychopathological disorders, obsessive-compulsive disorder (OCD) and major depression disorder (MDD), suggest the usefulness of distinguishing between two types of guilt: deontological guilt and altruistic guilt.

2 Obsessive-compulsive disorder

Obsessions are recurring and persistent thoughts or images, experienced in OCD as intrusive and undesirable and as the cause of marked anxiety or discomfort.

Roberto is obsessed by the doubt that he has not turned off the gas tap properly. This doubt implies strong anxiety linked to the fear that, if a gas leak occurred, there would be an explosion that could destroy the entire building where his apartment is located and kill a certain number of people. However, his main fear is that, if such an event occurred, it would be the result of his carelessness. To prevent this dramatic event, he checks the gas tap repeatedly and for a long time, often compulsively, in an attempt to eliminate any potential risk.

Claudio is obsessed by intruding thoughts of blasphemy that raise the doubt that he has intentionally offended God. To solve this problem, he engages in gruelling ruminations and mental compulsions, such as repeating the phrase 'I love God' several times.

Luigi is obsessed with order and symmetry. Before leaving the house, he must tidy up the objects placed on his desk. If he doesn't, he gets an intense feeling that things aren't as they should be and, more importantly, he deduces the likelihood of two negative consequences. The first is magical and superstitious by nature: 'If my objects are not ordered as they should be, something important to me will go wrong, and if something goes wrong, it will be my fault'. What could go wrong is likely to be an accident involving Luigi's wife. The second is subtler: 'if my objects are not right, then I am not right as a person', the whole self is imperfect in a moral sense.

Finally, Antonia is obsessed with the idea of being contaminated by her own and other people's excrement. This possibility does not arouse a fear related to health, but an unbearable feeling of disgust. To shake off this feeling, she engages in compulsive washing rituals.

Thoughts with the same obsession content are usually observed among the normal population (Berry and Laskey, 2012). Similarly, patients try to solve the problem aroused by obsessions the same way as everyone else's. For example, anyone might be afraid of leaving the gas tap open and, therefore, checks it. The difference lies in the importance attributed to obsessions and the severity/rigidity of the standard used to evaluate the results of the problem-solving process. What makes these possibilities so serious for obsessive patients? What are they really worried about?

Obsessions have a common denominator, the fear of being guilty. Claudio fears being guilty of disrespect towards God, Roberto fears the responsibility for having caused a gas explosion, Luigi is obsessed, ultimately, with the superstitious fear of not preventing an accident involving his wife. Obsessive patients tend to be prone to guilt, a sense of responsibility, and a fear of guilt to a greater extent than individuals extracted from the normal and clinical populations (Chiang et al., 2016; D'Olimpio et al., 2013; Mancini and Gangemi, 2011). Nakame et al. (2012) reported, in obsessive patients exposed to feared stimuli, a neural activation similar to that observed in anyone feeling guilty.

The reduction of responsibility, and therefore of the possibility of being guilty, both experimentally and therapeutically, reduces obsessive symptoms, while induction of a sense of responsibility and the fear of not being worthy of one's responsibility (i.e., induction of guilt) arouses controlling obsessive behaviour in non-clinical subjects. The same induction among obsessive patients, even patients with obsessions and compulsions related to the fear of contamination, activates controlling behaviour with higher obsessive characteristics than that observed in non-clinical subjects (for a summary of the studies, see Mancini, 2018).

Antonia's case is different. For her, being contaminated with substances such as excrement causes disgust, but not guilt or fear of guilt. Again, the literature supports the role of disgust in OCD. Bhikram et al. (2017) concluded from their review that "Recent research has identified the important role of disgust in obsessive-compulsive disorder (OCD) symptomatology. Exaggerated and inappropriate disgust reactions can drive some of the symptoms of OCD and, in some cases, can even outshine feelings of anxiety" (304).

Often, obsessive patients have symptoms related to both guilt and disgust and, even more frequently, they switch from one type of symptom to another during the course of the disorder.

Consequently, two questions emerge from clinical and empirical observations.

What kind of guilt is feared by obsessive individuals? It is usually assumed that to feel guilty, it is necessary to believe that you have deliberately acted or failed to act, causing harm or suffering to a victim, and that you have transgressed an internalized moral norm (Castelfranchi, 1994; Prinz and Nichols, 2010). Conversely, among patients with OCD, it is noted that they fear faults that do not harm anyone (for example, having blasphemous thoughts), being more concerned about the risk of having to blame themselves rather than the consequences for others. Roberto, for example, does not worry about the gas tap if the responsibility is not his, such as when he is not the last to leave the house. Luigi is not concerned about his wife having an accident for reasons beyond his responsibility. Thus, the sense of guilt feared by obsessives does not seem to be linked to the fate of the victim, but rather to the risk of having to blame themselves for not having done everything they could have done to fulfil their responsibilities.

With regard to OCD, therefore, two questions have arisen for the psychology of emotions. Is it possible to feel guilty only for the transgression of an internalized moral norm and not for the eventual harm to others? What is the relationship between guilt and disgust?

3 Major Depressive Disorder (MDD)

MDD is characterized by low mood (intense sadness) and a loss of interest in normal daily activities.

Martha is a 28-year-old woman who reports suffering from several depressive symptoms (e.g., fatigue, insomnia, anhedonia, chronic sadness, and guilt). She describes a very intimate and satisfying relationship with her mother, which has grown even stronger since her father died eight years ago. She describes herself as very caring and helpful towards her mother, a figure whom Martha perceives as emotionally vulnerable. On the contrary, she reports negative feelings about her sister, whom she considers irresponsible and a source of emotional distress for her mother. Thus, Martha reports the belief that she is the last chance to make her mother happy.

The depression started after Martha failed a university exam twice. Martha felt very guilty for failing because, in her opinion, this seriously undermined her goal of making her mother satisfied and happy. The depressive reaction was aggravated and maintained due to a vicious circle that exacerbated her feelings of guilt. Martha considered her depressive symptoms, in particular her loss of motivation and her propensity to cry and complain, as a further failure of her goal of making her mother happy. She feels more and more a burden to her mother and not a source of satisfaction.

It has recently been argued that at least one form of depression can be better defined as a disorder characterized by 'concern for others' rather than 'concern for self' (O'Connor et al., 2012). According to O'Connor et al. (2012), our understanding of depressive symptomatology thus appears to have suffered from a bias that overestimated the importance of motivation for self-centeredness and neglected the other set of motivational drives directed to others, including caring, altruism, and protection of the group. Recently, a growing body of empirical evidence has disproved these hypotheses, underlying the central role played by altruistic concerns in depression.

MDD suggests the hypothesis that it is possible to feel guilty, in a way that we could define as altruistic, resulting not from the transgression of a moral norm but the perceived failure of one's altruistic goals.

There thus emerges a question regarding the psychology of emotions, mirroring the question posed by OCD. Is it possible to have a sense of guilt essentially due to the failure of altruistic goals and not to the transgression of moral norms?

The view we advance in this chapter is that there are two essentially different types of guilt. For one, deontological guilt, awareness of having transgressed an internalized moral norm is necessary, but not the assumption of having harmed a victim. For the other, altruistic guilt, the conviction of having harmed a victim is necessary, but not the assumption of having transgressed an internalized moral norm. In most daily experiences of guilt, the two emotions coexist. Indeed, most moral norms are about respecting the good of the other. For example, six of the Ten Commandments concern the well-being of and respect for other people. However, in some cases, such as in the symptomatic domain of obsessive or depressed patients, only one form of guilt may emerge or assume a dominant role.

4 The altruistic guilt

To feel altruistic guilt, it is necessary to believe that you have failed to pursue an altruistic goal because of your own act or omission, whether real, planned, or desired. It must also be assumed that the conditions to act differently actually existed.

There are three defining elements of an altruistic goal. First of all, the content: the most obvious is linked to the good of the other. Another, less obvious content, which however appears evident in the case of sentimental relationships, is the desire to stand by another person in difficulty, even if that closeness is not useful or reassuring for the other (Parisi, 1977). A second element is that a goal, to be fully altruistic, must be pursued through sacrifice, that is, by putting the other's benefit before one's own. Common sense intuition indicates that an action is even more altruistic when it involves a cost to the actor, while it is not considered particularly altruistic to give the other something that is cost-free. The third element of an altruistic goal is that the good of the other and standing by him must be pursued in a disinterested way and not for one's own advantage.

Now, we would like to clarify one important misunderstanding that arises from the affirmation that being altruistic is in itself a moral norm. From this perspective, when one pursues the good of another, one respects the duty to be altruistic. To clarify this misunderstanding, we should start from an important premise: the psychological significance of an action depends on its subjective goal and not on its objective results. Thus, "*helping because you care is different, psychologically speaking, from helping because you think it is what morality demands*" (Prinz and Nichols, 2010: 113). Therefore, it is possible to pursue the good of another for at least two reasons. In the first place, to pursue an altruistic goal, that is, because one holds the good of the other as important in and of itself. Second, because of a sense of duty driven by the goal of respecting internalized moral norms, such as 'be charitable'. Thus, the statement 'be altruistic out of moral duty' is an oxymoron. One cannot be altruistic out of respect for one's moral duty, but certainly one can also pursue the good of the other out of moral duty.

Between these two ways of pursuing the good of another, out of altruism or out of a sense of moral duty, there is a great psychological difference. For example, let's imagine the case of a mother who realizes she doesn't love her children and feels guilty about it. In this case, her guilt would not be for the suffering of her children, which perhaps is even non-existent, but for her own inconsistency with the intuitive moral norm according to which a mother must love her children, otherwise, she violates the laws of nature.

The difference between other-directed behaviours motivated by altruism and those motivated by moral duty appears evident with a change of perspective. A few years ago, one of the authors clinically observed a young patient suffering from an acute depressive episode. A few months earlier, some days after her mother's death, while she was sorting out her mother's documents, she had found her mother's diary, written during the patient's childhood. In the diary, the mother often wrote about how little affection she felt for her children, how much she felt they were a burden, and how much she cared for them out of a sense of duty. This discovery surprised the patient, who had always had a completely different representation of her mother and her relationship with her children.

An intriguing question is whether altruistic goals, not instrumental to one's own advantage, actually exist, or whether, on the contrary, the good of the other is pursued only because of certain benefits to oneself. The answer lies in a long series of subtle experiments conducted by Batson, summarized in a chapter by Stich et al. (2010), and in other studies summarized by Warneken and Tomasello (2009): altruistic goals really exist. Human beings can pursue the good of another without any kind of personal advantage, even if there is no relationship with the other and even if the other is anonymous (i.e., a non-specific individual). People help others with a view to a truly altruistic goal, and not to reduce their discomfort induced by observing the difficulties of others, nor because they are afraid of being punished if they do not help, nor to avoid the pain associated with the sense of guilt they would experience if they did not help, nor in view of gratification, experienced as a positive sensation, which can derive from others or oneself (e.g., pride in having helped another), nor for the desire to feel the inner echo of the other's relief on being helped to overcome a source of suffering. Indeed, individuals care for each other, even though they know they will have no information on the effect of their help on the well-being of those they have helped (Stich et al., 2010). Furthermore, Tomasello's studies, summarized in Warneken and Tomasello (2009) and Tomasello (2016), found altruistic behaviours in very young children, around 2 years of age. According to the authors, this would suggest that the altruistic predisposition is innate and not a consequence of child rearing.

In support of the innate origin of altruism, some studies show monkeys and rats letting themselves starve if they associate eating to the suffering of another individual (Bekoff and Pierce, 2010). Thus, it seems that strictly (i.e., final) altruistic goals, pursued at a personal and likely innate cost, do indeed exist. This supports the idea that there is a possibility of feeling altruistic guilt.

It should be noted that altruistic guilt can arise from the failure of one of two altruistic goals. The first is closeness to the victim, which includes not only physical closeness to the victim but also the sharing of the respective ill-luck or misfortune or, where this is not possible, the participation in the suffering of the other. For example, if a good friend of mine is mourning the death of a parent, I am motivated to go to the funeral and show my emotional closeness and compassion for the friend's suffering, and therefore, for example, I may feel guilty if the evening after the funeral I go dancing. The second altruistic goal is, conversely, sharing one's joys with the other. I may feel selfish, and guilty about my selfishness, if I don't let my friends share in my joy, for example, in my wedding.

We report here two examples:

> I suffered from severe symptoms and was hospitalized. During this time, I shared a room with another person and we became friends. After three days, the doctor told me that I was fine and that I could go home. While I was packing my bags, my friend walked into the room. He was demoralized: the doctor told him he had cancer. Even today, I can't shake off the idea that I was going back to my life and he, instead, was going through a terrible experience. I felt guilty for not sharing his bad luck.
>
> *(Castelfranchi, 1991: 69)*

In this example, as in the following one, the sense of guilt arises from the failure of one of the two altruistic objectives, namely that of proximity to the victim, which includes not only physical proximity to the victim but also the sharing of the respective luck and misfortune, or, when this is impossible, of compassion for the pain of the other.

> I was on call in my hospital service when they called me from another service where my grandmother was hospitalized. A few minutes after I arrived, I realized my grandmother was in a coma and was about to die. I decided to return to my service to inform a patient that I could not speak to him that day. When I went back to my grandmother, I realized that in the meantime she died. Days later, I still feel guilty for not being near her and holding her hand while she was dying.

This is an example (from F.M.) of altruistic guilt due to affection, where guilt is aroused by not having been close to the victim. In both of these examples, the guilt stemmed from the failure of altruistic goals, particularly the goal of being close to the victim and sharing and participating in their pain. The transgression of a moral norm does not appear to be involved. Both protagonists wanted to stay close to the victim, not out of their sense of duty but out of their friendship and attachment, that is, for emotional and altruistic reasons.

The disposition to act out of altruistic guilt appears to be oriented in three directions: avoiding other altruistic faults, taking care of another's good by placing it before one's own, or maintaining a psychological closeness with the victim and, therefore, participating in the victim's suffering. This last case may then manifest itself as survivor guilt or guilt over getting better, even where one's good fortune is reduced. For example, someone might, without being aware of it, systematically block his efforts to achieve a goal because, if he were successful, the distance between him and, for example, a less fortunate sibling, would increase (Weiss, 1993). Therefore, systematic proneness to avoiding success, characteristic of those who feel altruistic guilt (Weiss and Sampson, 1986), does not appear to be motivated by a desire for atonement or the levelling of inequity (Castelfranchi, 1994; Mancini, 1997) but rather by the desire not to create further distance from the victim.

The facial expressions related to guilt are not known. Consequently, neither are those related to altruistic guilt. Verbal expressions, internal and external, refer to the victim, to his/her pain, his/her misfortune, and also to one's actions and omissions. For instance, in a study conducted by Basile and Mancini (2011), altruistic guilt was usefully elicited by sentences like the following: "How could I have left her alone?!", "She was suffering so much and I did nothing to help her!", "I left her alone with her difficulty", "I would have been able to help her and instead I didn't do anything". In brief, altruistic guilt also entails a distressing sense of pity for the victim, a proneness to saying "I'm sorry", to focusing attention on the suffering victim, a compassionate attitude towards the suffering other, and, finally, a proneness to relieving the victim's pain through personal sacrifices (Basile and Mancini, 2011).

5 The deontological guilt

Deontological guilt, as opposed to altruistic guilt, arises from the thought of having violated an internalized moral norm, and includes the feeling of being unworthy. Sometimes, one can find another or oneself guilty, even if no one has been harmed, not even oneself. Let's look at an example.

> Julie and Mark are brother and sister. They travel together in France during the summer holidays. One night, they are alone in a cabin near the beach. They decide it would be interesting and fun to try having sex. At least, it would be a new experience for both of them. Julie is already on birth con-

> trol pills, but Mark uses condoms too, just to be safe. They both enjoyed the experience but decide never to do it again. They will regard this night as a special secret that will bring them even closer to each other.
>
> *(Haidt, 2001: 814)*

This story has been told to thousands of individuals around the world, belonging to different cultures and religions, and most of them have found the incest between Julie and Mark to be morally blameworthy. Most people share this judgement even though the story makes it very clear that both are adults and consenting; both are mentally competent, that there is no risk of procreation; that there is no risk of psychological damage nor damage to their social image. The intuition that this behaviour is reprehensible is strong, as is the idea that everyone would feel guilty if they were the protagonists of the story. Let's imagine another example. A man had just graduated from medical school and just started being on call at a clinic. One evening, being on call, he found a patient in a coma due to final-stage intestinal cancer. Even in this state of unconsciousness, the patient complained of pain. The service manager told him to administer a strong dose of morphine, which would reduce the pain and speed up death. He was about to inject the morphine, but a thought came to his mind: "Who am I to decide this person's life and death? Who gives me the authority to take this action and replace God?" He then removed the needle; otherwise, he would have felt too guilty. In this example, the moral obstacle that stopped the young doctor also involved unnecessary pain for the poor patient. Therefore, feelings of guilt can exist independently of the well-being of others.

The feeling of deontological guilt is based on the conviction of having transgressed an internalized moral norm. In other words, the individual has the goal of respecting the norm and this is an ultimate goal. Both conditions are necessary but not sufficient. To feel ethical guilt, other conditions must also be met. One must believe that he could have acted differently, that is, that he was free from constrictions and was not obliged to act as he did. We can also feel guilty for intentions, desires, or dispositions to act, even if they are not put into action. For example, one might feel guilty, and morally unworthy, for having paedophiliac desires, even if they are not pursued, but on condition of assuming that one did not do everything in his power to free himself of those desires.

The impulse to action in deontological guilt appears to be directed in three directions: to constrain one's self, by signalling a renewed willingness to submit and obey through confession, apology, and penance; to prevent other potential faults, including the search for justifications; to purify oneself, for example, through washing rituals (Lee and Schwarz, 2011; Zhong and Liljenquist, 2006). It is no coincidence that, in every religion, ritualistic body washing is used to free the conscience from sin. Baptism is a washing with which one purifies oneself from original sin, that is, from deontological guilt par excellence, from an act of pure disobedience to God, that is, hubris.

5.1 Psychological characteristics of internalized moral norms

But when we speak of moral norms regarding deontological guilt, what exactly are we referring to and how do such norms differ from conventional norms?

Moral norms are deontic norms and, as such, they limit the range of possible choices. Traditionally, moral norms are considered to be different from other ethical norms, such as the conventional norms of good manners or the rules of billiards, for four reasons related to the so-called moral signature (Haidt and Joseph, 2004). Moral norms are experienced as (1) universal and (2) unchangeable; (3) their transgression is usually considered more serious than the transgression of conventional norms; and, finally, (4) they regard the well-being of and respect for others.

Moral norms are considered universal, because they are valid for everyone. A norm *ad* or *contra personam* is not a moral norm. Moral norms are considered immutable. For example, paedophilia would be considered immoral, even if we observed it in a culture that admits it. The fact that they are considered universal and unchangeable leads to experiencing moral norms as if these were natural laws. Their transgression is considered more serious than the transgression of conventional norms and, finally, moral norms refer only to the well-being of others.

Conventional norms, on the contrary, are contingent, that is, dependent on the sociocultural environment. For example, burping while eating is reprehensible in our culture, but the Eskimos seem to see it as an adequate way for a guest to express his appreciation for the host's food. Conventional norms are modifiable. For instance, the rules of billiards can be modified by an agreement between players. The transgression of conventional norms is not habitually considered serious. For instance, burping while eating may elicit criticism or hilarity but not a moral condemnation. Coherently with the Moral Signature, conventional norms are not related to the well-being of others. For instance, the norm "While eating, no elbows on the table", defends the space of the other diners, but saying that it defends their well-being would be an exaggeration.

Yet, are Moral Standards universal? Some studies seem to dispute the idea that internalized moral norms are perceived as universal. For example, Kelly et al. (2007) have shown that an officer on an oil tanker who inflicts severe corporal punishment on a sailor who fell asleep while on watch is judged morally guilty, while that same officer would be held not guilty, or less guilty, if he were commanding a sailing ship in the 1600s, when such punishments were usual. However, these data do not sufficiently question the idea that moral norms are considered universal. It is pertinent to distinguish two types of sentences: it is one thing to say that, in the seventeenth century, it was right to administer severe corporal punishment while today it is not; it is quite another to affirm that the seventeenth-century officer was not morally guilty because he was convinced, sincerely trusting in the fairness of his decision, that it was consistent with the morals of his time. But this second judgement does not claim that the moral principles of this period were 'right'. It is plausible that the answers given by the participants in Kelly's study belonged to this second type. The first judgement would imply that the moral norm could be put into perspective, while the second would put the judgement on the officer into perspective, taking into consideration what seemed right to him, but not implying that the officer's behaviour was inherently right.

It is probably more pertinent to reverse the question: who is authorized to change the rules and under what conditions? The appropriateness of this question is suggested by the comparison between two kinds of findings. From the studies by Kelly et al. (2007), it appears that the oil tanker officer described previously would have been found not guilty or less guilty if he had inflicted corporal punishment in carrying out his superior's order. Milgram's famous studies (e.g., 1974) confirm that authoritativeness, embodied in a scientist, can make harmful behaviour morally permissible for others. This seems to suggest that a human authority can modify moral norms and, therefore, that moral and conventional norms are similar, at least in this respect. Conversely, other findings suggest that moral norms cannot be changed by human authority. For example, the studies by Turiel and Nucci (1978) and Nichols (2004) show that children do not recognize the authority, for example, of their teacher, to change moral norms (do not harm a friend), while they do recognize the teacher's authority to change conventional norms (e.g., do not chew chewing gum in class). The conflicting nature of the data can probably be resolved by considering the relationship between the stature of the authority and the moral importance of the norm. The moral importance of a norm seems to depend on how much the transgression of the norm disturbs what appears to be the natural order. The stature of the authority is linked to how much the authority's directive appears to be with the natural order, traditions, and God's will.

The Pope has the right to modify the moral norm not to kill and command the Crusaders to exterminate infidels, if it is assumed that he is acting on behalf of God. On the other hand, the teacher is not recognized as having the authority to change the moral norm "Don't pull your friend's hair" but only to change the conventional norm, "Don't chew gum in class". Thus, the different modifiability of moral and conventional norms appears related to the authority recognized in those who change the norm and to the moral importance of the norm. Furthermore, the modifiability of a norm appears to be related to whether the transgression of the norm appears to be caused by the hubris or arrogance that leads human beings to assume their power and rebel against the given order – divine, human, or natural. In short, does the transgression show lack of respect for the norm Don't play God/ Don't tamper with nature?

Does the content of internalized moral norms only concern the good of others? In effect, many internalized moral norms do concern the good and the rights of others, for example, do not kill, do not steal, do not inflict useless pain. Others, however, though they too may be internalized, are not linked to our relationships with others (see Moral Foundation Theory – MFT – Haidt and Joseph, 2004; Graham and Haidt, 2012). For example, the first three of the Ten Commandments regulate, explicitly and exclusively, the relationship with the divinity, and not relationships with other people: (1) I am the Lord thy God, and thou shalt not have strange gods before me. (2) Thou shalt not take the name of the Lord thy God in vain. (3) Remember the Sabbath day, to keep it holy. Similarly, there are internalized moral norms that prohibit sexual behaviour that does not harm or violate anyone, such as coupling with animals, incest between consenting adults even without any risk of procreation, or masturbation.

6 Empirical evidence of the difference between altruistic and deontological guilt, and more generally between the two moralities

Various studies have demonstrated that altruistic guilt and deontological guilt are distinct from both behavioural and neurological points of view. An initial series of studies on moral choices was conducted by using the 'trolley car dilemma' (Foot, 1967). In its original form, the trolley dilemma asks participants to imagine that a trolley car is careening out of control on a track with five persons on it who, if the trolley continues on its course, will be run over and killed. Participants are then asked if they would pull an exchange lever, sending the trolley down another track where, however, there is another person who will certainly be hit and killed. This dilemma is especially interesting for the distinction between the two types of guilt. Indeed, it requires participants to choose between two incompatible options, which in light of what has been said so far can be defined as altruistic/humanitarian versus deontological. The altruistic/humanitarian option consists in moving the lever to cause the death of one person in order to save five, thus reducing as much as possible the overall suffering and harm. Nevertheless, moving the lever amounts to assuming responsibility for changing the course of events decided by fate, or for believers, by God. The deontological option consists in omitting to move the lever and allowing the five people to die, but not taking the responsibility to change the natural course of events and thus respecting the deontological principle *Do Not Play God*. According to Sunstein (2005), this principle is capable of explaining why, all things being equal, omission tends to be considered less grave than action. In line with these studies, Gangemi and Mancini (2013) have shown that the people who choose not to act tend to justify their choice on the *Do Not Play God* principle (for example, "Who am I to decide who lives and who dies?), while those who choose to act, appeal to the minimization of others' pain and suffering, and thus to an altruistic/humanitarian principle (for example, "Better that only one person die rather than five"). Furthermore, the induction of deontological guilt implies a preference for not moving the lever, while the induction of altruistic guilt implies moving it (Mancini and Gangemi, 2015). A study by D'Olimpio and Mancini (2016) confirmed this finding, adding the evidence that a preference for omissive choices is ascribable to deontological guilt and not to shame. Another study highlighted that the deontological choice is more frequent if participants are asked to imagine being next to the exchange and to have nearby a figure who represents a moral authority, such as a judge or a police officer. The contrary happens when participants are asked to imagine themselves next to the lever and therefore close to the five people. The first situation plausibly induces respect for authority and therefore for the *Do Not Play God* principle, while the second activates empathy and, in turn, an altruistic/humanitarian impulse (Gangemi and Mancini, 2013).

Other researchers have found that respect for the moral norm "Do not tell lies" can even restrain the telling of white lies that would create a benefit for the deceived and small harm for the deceiver, and Pareto lies in which both the deceived and the deceiver would benefit. Respect for the moral norm, therefore, seems to be able to win out over the effect of the altruistic and cooperative disposition (Biziou-van-Pol et al., 2015).

Some findings seem to suggest that deontological guilt, but not altruistic guilt, reduces the moral authority that one recognizes in oneself. For example, the induction of deontological guilt reduces refusals of unjust offers in the three-person *Ultimatum Game*, unlike what happens with the induction of altruistic guilt (Mancini and Mancini, 2015). This suggests that induction of deontological guilt lessens the feeling of being entitled to make justice prevail.

Basile and Mancini (2011) activated the two senses of guilt separately by using as stimuli facial expressions of basic emotions (i.e., Ekman photos) accompanied by internal dialogue phrases typically associated with the two types of guilt feelings. For example, for deontological guilt, angry and contemptuous faces together with phrases such as "How could I have done that!", while for altruistic guilt, sad faces with phrases such as "How could I have left her alone!". Moreover, in a study using functional magnetic resonance imaging (fMRI) to identify the neural substrate of the two guilt feelings, Basile et al. (2011) found activation of the insula and the anterior cingulate cortex in the condition of deontological guilt and activation of medial prefrontal areas in the condition of altruistic guilt. These findings appear to be particularly interesting, not only because they demonstrate that the two guilt feelings can be "traced" to different cerebral circuits, but also for the specific areas involved. The medial prefrontal areas, which are activated by altruistic guilt, are normally activated by the theory of mind tasks and are associated with the representation of others' intentions (Blair, 1995; Shallice, 2001) and with the experience of empathy and compassion. Therefore, they are areas involved in the understanding of the mind of the victim (Moll et al., 2005). On the other hand, the insula, which is activated by deontological guilt, is associated with the experience of disgust and self-blame (Rozin et al., 2000).

7 Deontological guilt and disgust

In general, starting from the observation that, in all religions, sins soil the conscience and washing purifies it, the scientific literature has suggested the existence of a strong relationship between guilt and disgust (Lee and Schwarz, 2011). For example, several studies have confirmed the relationship between the physical component of disgust, the contamination of moral evil, and the need to wash (Doron et al., 2012). In this regard, Zhong and Liljenquist (2006) have described the 'Lady Macbeth' effect, in which a threat to moral purity implies the need to wash and that physical washing provides relief from the consequences of immoral behaviour and reduces the threat to one's moral image (Lee and Schwarz, 2011). However, several studies have not replicated this effect (e.g., Earp et al., 2014). The diversity of findings can be explained if it is considered that the Macbeth effect is solely due to the deontological component of guilt and not due to the altruistic one. In fact, in each of the studies cited, the two components, altruistic and deontological, were not controlled, but a general sense of guilt was induced. In fact, in a recent study, the induction of deontological but not altruistic guilt led to the 'Lady Macbeth' effect (D'Olimpio and Mancini, 2014). This study was replicated (Ottaviani et al., 2018) to confirm that the induction of deontological, but not altruistic, guilt provokes, in addition to thorough washing, the typical physiological activation observed by way of *Heart Rate Variability*.

These findings are supported by another study that used tDCS (transcranial direct current stimulation) (Ottaviani et al., 2018). Stimulating the insula cortex activates the parasympathetic nervous system in a way compatible with the activation of disgust, increases disposition to words related to cleaning, and induces the tendency to feel disgust. Above all, the subject himself judges transgressions of moral norms to be more serious when the insula cortex is activated compared to when it is not. In situations like, by way of example, "you see a politician use tax revenues to construct an addition to his own home". Whereas activation of the insula cortex does not induce changes in altruistic judgements, such as "you see a boy set up a series of traps to kill stray cats in his neighbourhood".

We have found additional evidence of a close relationship between ethical guilt and disgust. Both disgust and guilt reduce self-rank in the social cognitive chain of being (SCCB). The SCCB represents the propensity of human beings to organize their moral world along a vertical axis, with those deserving obedience and respect in a higher position, those who must give respect and obedience in a lower position, and those who deserve contempt in the lowest position (Brandt and Reyna, 2011). But there may be a specific relationship between deontological, but not altruistic, guilt and rank in the SCCB. Induction of deontological guilt reduces the rejection of unfair offers in the Ultimatum Game, in contrast with what occurs if altruistic guilt or shame is induced (Mancini and Mancini, 2015). This suggests that inducement of deontological guilt reduces the rank of those who identify with the SCCB and feel less empowered to enforce justice.

8 Deontological guilt and OCD

Some studies suggest that the guilt feared by the obsessive patient is predominantly deontological and that obsessive patients are more sensitive to ethics than non-obsessive subjects (for a review, see Gangemi and Mancini, 2017). Mancini and Gangemi (2015) found that OC patients almost always solved the trolley dilemma with an omission, thus avoiding deontological guilt, while healthy controls and patients with anxiety disorders almost always solved the dilemma by shifting the lever, thus avoiding altruistic guilt. Franklin et al. (2009) studied moral choices using the trolley car dilemma, showing that in patients with OC, preference for action was inversely related to the severity of their symptoms. Giacomantonio et al. (2019) documented that in a condition of uncertainty, individuals without a psychiatric diagnosis spent more time in obsessive checks when they experienced deontological rather than altruistic guilt. In two previously cited studies (D'Olimpio and Mancini, 2014; Ottaviani et al., 2018), the results showed that, in non-clinical participants, the induction of ethical guilt led to obsessive control and washing behaviours to a greater extent than the induction of altruistic guilt. In OC patients, the 'Lady Macbeth' effect is significantly higher than in non-OC participants (Reuven et al., 2013).

Several studies with functional magnetic resonance imaging (e.g., Mataix-Cols et al., 2005; Rauch et al., 1998) have shown that, during a symptom-inducing activity, OC patients show the same activation, i.e., similar areas of the brain (e.g., anterior cingulate cortex and insulae), as that shown by healthy individuals who experience deontological guilt (Basile et al., 2011). This overlap would suggest that patients may experience deontological guilt when provoking symptoms. These results are in line with those found in an fMRI study (Basile et al., 2013), in which the authors examined the brain responses of obsessive patients while processing deontological guilt and altruistic guilt stimuli. During deontological guilt processing, OC patients showed decreased activation in the anterior cingulate cortex, insula, and precuneus, compared with healthy controls. There were no differences between the two groups when processing altruistic cues for guilt, anger, or sadness. According to the neuro-efficiency hypothesis (Neubauer and Fink, 2009), this reduced activation would suggest the brain efficiency of patients, due to their frequent exposure to deontological guilt feelings (Carnì et al., 2013).

9 Altruistic guilt and major depression disorder

In 2013, Schreiter, Pijnenborg, and aan het Rot performed a systematic review to shed light on the controversial relationship between depression and empathy. Their meta-analysis showed that depression was related to the empathic stress component of affective empathy. Most other subsequent studies have brought consistent additional evidence showing an association between high levels of empathic stress and depressive symptoms (Ekinci and Ekinci, 2016; Gambin and Sharp, 2018; Guhn et al., 2020; Kim and Han, 2018; Tone and Tully, 2014).

Stimulating findings in neuroscience also illuminate the abnormal empathic profile of depressed individuals. Fujino et al. (2014), comparing the hemodynamic responses to the visual pain stimuli of others in depressed and healthy participants, highlighted a reduced activation of the left inferior frontal gyrus (which represents the evaluation component of others' pain) and increased activation of the emotional correlates of these processes. Together with some convergent evidence gathered among the healthy population (Berna et al., 2010), this is in line with the hypothesis that depressed individuals experience intense and downregulated negative arousal in response to others' pain (i.e., empathic distress).

Furthermore, Pulcu et al. (2014) observed hypersensitivity in individuals with MDD of the subgenual septal cingulate cortex (sgACC) region in response to altruistic actions. This region was first identified as abnormal in depression (e.g., Greicius et al., 2007) but more recently has also been related to altruistic decision-making (e.g., Cutler and Campbell-Meiklejohn, 2019) and both empathic distress and altruistic guilt (Basile et al., 2011; Pulcu et al., 2014).

Strong evidence of abnormal empathic capacity among depressed individuals has led some authors to advance the hypothesis that this disorder could be better understood as a form of pathological altruism (O'Connor et al., 2012). The first real study to shed light on altruistic ecological behaviours related to depression was that of Fujiwara (2009). The results, checked for a large number of potential confounding demographic variables, showed that charitable support was able to predict the onset of MDD longitudinally.

Preliminary evidence from the field of developmental psychopathology has reported that an unusually early appearance of the theory of mind among girls predicts high levels of altruistic guilt in adolescence which, in turn, would predict the onset of depression (Rasco, 2004).

According to O'Connor, the fundamental determinant linking empathy dysregulation and depression is pathological altruistic guilt, primarily in its survivor components. Survivor's guilt is fundamentally interpersonal, focused on others and devoid of culpability. Another central feature of the pathological aspect of survivor's guilt can be found in the pervasive nature of the underlying goals rigidly pursued by the individual and which, consequently, would inhibit the pursuit of other healthy life goals (O'Connor et al., 2012).

In support of these hypotheses, studies have reported a positive and significant association between the severity of depressive symptoms and survivor's guilt. Furthermore, this result was found to be stable in all countries (Japan, Sweden, and Germany) and several ethnic groups living in the United States (O'Connor et al., 2007). Furthermore, depressed individuals have been shown to score higher in these subscales than healthy controls (O'Connor et al., 2002) and this result was replicated with a fully remitted MDD sample (Green et al., 2012). Additionally, Neelapaijit et al. (2017) reported higher beliefs related to omnipotent guilt and survivor's guilt among depressed individuals compared to healthy subjects. Finally, correlates of depression such as pessimistic thinking have been found to correlate with survivors' guilt levels (Menaker, 1995). Recently, Gambin and Sharp (2018), in a study of depressed adolescent in-patients, partially replicated and extended these results. Specifically, they demonstrated that generalized (but not contextual) guilt mediated the path that led from affective empathy to depression.

10 Conclusions

The study of two psychopathological disorders, OCD and MDD, offers the opportunity to distinguish two types of guilt, deontological and altruistic, independent and unrelated. Deontological guilt arises from the transgression of internalized moral norms. Moreover, deontological transgressions are ultimately caused by Hybris, or the lack of respect for moral authority, which is usually identified by children in parents, by believers in divinities, and by non-believers in what appears to be the natural order. Altruistic guilt is experienced when one believes that one has acted inconsistently with one's altruistic motives. Altruistic guilt is related to empathy and affection, and is experienced when the sufferer is close. Our proposal is similar to previous psychological approaches to guilt because it considers the presence of two elements necessary to guilt: harm to a victim and the transgression of an internalized moral norm. It differs from previous approaches because it posits the possibility of experiencing guilt even if only one of these two components is present, insofar as the two types of guilt are independent of each other. This approach eliminates the need to demonstrate that the basis of any internalized moral norm is an altruistic/humanitarian goal and that the basis of every altruistic act is the goal of respecting a moral norm.

Note

1 An earlier version of the sections devoted to deontological guilt, altruistic guilt, and the proof of their differences has been published, in Italian, in the Giornale Italiano di Psicologia: Mancini, F. and Gangemi, A. Senso di colpa deontologico e senso di colpa altruistico: una tesi dualista. Giornale italiano di psicologia, 3 September 2018, doi: 10.1421/92800.

References

Basile, B., and Mancini, F. (2011). Eliciting guilty feelings: A preliminary study differentiating deontological and altruistic guilt. *Psychology*, 2, 98–102.

Basile, B., Mancini, F., Macaluso, E., Caltagirone, C., and Bozzali, M. (2013). Abnormal processing of deontological guilt in obsessive-compulsive disorder. *Brain Structure and Function*, 219(4), 1321–1331.

Basile, B., Mancini, F., Macaluso, E., Caltagirone, C., Frackowiak, R. S., and Bozzali, M. (2011). Deontological and altruistic guilt: Evidence for distinct neurobiological substrate. *Human Brain Mapping*, 32(2), 229–239.

Baumeister, R. F., Stillwell, A. M., and Heatherton, T. F. (1994). Guilt: An interpersonal approach. *Psychological Bulletin*, 115, 243–267.

Bekoff, M., and Pierce, J. (2010). *Wild justice: The moral lives of animals*. Chicago, IL: University of Chicago Press.

Berna, C., Leknes, S., Holmes, E. A., Edwards, R. R., Goodwin, G. M., and Tracey, I. (2010). Induction of depressed mood disrupts emotion regulation neurocircuitry and enhances pain unpleasantness. *Biological Psychiatry*, 67, 1083–1090.

Berry, L.-M., and Laskey, B. (2012). A review of obsessive intrusive thoughts in the general population. *Journal of Obsessive-Compulsive and Related Disorders*, 1(2), 125–132.

Bhikram, T., Abi-Jaoude, E., and Sandor, P. (2017). OCD: Obsessive-compulsive . . . disgust? The role of disgust in obsessive-compulsive disorder. *Journal of Psychiatry and Neuroscience*, 42(5), 300–306.

Biziou-van-Pol, L., Haenen, J., Novaro, A., Liberman-Occhipinti, A., and Capraro, V. (2015). Does telling white lies signal pro-social preferences? *Judgment and Decision Making*, 10, 538–548.

Blair, R. (1995). A cognitive developmental approach to morality: Investigating the psychopath. *Cognition*, 57(1), 1–29.

Brandt, M. J., and Reyna, C. (2011). The chain of being: A hierarchy of morality. *Perspectives on Psychological Science*, 6, 428–446.

Carnì, S., Petrocchi, N., Del Miglio, C., Mancini, F., and Couyoumdjian, A. (2013). Intrapsychic and interpersonal guilt: A critical review of the recent literature. *Cognitive Processing*, 14(4), 333–346.

Castelfranchi, C. (1994). I sensi di colpa. In C. Castelfranchi, R. Conte, and R. D'Amico (a cura di), *I sensi di colpa*. Firenze: Giunti.

Chiang, B., Purdon, C., and Radomsky, A. S. (2016). Development and initial validation of the Fear of Guilt Scale for obsessive-compulsive disorder (OCD). *Journal of Obsessive-Compulsive and Related Disorders*, 11, 63–73.

Cutler, J., and Campbell-Meiklejohn, D. (2019). A comparative fMRI meta-analysis of altruistic and strategic decisions to give. *NeuroImage*, 184, 227–241.

D'Olimpio, F., Cosentino, T., Basile, B., Tenore, K., Gragnani, A., and Mancini, F. (2013). Obsessive-compulsive disorder and propensity to guilt feeling and to disgust. *Clinical Neuropsychiatry*, 10(3), 1, 20–39.

D'Olimpio, F., and Mancini, F. (2014). Role of deontological guilt in obsessive-compulsive disorder-like checking and washing behaviors. *Clinical Psychological Science*, 1–13.

D'Olimpio, F., and Mancini, F. (2016). "Don't Play GoD!": Is inaction preference linked to obsessive compulsive characteristics? *Clinical Neuropsychiatry*, 13(6), 122–129.

Doron, G., Sar-el, D., and Mikulincer, M. (2012). Threats to moral self-perceptions trigger obsessive compulsive contamination related behavioral tendencies. *Journal of Behavior Therapy and Experimental Psychiatry*, 43, 884–890.

Earp, B. D., Everett, J. A. C., Madva, E. N., and Hamlin, J. K. (2014). Out, damned spot: Can the'Macbeth Effect' be replicated? *Basic and Applied Social Psychology*, 36, 91–98.

Ekinci, O., and Ekinci, A. (2016). Relationship between empathic responding and its clinical characteristics in patients with major depressive disorder. *Dusunen Adam*, 29(2), 145–154.

Foot, F. (1967). The problem of abortion and the doctrine of the double effect in virtues and vices. *Oxford Review*, 5, 5–15.

Franklin, S. A., McNally, R. J., and Riemann, B. C. (2009). Moral reasoning in obsessive-compulsive disorder. *Journal of Anxiety Disorders*, 23, 575–577.

Fromm, E. (1985). *Etica y Psychoanalysis*. Madrir: Fondo De Cultura Economica. (Original work published 1947.)

Fujino, J., Yamasaki, N., Miyata, J., Kawada, R., Sasaki, H., Matsukawa, N., Takemura, A., Ono, M., Tei, S., Takahashi, H., Aso, T., Fukuyama, H., and Murai, T. (2014). Altered brain response to others' pain in major depressive disorder. *Journal of Affective Disorders*, 165, 170–175.

Fujiwara, T. (2009). Is altruistic behavior associated with major depression onset? *PLoS One*, 4, e4557.

Gambin, M., and Sharp, C. (2018). The relations between empathy, guilt, shame and depression in inpatient adolescents. *Journal of Affective Disorders*, 241, 381–387.

Gangemi, A., and Mancini, F. (2013). Moral choices: The influence of the do not play God principle. In M. Knauff, M. Pauen, N. Sebanz, and I. Wachsmuth (Eds.), *Cooperative minds: Social interaction and group dynamics. Proceedings of the 35th annual meeting of the Cognitive Science Society* (pp. 2973–2977). Austin, TX: Cognitive Science Society.

Gangemi, A., and Mancini, F. (2017). Obsessive patients and deontological guilt: A review. *Journal of Experimental Psychopathology*, 4(2), 155–168.

Giacomantonio, M., Salvati, M., and Mancini, F. (2019). Am I guilty or not? Deontological guilt, uncertainty, and checking behavior. *Applied Cognitive Psychology*, 33(6), 1279–1287.

Graham, J., and Haidt, J. (2012). Sacred values and evil adversaries: A moral foundations approach. In P. Shaver and M. Mikulincer (Eds.), *The social psychology of morality: Exploring the causes of good and evil* (pp. 11–31). New York: APA Books.

Green, S., Lambon, R. M. A., Moll, J., Deakin, J. F., and Zahn, R. (2012). Guilt-selective functional disconnection of anterior temporal and subgenual cortices in major depressive disorder. *Archives of General Psychiatry*, 69, 1014–1021.

Greicius, M. D., Flores, B. H., Menon, V., Glover, G. H., Solvason, H. B., Kenna, H. et al. (2007). Resting-state functional connectivity in major depression: Abnormally increased contributions from subgenual cingulate cortex and thalamus. *Biological Psychiatry*, 62, 429–437.

Guhn, A., Merkel, L., Hübner, L., Dziobek, I., Sterzer, P., and Köhler, S. (2020). Understanding versus feeling the emotions of others: How persistent and recurrent depression affect empathy. *Journal of Psychiatric Research* (In press).

Haidt, J. (2001). The emotional dog and its rational tail: A social intuitionist approach to moral judgment. *Psychological Review*, 108, 814–834.

Haidt, J., and Joseph, C. (2004). Intuitive ethics: How innately prepared intuitions generate culturally variable virtues. *Daedalus*, 133, 55–66.

Hoffman, M. L. (1982). Development of prosocial motivation: Empathy and guilt. In N. Eisenberg (Ed.), *The development of prosocial behavior* (pp. 218–231). New York: Academic Press.

Hoffman, M. L. (1998). Varieties of empathy-based guilt. In J. Bybee (Ed.), *Guilt and children* (pp. 91–112). San Diego: Academic Press.

Kelly, D., Stich, S., Haley, K. J., Eng, S. J., and Fessler, D. M. T. (2007). Harm, affect, and the moral/conventional distinction. *Mind and Language*, 22, 117–131.

Kim, H., and Han, S. (2018). Does personal distress enhance empathic interaction or block it? *Personality and Individual Differences*, 124, 77–83.

Kubany, E. S., and Watson, S. B. (2003). Guilt: Elaboration of a multidimensional model. *The Psychological Record*, 53, 51–90.

Kugler, K., and Jones, W. H. (1992). On conceptualizing and assessing guilt. *Journal of Personality and Social Psychology*, 63, 318–327.

Lee, S. W. S., and Schwarz, N. (2011). Clean slate effects: The psychological consequences of physical cleansing. *Current Directions in Psychological Science*, 20, 307–311.

Mancini, F. (1997). Il senso di colpa. *Psicoterapia*, 9, 12–27.

Mancini, F. (2018). *The obsessive mind*. Abingdon-on-Thames: Routledge.

Mancini, F., and Gangemi, A. (2011). Fear of deontological guilt and fear of contamination in obsessive-compulsive disorder. *Journal of Behavior Therapy and Experimental Psychiatry*, 49, 157–163.

Mancini, F., and Gangemi, A. (2015). Deontological guilt and obsessive compulsive disorder. *Journal of Behavior Therapy and Experimental Psychiatry*, 49, 157–163.

Mancini, F., and Mancini, A. (2015). Do not play God: Contrasting effects of deontological guilt and pride on decision-making. *Frontiers in Psychology*, 6, 1251.

Mataix-Cols, D., Rosario-Campos, M. C., and Leckman, J. F. (2005). A multidimensional model of obsessive-compulsive disorder. *American Journal of Psychiatry*, 162, 228–238.

Menaker, A. (1995). *The relationship between attributional style and interpersonal guilt*. Doctoral Dissertation, California School of Professional Psychology, Alameda, CA.

Milgram, S. (1974). *Obedience to authority: An experimental view*. New York: Harper and Row.

Moll, J., de Oliveira-Souza, R., Moll, F. T., Ignàcio, F. A., Bramati, I. E., Caparelli-Dàquer, E. M., and Eslinger, P. J. (2005). The moral affiliations of disgust: A functional MRI study. *Cognitive Behavioral Neurology*, 18, 68–78.

Nakame, T., Narumoto, J., Sakay, Y., Nishida, S., Yamada, K., and Fukui, K. (2012). The neural basis of dysfunctional beliefs in non-medicated patients with obsessive-compulsive disorder. *Progress in Neuro-Psychopharmacology and Biological Psychiatry*, 37(1), 22–25.

Neelapaijit, A., Wongpakaran, T., Wongpakaran, N., and Thongpibul, K. (2017). Pathogenic beliefs among patients with depressive disorders. *Neuropsychiatric Disease and Treatment*, 13, 1047–1055.

Neubauer, A. C., and Fink, A. (2009). Intelligence and neural efficiency: Measures of brain activation versus measures of functional connectivity in the brain. *Intelligence*, 37(2), 223–229.

Nichols, S. (2004). *Sentimental rules: On the natural foundations of moral judgement*. Oxford: Oxford University Press.

O'Connor, L. E., Berry, J. W., Lewis, T., Mulherin, K., and Crisostomo, P. S. (2007). Empathy and depression: The moral system on overdrive. In T. Farrow and P. Woodruff (Eds.), *Empathy in mental illness* (pp. 49–75). Cambridge: Cambridge University Press.

O'Connor, L. E., Berry, J. W., Lewis, T. B., and Stiver, D. J. (2012). Empathy-based pathogenic guilt, pathological altruism, and psychopathology. In B. Oakley, A. Knafo, G. Madhavan, and D. S. Wilson (Eds.), *Pathological altruism* (pp. 10–30). Oxford: Oxford University Press.

O'Connor, L. E., Berry, J. W., Weiss, J., and Gilbert, P. (2002). Guilt, fear, submission, and empathy in depression. *Journal of Affective Disorders*, 71(1–3), 19–27.

Ottaviani, C., Mancini, F., Provenzano, S., Collazzoni, A., and D'Olimpio, F. (2018). Deontological morality can be experimentally enhanced by increasing disgust: A transcranial direct current stimulation study. *Neuropsychologia*, 119, 474–481.

Parisi, D. (1977). Affetto. *Giornale Italiano di Psicologia*, 5, 127–142.

Prinz, J., and Nichols, S. (2010). Moral emotions. In J. Doris (Ed.), *Moral psychology handbook* (pp. 111–148). Oxford: Oxford University Press.

Pulcu, E., Lythe, K., Elliott, R., Green, S., Moll, J., Deakin, J. F. W., and Zahn, R. (2014). Increased amygdala response to shame in remitted major depressive disorder. *PLoS One*, 9(1).

Rasco (2004), cited in O'Connor, L. E., Berry, J. W., Lewis, T., Mulherin, K., and Crisostomo, P. S. (2007). Empathy and depression: The moral system on overdrive. In T. Farrow and P. Woodruff (Eds.), *Empathy in mental illness* (pp. 49–75). Cambridge: Cambridge University Press.

Rauch, S. L., Dougherty, D. D., Shin, L. M., Alpert, N. M., Manzo, P., Leahy, L., Fischman, A. J., Jenike, M. A., and Baer, L. (1998). Neural correlates of factor-analyzed OCD symptom dimensions: A PET study. *CNS Spectrums*, 3, 37–43.

Reuven, O., Liberman, N., and Dar, R. (2013). The effect of physical cleaning on threatened morality in individuals with obsessive-compulsive disorder. *Clinical Psychological Science*, 1–6.

Rozin, P., Haidt, J., and McCauley, C. R. (2000). Disgust. In M. Lewis and J. Haviland-Jones (Eds.), *Handbook of emotions* (2nd ed., pp. 673–653). New York: Guilford Press.

Schreiter, S., Pijnenborg, G. H. M., and aan het Rot, M. (2013). Empathy in adults with clinical or subclinical depressive symptoms. *Journal of Affective Disorders*, 150(1), 1–16.

Shallice, T. (2001). Theory of mind and the prefrontal cortex. *Brain*, 124, 247–248.

Stich, S., Doris, J. M., and Roedder, E. (2010). Altruism. In J. M. Doris and The Moral Psychology Research Group (Eds.), *The moral psychology handbook* (pp. 147–205). Oxford: Oxford University Press.

Sunstein, C. (2005). Moral heuristic. *Behavioral and Brain Sciences*, 28, 531–573.

Tomasello, M. (2016). *A natural history of human morality*. Cambridge, MA: Harvard University Press.

Tone, E. B., and Tully, E. C. (2014). Empathy as a "risky strength": A multilevel examination of empathy and risk for internalizing disorders. *Development and Psychopathology*, 26(4, Pt 2), 1547–1565.

Turiel, E., and Nucci, L. (1978). Social interactions and the development of social concepts in preschool children. *Child Development*, 49, 400–407.

Warneken, F., and Tomasello, M. (2009). The roots of human altruism. *British Journal of Psychology*, 100, 455–471.

Weiss, J. (1993). *How psychotherapy works: Process and technique*. New York: Guilford Press.

Weiss, J., and Sampson, H. (1986). *The psychoanalytic process: Theory, clinical observation and empirical research*. New York: Guilford Press.

Zhong, C. B., and Liljenquist, K. (2006). Washing away your sins: Threatened morality and physical cleansing. *Science*, 313, 1451–1452.

6

THE NARRATIVE SELF IN SCHIZOPHRENIA AND ITS COGNITIVE UNDERPINNINGS

Ines Adornetti and Francesco Ferretti

1 Introduction: schizophrenia as a disorder of the self

Although more than a century has passed since schizophrenia was first documented as a peculiar set of disorders with the description of *dementia praecox* by Kraepelin, its aetiology, essential symptomatology, and natural course remain elusive. Indeed, despite the availability of criteria established for diagnostic identification, such as those included in the latest editions of *Diagnostic and Statistical Manual of Mental Disorders* (APA, 2013)[1] and the *International Classification of Disease* (ICD-11),[2] schizophrenia is still a broad clinical syndrome defined by reported subjective experiences (symptoms), loss of functions (behavioural impairments), and variable patterns of course (Jablensky, 2010). If on the one hand scholars are faced with a variety of phenotypic expressions, on the other hand almost everyone agrees that a disturbance in the sense of self is a universal feature characterizing the lives of persons with schizophrenia (e.g., Lysaker and Lysaker, 2002, 2010; Sass and Parnas, 2003; Kean, 2009; Henriksen and Nordgaard, 2014; Davidson, 2020).

Since the time of Kraepelin (1919) and Bleuler (1911), schizophrenia has been associated with specific alterations in the dimension of personal identity. Although dedicating little space to self-experience, Kraepelin acknowledges that abnormalities in this dimension are a central aspect of the disorder. He writes that "dementia praecox consists of a series of states, the common characteristic of which is a peculiar destruction of the internal connection of the psychic personality" (1919: 3). In his revision of Kraepelin's work, Bleuler (1911) closely ties this disorder to a loss of, or alteration in, persons' basic sense of self. In *Dementia Praecox and the Group of Schizophrenia*, the Swiss psychiatrist explains that he replaced the expression 'dementia praecox' with the term 'schizophrenia' because of the importance of the splitting of the different psychic functions. He states that, "If the disease is marked, the personality loses its unity; at different times, different psychic complexes seem to represent the personality" (9) and highlights that persons with schizophrenia struggle to recognize themselves as subjects of their own experiences and agent of their own actions. These phenomena are particularly evident, for example, in individuals suffering from thought insertion as they believe that some of the thoughts that they experience are not their own. As an illustration of this, consider the following first-person accounts:

> I look out the window and I think that the garden looks nice and the grass looks cool, but the thoughts of Eammon Andrews come into my mind. . . . He treats my mind like a screen and flashes his thoughts onto it like you flash a picture.
>
> *(Mellor, 1970: 17, reported in O'Brien and Opie, 2003: 107)*

Another impressive example illustrating the dissolution of the first-person perspective in schizophrenia is provided by Elyn Saks (2007) in her autobiography *The Center Cannot Hold: My Journey through Madness*. She writes:

> And then something odd happens. My awareness (of myself, of him, of the room, of the physical reality around and beyond us) instantly grows fuzzy. Or wobbly. I think I am dissolving. I feel – my mind feels – like a sand castle with all the sand sliding away in the receding surf.
>
> *(Saks, 2007: 12)*

After Kraepelin and Bleuler, the idea that schizophrenia involves the experience of a fragile and instable sense of identity has been acknowledged by authors from a wide range of disciplines, including (but not limited to) existential psychiatry (e.g., Laing, 1978), psychoanalysis (e.g., Freud, 1957; Frosch, 1983), and phenomenology (e.g., Minkowski, 1987; Blankenburg, 2001; Sass and Parnas, 2002). For example, within the framework of existential psychiatry, Laing (1978) describes persons with this disorder as fundamentally alienated and as experiencing disrupted relations with the world and themselves. As an illustration, the author provides the following speech sample of a person with schizophrenia:

> These thoughts go on and on, I am going over the border. My real self is a way down – it used to be just at my throat but now it has gone down further. I'm losing myself. It's getting deeper and deeper. I want to tell you things, but I'm scared. My head is full of thoughts, fears, hates, jealousies. My head can't grip them; I can't hold onto them.
>
> *(Laing, 1978: 151, quoted in Lysaker and Lysaker, 2010: 333)*

Further examples of first-person accounts illuminating the alterations of the self in schizophrenia are offered by Frosch (1983), in the context of a psychoanalytic description of the disorder, and by Stanghellini (2004) within a phenomenological perspective.

> I become everything I experience to a point where it ultimately resolves into a state of considering myself the universe. I can open myself completely. My mind withdraws from anything that is directly dangerous to my body. . . . It means my sense of identity is expanded and there is no longer a me.
>
> *(Frosch, 1983: 261, quoted in Lysaker and Lysaker, 2010: 334)*

> I feel lifeless. I have this 'feeling of vagueness' especially at sunset hours. I see colors as brighter. All sensations seem to be different from usual and to fall apart. My body is changing, my face too. I feel disconnected from myself, from my muscles, as if they were cropped up in an outer space. . . . It also occurs that in this state I get lost when I stay with others. What I lack is the common thought. I have nothing to share with them. In this way, the others become incomprehensible and scaring.
>
> *(Stanghellini, 2004: 126, quoted in Lysaker and Lysaker, 2010: 336)*

Recently, the disturbances in self-experience characterizing schizophrenia have drawn the attention of cognitive scientists (e.g., Frith, 1992; Gallagher, 2000; Jeannerod, 2009; Cermolacce et al., 2007). This interest can be traced back to a more general theoretical orientation that has emerged over the past two decades characterized by a convergence in the topics of research and methods of cognitive sciences and psychiatry (e.g., Di Francesco et al., 2016). On the one hand, cognitive psychologists and cognitive neuroscientists, in an attempt to shed light on the functioning of human mind, have progressively tried to model various forms of psychopathology. On the other hand, psychiatrists have gradually taken interest in the methodologies and assumptions of the cognitive sciences in order to elaborate patterns of explanation of mental disturbances in compliance with knowledge about processing systems (Cratsley and Samuels, 2013). In this chapter, we explore the alterations in the dimension of the self in schizophrenia within the conceptual framework of cognitive sciences. Specifically, we employ the conceptual tools and empirical findings of cognitive sciences to investigate a specific aspect of the alteration of personal identity in schizophrenia: the relationship between the unity of the self and narrative. We suggest this approach is very effective to discuss one of the main issues characterizing such a relationship: whether narrative depends on language – and therefore whether the unity of the self depends on narrative language. Analysing the proprieties and the cognitive systems involved in narrative processing, we propose that the ability to tell stories, rather than on language, relies on cognitive devices (those constituting the 'narrative brain') operating at a deeper level than the devices that process linguistic information. To corroborate this view, we take into account the defining features of narrative and the cognitive architectures involved in their processing. Against the standard view according to which the narrative self depends on the proper functioning of language, we propose that the structure of narrative discourse is a surface effect of a deeper process that acts primarily on the way the sequences of thoughts are organized, rather than on the way thoughts are expressed. In the light of these considerations, we propose that the disturbances characterizing the construction of the narrative self in schizophrenia have to be attributed primarily to cognition, rather than language.

2 The narrative self in schizophrenia

As mentioned previously, in recent years, a growing number of studies have been investigating the phenomena characterizing the sense of self in both healthy individuals and pathological populations from a perspective aiming to integrate philosophical models with the data coming from cognitive sciences (e.g., Bermúdez, 1998; Gallagher, 2000; Zahavi, 2005; Musholt, 2015; Di Francesco et al., 2016; Marraffa and Paternoster, 2016). Against this background, a major tendency has been that of assuming minimal forms of self as the foundation of more advanced and organized forms (e.g., Gallagher, 2000; Gallagher and Zahavi, 2015; Prebble et al., 2013). In this regard, summarizing a long theoretical tradition dating back to William James (1950), Gallagher, and Zahavi have identified two specific forms of selfhood: the *minimal self* and the *narrative self* (Gallagher, 2000; Gallagher and Zahavi, 2015; Zahavi, 2010, 2014). The minimal self pertains to what is accessible to immediate self-awareness: it is "a consciousness of oneself as an immediate subject of experience, unextended in time" (Gallagher, 2000: 15). The main aspects of the minimal self are ascribable to the context of motor action and involve the senses of ownership – the sense that it is my body that is moving – and agency – the sense that I am the originator or the source of the action. Within this framework, phenomena such as delusions of control or thought insertions affecting people with schizophrenia are interpreted as involving problems with the sense of agency, as patients make mistakes about the agency of various bodily movements (Gallagher, 2000). Indeed, individuals who show these symptoms wrongly attribute their experience to other people as regards agency (they state that someone else caused the action); with respect to ownership, they instead are capable of correctly self-attributing the experiences (they recognize that they themselves are the ones who undergo the action). Within this framework, it is also suggested that the presence of a minimal self is independent of the possession of linguistic and conceptual abilities. Conversely, according to Gallagher, linguistic capacities are required for the more elaborate levels of selfhood, such as the narrative self. The narrative self is the dimension of the self that is extended in time – the dimension providing a sense of continuity and coherence to the self across time (Baerger and McAdams, 1999). Gallagher (2000: 15) defines it as "a more or less coherent self (or self-image) that is constituted with a past and a future in the various stories that we and others tell about ourselves". In other words, from this perspective, the temporal dimension of the self is a product of narrative language: without the ability to tell stories, it is not possible to have a self that is extended in time.

A growing body of investigations has been analysing the *life stories* of patients with schizophrenia (e.g., Gallagher, 2003; Phillips, 2003; Raffard et al., 2010; Allé et al., 2015; Allé et al., 2016; Holm et al., 2016), which are supposed to shed light on the process constituting the individual's narrative self. Indeed, the construction of a *coherent* life narrative by integrating personal past, present, and future in a story is thought to reflect self-continuity over time (McAdams, 1996), namely the feeling of being the same person across time, despite life's many changes (Habermas and Köber, 2014). To construct a global coherent life story, it is necessary to establish temporal order of events, explaining causal connections between those events and evaluating how events have influenced the self (Habermas and Bluck, 2000; Holm et al., 2016). Research has shown that processes of this kind are disrupted (to various degrees) in schizophrenia. In this regard, consider the following case history reported by Phillips (2003) illustrating an impoverished and fragmented self-narrative in a man, Mr. B, with long-standing chronic schizophrenia. Mr. B experienced his first schizophrenic breakdown in his early 20s after he got married and became a father for the first time. Over the years, he struggled to work despite repeated psychotic collapses (i.e., hallucinatory and delusional experiences) and hospitalizations. Gradually, Mr. B assumed a disabled status and remained at home for most of two decades, limiting himself to doing minor household chores. The situation worsened when Mr. B suddenly decided to stop taking his medication. This decision caused a crisis in the home leading his wife to institute divorce proceedings and forcing Mr. B to return to his parents' house. Phillips (2003) narrates that on a few occasions he asked Mr. B about his view of his self, but he replied by laughing and telling him not to ask senseless questions. The psychiatrist describes the self-narrative of his patient in the following way:

> Mr. B has always . . . been unable to present a coherent life narrative or sense of self. . . . The dimension of constructed or fictive self is occasional, unpredictable, fragmented, at times delusional, and not very coherent. It contains the burning at the stake, the various moments at which the illness started, and the frequent, imagined accusations toward his wife. It does not involve the projection of an imagined future that connects with the present and past in a constructive and hopeful manner. The integration of future into his narrative has always been minimal. When he thinks about it, he imagines a future in which he will be living on the street, or more positively, in which he will simply be living comfortably in a hospital. His efforts to locate a self that is not that of the mentally ill man take the form of occasional pathetic denials of his illness and the insistence that he is more himself off the medication, whatever the devastations that occur in that state. . . . With his fragmented and impoverished self-narrative, Mr. B presents a self that is barren and minimally unified.
>
> *(Phillips, 2003: 329)*

These observations have been corroborated in subsequent experimental studies that have systematically investigated the features of life narratives in people with schizophrenia. Allé and colleagues (2015), for example, analysed the life stories and the ability to integrate and connect personal memories into a coherent narrative in 27 stabilized outpatients with schizophrenia and 26 healthy participants. The life narratives were elicited through an experimental protocol drawn up by Habermas and de Silveira (2008). Participants were asked to remember the seven most important events in their lives and to write them down on cards. Then, they had to narrate their life story in 20 minutes, explaining how they had become the persons they are today. Participants were also asked to date the memories. Analyses were conducted on many parameters. For the aims of our argument, the most important of them were the indicators of *causal-motivational*, *thematic*, and *temporal coherence*. Causal-motivational coherence refers to arguments relating to personal change and includes descriptions of how events determine other events and influence one's personality evolution. Thematic coherence is supported by arguments which explain an action with reference to an enduring personality trait; it is a way of knowing what is stable in the narrator's life across several life themes. Eventually, temporal coherence reflects the narrator's ability to locate events chronologically across the course of the story. The results revealed that indicators of causal-motivational, thematic, and temporal coherence were significantly lower in the group of patients compared to controls. Specifically, "Patients with schizophrenia made fewer comments on changes that occurred throughout their life and to explain how these events have influenced the person they are today, which was reflected in a reduced global causal-motivational coherence" (Allé et al., 2015: 7). As for temporal coherence, patients produced a significantly higher number of anachronies (i.e., deviations from the temporal order of events) compared to the control group, making it more difficult to understand the temporal locations of the memories.

These findings are in line with the results of other studies showing that persons with schizophrenia are impaired in the ability to connect past experiences to the current self and to extract meaning from their memories (D'Argembeau et al., 2008; Dimaggio et al., 2012; Raffard et al., 2009; Raffard et al., 2010; Allé et al., 2016; Malek et al., 2019). In an investigation by Raffard and colleagues (2010), 81 outpatients with schizophrenia were asked to respond to a questionnaire that concerned the descriptions of 'self-defining memories', namely exemplar self-narratives of events that according to the individuals give essence to their sense of identity (Singer and Salovey, 1993). The self-narratives were analysed with respect to different indicators: meaning-making (what the individual learns or understands from the event), self-event connections (points in the stories where the narrator binds some aspect of the event to some aspect of the self), and narrative coherence. The latter indicator was coded along three dimensions: context, which concerned information such as time, location, and characters involved in the event; chronology, i.e., the temporal order of the narrative; theme, which was evaluated with reference to the extent to which the subject maintained the topic throughout the narrative, developed the topic, made causal connections, elaborated the details, and inserted personal evaluations. The results revealed that patients with schizophrenia made fewer meaning-making (see also Berna et al., 2011) and self-event connections than the control groups composed of 50 healthy individuals.

Moreover, patients produced narratives that were less coherent, i.e., less contextualized, less temporal ordered, and thematically less developed than those of the controls, thus corroborating the view that persons with schizophrenia exhibit a specific impairment in the ability to create coherent narratives of their lives by linking together important events to their self.

The observations made so far allow us to stress a significant aspect characterizing the narrative self in schizophrenia. The reduced coherence of patients' life stories appears to be the product of a twofold difficulty: on the one hand, schizophrenic patients show an inability to temporally organize the events that contributed to determine their personal identity; on the other hand, they are not able to extract meaning from these events or reflect on how they have contributed to shaping their subjectivity. That said, the next step is to determine whether the difficulty in constructing a coherent temporally extended self is the result of language impairments, narrative impairments to be exact, or not. In other words, the next move is to evaluate whether the deficit in storytelling in schizophrenic patients might be considered the product of a deeper impairment relating to the ability to structure (causally and temporally) the sequences of events constituting a narrative.

From the considerations made so far and from the empirical findings discussed, we have highlighted the key role of narrative in the construction of the self. In doing so, we are in line with the standard view of cognitive sciences. However, differently from this view, we propose an alternative hypothesis to account for such a role. Scholars adhering to the standard view suggest that narrative is a product of language and, therefore, the alterations in the dimension of the self in individuals with schizophrenia are strongly connected to alterations in language use (e.g., Gallagher, 2000, 2003). According to an alternative hypothesis, the disorders of the self in schizophrenia largely reflect dysfunctions in cognitive processes that underlie both narrative and language (Cosentino, 2011; Cosentino and Ferretti, 2015). As is evident from these considerations, investigating these issues means not only explaining the disturbances of the self in schizophrenia, but more generally providing an account of how human beings construct their own subjectivity and how and why narrative plays a pivotal role in such a process. Although the debate is far from being conclusive, in this chapter we adhere to a hypothesis alternative to the standard view.

3 'Delinguisticizing' the narrative self

As mentioned previously, when delineating the notion of the narrative self, Gallagher (2000) adheres to the view according to which language represents the core constituent of human identity. The author suggests that human beings have a sense of a coherent and continuous self because they have language; more specifically, because they have the ability to tell stories. In his words: "We use words to tell stories, and in these stories we create what we call our selves" (19). In supporting such a view, which has a long philosophical and psychological tradition, Gallagher follows the account of human subjectivity elaborated by Daniel Dennett (1991).

According to Dennett, personal identity must be interpreted as a *centre of narrative gravity*: human beings cannot prevent themselves from inventing their selves; once they have become language users, humans are trapped in the web of language and begin assembling their own stories, which end up controlling their creators. As the author writes:

> And just as spiders don't have to think, consciously and deliberately, about how to spin their webs, and just as beavers, unlike professional human engineers, do not consciously and deliberately plan the structures they build, we (unlike professional human storytellers) do not consciously and deliberately figure out what narratives to tell and how to tell them. Our tales are spun, but for the most part we don't spin them; they spin us. Our human consciousness, and our narrative selfhood, is their product, not their source.
>
> *(Dennett, 1991: 418)*

This quotation offers many points for reflection. For example, from it emerges the idea that the narrative self is not real, but an empty abstraction, given that our narrative selfhood is the product of the stories we tell. In fact, from Dennett's perspective, the individual self can be considered as a movable and abstract point where the various narratives that the subject tells about herself, or that others have told about her, meet up. Although this eliminative view deserves a more in-depth analysis, we intend to focus our discussion on another point characterizing Dennett's account of human subjectivity. Specifically, we want to stress that this perspective is based on a more general idea of the relationship between narrative and language, an idea according to which language represents a necessary condition (both logically and temporally) for the ability to tell stories. This idea is a major tenet of the constructivist perspective of narrative (Bruner, 1990, 1991; Dautenhahn, 2002; Hutto, 2009), of which the psychologist Jerome Bruner is the main representative. In line with culturalist constructivism, according to Bruner, the ability to tell stories has to be viewed as the result of forms of social apprenticeship characterizing the individual's development within a social group. Internal cognitive systems are not relevant for narrative competence; all that matters is this process of internalization of social and cultural factors.

The issue of the relationship between narrative and language is the key point to clarify our hypothesis on the connection between self and narrative. In order to state that narrative is the product of language, it is necessary to identify the properties characterizing the narrative dimension and ask whether they are reducible to language abilities or not. Although scholars of narratology have different opinions about the nature and number of these properties, there is convergence, however, on the fact that 'global coherence' is one of the main features of a narrative. Such a property is relevant to our argument because, as we have already seen, schizophrenic patients have difficulties in the construction of coherent life narratives. If we take global coherence as a litmus test to study the relationships between language, narrative, and construction of the self, the first step is that of investigating the nature of this property; more in detail, the first move is asking whether global coherence can be reduced to the functioning of linguistic systems or not. The possibility of accounting for the role of narrative in the construction of the self depends on the way we answer this question.

The studies attesting the irreducibility of coherence to linguistic cohesion allow us to corroborate the independence and autonomy of narrative from language. As we have already seen, the coherence of a narrative depends, at least in part, on the speaker's ability to maintain thematic unity and to establish causal and temporal connections between the events constituting a story. According to a prominent tradition within linguistics, the coherence of a narrative or a discourse depends on the grammatical and lexical linear relations between adjacent sentences, that is to say on cohesion between pairs of consecutive statements (e.g., Bublitz, 2011; Daneš, 1974; Halliday and Hasan, 1976). As in the following text where the sentences are connected through lexical items (in italics):

> After the forming of the *sun* and the *solar system*, our *star* began its long existence as a so-called *dwarf* star. In the *dwarf phase* of its life, the energy that the *sun* gives off is generated in its core through the fusion of hydrogen into helium.
>
> *(Berzlánovich, 2008: 2)*

Although cohesive relations (grammatical and lexical) have an important role in the expression and recognition of coherence relations, theoretical arguments (Giora, 1985) and empirical findings (for a discussion, Adornetti, 2015) show that cohesion between consecutive sentences is not a necessary or sufficient condition for the coherence of utterances in the flow of speech. In this regard, a crucial distinction is that between global and local coherence. Global coherence refers to the relationship between the content of a verbalization with that of the general topic of conversation; local coherence concerns the conceptual links between individual sentences or propositions that maintain meaning in a text or narrative discourse (Glosser and Deser, 1990). While local coherence is made possible by cohesion relationships, global coherence is independent from linguistic devices (it is independent from cohesion). Schizophrenic patients represent a prototypical example in this regard. In spite of being able to process the lexical and syntactical aspects of individual sentences, these patients have problems in coherently connecting sentences during the flow of discourse (e.g., Marini et al., 2008). Because of this, their narratives can be affected by several kinds of impoverishment, which include *derailment* – sudden switching of topic with no obviously apparent logic or segues, *tangentiality* – oblique or irrelevant reply to questions, and *loss of goal* –failure to follow a chain of thought through to its natural conclusion (e.g., Andreasen, 1979; Frith, 1992; Kuperberg, 2010; McKenna and Oh, 2005; Pauselli et al., 2018). Consider the following example of schizophrenic derailment:

> Then, I always liked *geography*. My last teacher in the *subject* was *Professor* August A. He was a *man* with *black eyes*. I also like *black eyes*. There are also blue and gray *eyes* and other sorts, too. I have heard it said that snakes have green *eyes*. All people have *eyes*.
>
> *(Bleuler, 1911)*

Although in this text the sentences are locally coherent because they are connected through lexical cohesion (in italics), at the global level the discourse lacks coherence: it is not possible to recognize a central topic unifying the sentences constituting the text. For that, it has been suggested that the derailment of the discourse in schizophrenic patients does not depend on poor linguistic abilities (it is not a language disorder in a strict sense) but represents the surface expression of deeper cognitive deficits (Kuperberg, 2010; Stirling et al., 2006, Boudewyn et al., 2012; for a different perspective on schizophrenic language, see Cardella, 2017).

That said, if coherence is primarily a property of the cognitive dimension (a property relating to the way humans represent reality) and only secondarily a linguistic manifestation, then it makes sense to argue that narrative has only an indirect and secondary effect on the construction of the self: the causal processes that allow a narrative to act as a connection tool for the construction of the narrative self are the systems that process global coherence, which is a property referable to the cognitive level. The verification of this hypothesis passes through the identification of the cognitive systems at the basis of the processing of global coherence; above all, such verification depends on the fact that these systems, although involved in narrative processing, are autonomous and independent from language functioning. How to prove this hypothesis? The first thing to say is that the narrative dimension implies different processing systems and that global coherence is not a property that can be reduced to the functioning of a single cognitive device (for a discussion, see Ferretti, 2021; Ferretti and Adornetti, 2020). For space reasons and given the importance of the time factor in the construction of coherent self narratives, in this chapter we only focus on the systems that govern the ability to project in time. Our hypothesis is founded on two argumentative steps: the idea that the systems underlying the projection in time have a role in the construction of the self; the idea that these systems have a role in the processing of narrative discourse. Providing empirical foundation for this hypothesis means stating that the role of narrative in the construction of the self is a by-product of processing systems not specific for language. As such, it turns out to be a significant point to investigate the relationship between language and schizophrenia.

4 Mental time travel and self-continuity

One of main cognitive systems that allows humans to represent time is Mental Time Travel (MTT) (Tulving, 1985, 2005; Suddendorf and Corballis, 2007), the device underlying the ability to project into past and future. MTT is composed of two subsystems: *episodic memory* (EM), which is responsible for remembering past events (Tulving, 1985, 2005), thus contributing to important aspects of autobiographical memory; *episodic future thinking* (EFT) (Atance and O'Neill, 2001), which allows envisioning possible future personal experiences. Several lines of investigation have shown that EM and EFT are strongly connected to each other. Studies on individuals with acquired amnesia revealed that these patients are unable to project themselves into personal past and exhibit an equivalent deficit in imagining future personal experiences (Klein et al., 2002; Tulving, 1985). These observations go hand in hand with neuroimaging research that found that many of the same brain regions – medial temporal and frontal lobes, posterior cingulate, and retrosplenial cortex, as well as lateral, parietal, and temporal areas – are active both when remembering the past and when envisioning the future (e.g., Addis et al., 2007; Hassabis et al., 2007).

For our argument, it is important to highlight that the cognitive system underlying the human ability to mentally project in time evolved independently from language. In fact, comparative studies have shown that non-human animals, such as great apes, corvid, and rats, can to a greater or lesser extent remember past episodes and anticipate future needs (e.g., Clayton and Dickinson, 1998; Mulcahy and Call, 2006; Lu et al., 2012; Kano and Hirata, 2015). For example, a study by Kano and Hirata (2015) conducted with chimpanzees and bonobos revealed that these primates exhibit quite detailed memory for single events and an investigation by Mulcahy and Call (2006) attested foresight abilities in bonobos and orangutans. That precursors of MTT are present in animals that cannot talk (the fact that MTT is autonomous from the proper functioning of verbal abilities) allows us to advance the hypothesis that language abilities are not a necessary condition (logically or temporally) for the functioning of this cognitive system. Since it is our claim that MTT has a crucial role both in the construction of important aspects of the self – those providing a sense of continuity across time – and in the processing of significant properties of narrative discourse – global coherence – the fact that such a system is independent from language opens the way to the possibility of ensuring a cognitive foundation for these two processes.

To disentangle the role of MTT in the construction of self, it is important to clarify the meaning of the term 'episodic' characterizing its two subcomponents: episodic memory and episodic future thinking. In fact, this term denotes one of the most remarkable features of MTT: its *subjective character*. Tulving (2005) suggests that the ability to travel mentally in time implies a form of autonoetic consciousness, the consciousness involving explicit memory that requires self-awareness. From this view, EM and EFT are responsible for an individual's awareness of his or her existence and identity in time, from the personal past to the personal future.

This means that the process of MTT does not merely reflect the extraction of a specific meaning or knowledge, which depends on semantic memory (the memory that deals with general knowledge of one's environment, such as facts and rules); rather, it also involves the retrieval of one's personal episodes, as well as the generation of potential future ones (Schacter and Addis, 2007). As Tulving (2005: 9) states: "mental time travel allows the 'owner' of episodic memory ('self'), through the medium of autonoetic awareness, to remember one's own previous 'thought- about' experiences, as well as to 'think about' one's own possible future experiences". Similarly, according to Buckner and Carroll (2007), MTT can be defined as a process of "self-projection", namely as a shift of perception from the immediate environment to an alternative and imagined one, with the imagined event referenced to oneself. For this, it has been suggested that the two mechanisms constituting MTT are crucial for self-continuity as they are responsible for forming a 'diachronic unit' (Prebble et al., 2013). Indeed, being able to recall personal memories or anticipate possible personal future events allows individuals to form representations of themselves as unique beings who exist with meaningful continuity over time.

Some investigations have highlighted that in schizophrenic patients there are abnormalities in the neural circuits typically associated with MTT, among which are the ventromedial prefrontal cortex, the precuneus, and the hippocampus (Fornara et al., 2017). In support of this, behavioural studies have revealed that persons with schizophrenia show reduced ability to both retrieve specific events from their personal past and imagine possible scenarios that might happen in their personal future (e.g., Cuervo-Lombard et al., 2007; Danion et al., 2007; D'Argembeau et al., 2008; Raffard et al., 2013; Chen et al., 2016; Lyons et al., 2016; Fornara et al., 2017; Yang et al., 2018; Malek et al., 2019). It has been shown that patients with schizophrenia recall fewer autobiographical memories, namely memories involving information related to the self, than control participants (Elvevåg et al., 2003) and that these memories lack contextual details and are less specific (i.e., referring to events that occurred at a particular time and place and lasted less than a day) compared to control groups (Berna et al., 2016). Similarly, they suffer from difficulties in imagining future events (D'Argembeau et al., 2008; Chen et al., 2016). D'Argembeau et al. (2008) found that patients not only recalled fewer specific past events than healthy controls but were also more impaired in generating specific future events. For example, they exhibited difficulties when asked to describe general situations or emotional states that could potentially be associated with specific events such as feeling guilty about something or feeling relaxed. More recently, these results have been confirmed by Potheegadoo and colleagues (2013) and Wang and colleagues (2017). Interestingly, the authors of these two investigations also showed that during MTT, schizophrenic patients are inclined to adopt an observer perspective (seeing the event from the outside as an observer) rather than a field perspective (seeing what happens through the individual's own eyes), which suggests self-impairment. Indeed, the fact that patients assume field perspectives less frequently than participants of the control groups may reflect "a weakened sense of the individual of being an actor of his past events, and hence to a reduced sense of self" (Potheegadoo et al., 2013: 88).

From these considerations some important data emerge for the purposes of our argument. The first is that the processing of the time factor is based on systems that are autonomous and independent from those governing language processing and that such systems have important effects on the processes underlying the construction of the narrative self. The second point is that the abilities made possible by these systems – projecting oneself in time – are severely compromised in schizophrenia. Showing that the deficits in the representation of time affect the construction of the self in schizophrenia is a first important result for the purposes of our hypothesis: if MTT is largely independent from language, then deficits characterizing the temporal dimension of the self in schizophrenia do not depend on language. That said, there is one last point that has to be addressed: showing that the impairments in MTT also have an impact on narrative processing.

5 Mental time travel and narrative processing

Accumulating investigations reveal that the processes responsible for remembering the past and envisioning the future are also involved in the production of coherent narratives (for a discussion, see Corballis, 2017; Ferretti and Adornetti, 2020). Relevant in this regard are studies conducted on individuals with autism spectrum disorder (ASD) and amnesic patients with damage to the hippocampus. Like schizophrenic patients, a growing number of investigations report that also persons with ASD have impairments both in episodic memory (e.g., Crane and Goddard, 2008) and in projecting themselves into the future (e.g., Lind and Bowler, 2010; Marini et al., 2016). Recently, it has been suggested that these impairments are also responsible for some of the narrative difficulties often reported in this clinical population (Ferretti et al., 2018; Marini et al., 2019). In a study by Ferretti and colleagues (2018), children with ASD were administered a task aimed at assessing EFT: they were asked to imagine themselves in a possible future scenario (e.g., a snowy landscape) and to choose an item they would take with themselves (i.e., a coat) anticipating a potential future need (Atance and Meltzoff, 2005). Thereafter, participants were asked to generate episodes of a narrative discourse along two conditions: future generation and past generation. In the future generation task, the children were administered coloured drawings that portrayed the beginning of a story and were asked to continue it. In the past generation condition participants saw coloured pictures that depicted the end of a story and had to describe what was likely to have happened earlier. The performance of the children with ASD was compared to that of a group of children with typical development. The results revealed that an impairment in the ability to project themselves into the future also affected the generation of coherent fictional stories. Indeed, from the findings, it emerged that EFT skills were impaired only in a subgroup of children with ASD and that such a subgroup performed significantly worse on the narrative production task than both ASD participants with good EFT skills and participants with typical development. In particular, the subgroup of children with ASD with impaired EFT produced narratives that were globally less coherent than those generated by the other groups. According to the authors, these results allow supporting the view that

> the ability to tell stories relies on cognition more than cognition relies on language. In this sense, it is certainly true that, through stories, humans can extend themselves in the time and space dimensions, but it is primarily true that without time navigation capabilities, humans could never have had the ability to tell stories.
>
> *(Ferretti et al., 2018: 13)*

Relevant for our argument are also the studies on amnesic patients with damage to the hippocampus, a brain structure embedded deep in the temporal lobe, which has been proposed as one of main neural substrates of mental time travel (e.g., Maguire et al., 2016). Although linguistic functions such as lexical and grammatical processing are mainly unimpaired in these patients (e.g., Kensinger et al., 2001), recent research suggests that hippocampal disruption affects qualitative aspects of language production, particularly when creating detailed and complex narratives that unfold over time (e.g., Duff et al., 2009; Race et al., 2015; Hilverman et al., 2016). For example, a study by Race and colleagues (2015) showed that the hippocampus is involved not only in the generation of coherent fictional narratives (i.e., verbal narratives about pictures), but also in the production of discourse about future and past events, namely when participants had to imagine specific personal events about the future (e.g., winning the lottery) and recall specific personal events about the past (e.g., graduation ceremony). From the results it emerged that amnesic patients' descriptions of the past and future were reduced in higher level measures of linguistic integration, such as global coherence. As discourse coherence reflects the degree to which the speaker stays on topic and develops a global theme using causal linkages and elaborations, these results suggest that the hippocampus plays a critical role in the creation of narrative context by structuring linguistic elements around temporally specific details. Findings of this kind are particularly interesting to shed new light on the narrative deficits affecting patients with schizophrenia. Indeed, there is evidence that not only are these patients characterized by structural abnormalities in the hippocampus (Kalus et al., 2004; Hanlon et al., 2011), but also that such abnormalities (i.e., decreasing in volume) are linked to some of their discourse production impairments (Spalletta et al., 2010).

6 Conclusions

In this chapter, we have suggested that construction of the self that is extended in time is largely the result of a process governed by narrative. Following this thesis, it is possible to consider the difficulty of schizophrenics in the construction of a unitary self as a disorder largely linked to narrative deficits. Considerations of this type, which are the standard hypothesis in cognitive science, are widely shared in the contemporary debate. Although we share the main tenet of hypothesis – the idea that narrative plays a central role in the construction of the self – we diverge from the standard view with respect to the way of explaining 'how' and 'why' narrative has such a role. To this aim, we have investigated the nature of narrative and the functioning of the systems underlying the processing of the narrative dimension. From this analysis, it has emerged that narrative is independent from language and that the ability to tell stories relies on cognition more than on language. From the point of view of cognitive architectures, in fact, we have shown that the systems that process the narrative dimension – mental time travel – despite having a strong impact on language functioning, evolved in contexts different from that of linguistic communication. From the point of view of properties, we have stressed that global coherence governs the construction of temporal and causal sequences of events at the level of thought, before that of the expression of thought. From these considerations, a new way of conceiving the relationship between narrative and the construction of the self emerges. If for the proponents of the standard view the role of narrative depends almost exclusively on language (given that narrative capacity is the apical development of linguistic competence), from our point of view narrative is first and foremost the product of cognitive systems not specific for language. In a perspective of this kind, studies on the disorders of the self in schizophrenia also acquire new light. If narrative is a by-product of the role played by the systems that process the causal and temporal sequence of events, then the difficulties of constructing a self that is extended in time by individuals with schizophrenia is a process largely independent from language. The narrative deficits of schizophrenics are a surface effect of what happens on a deep cognitive level. In a perspective of this type, the study of such deficits turns out to be a useful test for analysing, in addition to the processes of the construction of the self, also the nature of narrative and, in this way, the proper nature of human language.

Authors contribution

For the specific constraints of the Italian Academy, we specify that Ines Adornetti wrote Sections 1, 2, 3, and 4; Francesco Ferretti wrote Sections 3, 5, and 6.

Notes

1 According to the DSM-5, a diagnosis of schizophrenia can be made if two (or more) of the following symptoms are present for a significant portion of time during a one-month period: delusions, hallucinations, disorganized speech, grossly disorganized or catatonic behavior, and negative symptoms. At least one of the symptoms occurring in the one-month period must be delusions, hallucinations, or disorganized speech.

2 According to the ICD-11, schizophrenia is characterized by multiple disorders, such as thinking disturbances (e.g., delusions, thought disorganization), perception (e.g., hallucinations), self-experience (e.g., the experience that one's feelings, thoughts, or behavior are controlled by an external force), cognition (e.g., impaired attention, social cognition), volition (e.g., loss of motivation), affect (e.g., blunted affect), and behavior (e.g., bizarre

or purposeless). Psychomotor disturbances may be also present. Core symptoms are persistent delusions, persistent hallucinations, thought disorder, and experiences of influence, passivity, or control. A diagnosis of schizophrenia is made when symptoms have persisted for at least one month.

References

Addis, D. R., Wong, A. T., and Schacter, D. L. (2007). Remembering the past and imagining the future: Common and distinct neural substrates during event construction and elaboration. *Neuropsychologia*, 45(7), 1363–1377.

Adornetti, I. (2015). The phylogenetic foundations of discourse coherence: A pragmatic account of the evolution of language. *Biosemiotics*, 8(3), 421–441.

Allé, M. C., d'Argembeau, A., Schneider, P., Potheegadoo, J., Coutelle, R., Danion, J. M., and Berna, F. (2016). Self-continuity across time in schizophrenia: An exploration of phenomenological and narrative continuity in the past and future. *Comprehensive Psychiatry*, 69, 53–61.

Allé, M. C., Potheegadoo, J., Köber, C., Schneider, P., Coutelle, R., Habermas, T., . . . and Berna, F. (2015). Impaired coherence of life narratives of patients with schizophrenia. *Scientific Reports*, 5, 12934.

American Psychiatric Association (APA). (2013). *Diagnostic and statistical manual of mental disorders* (5th ed.). Washington, DC: American Psychiatric Publishing.

Andreasen, N. C. (1979). Thought, language and communication disorders: II diagnostic significance. *Archives of General Psychiatry*, 36, 1325–1330.

Atance, C. M., and Meltzoff, A. N. (2005). My future self: Young children's ability to anticipate and explain future states. *Cognitive Development*, 20(3), 341–361.

Atance, C. M., and O'Neill, D. K. (2001). Episodic future thinking. *Trends in Cognitive Sciences*, 5(12), 533–539.

Baerger, D. R., and McAdams, D. P. (1999). Life story coherence and its relation to psychological well-being. *Narrative Inquiry*, 9(1), 69–96.

Bermúdez, J. (1998). *The paradox of self-consciousness*. Cambridge, MA: MIT Press.

Berna, F., Bennouna-Greene, M., Potheegadoo, J., Verry, P., Conway, M. A., and Danion, J. M. (2011). Impaired ability to give a meaning to personally significant events in patients with schizophrenia. *Consciousness and Cognition*, 20(3), 703–711.

Berna, F., Potheegadoo, J., Aouadi, I., Ricarte, J. J., Alle, M. C., Coutelle, R., . . . and Danion, J. M. (2016). A meta-analysis of autobiographical memory studies in schizophrenia spectrum disorder. *Schizophrenia Bulletin*, 42(1), 56–66.

Berzlánovich, I. (2008). *Lexical cohesion and the organization of discourse*. www.rug.nl/let/onderzoek/onderzoekinstituten/clcg/berzlanovich.pdf

Blankenburg, W., and Mishara, A. L. (2001). First steps toward a psychopathology of "common sense". *Philosophy, Psychiatry, and Psychology*, 8(4), 303–315.

Bleuler, E. (1911). *Dementia praecox or the group of schizophrenias*. Translated by J. Zinkin. New York: International Universities Press, 1950.

Boudewyn, M. A., Carter, C. S., and Swaab, T. Y. (2012). Cognitive control and discourse comprehension in schizophrenia. *Schizophrenia Research and Treatment*, article 484502.

Bruner, J. (1990). *Acts of meaning*. Cambridge, MA: Harvard University Press.

Bruner, J. (1991). The narrative construction of reality. *Critical Inquiry*, 18(1), 1–21.

Bublitz, W. (2011). Cohesion and coherence. In J. Zienkowski, J. Östman, and J. Verschueren (Eds.), *Discursive pragmatics* (pp. 37–49). Amsterdam/Philadelphia: John Benjamins Publishing Company.

Buckner, R. L., and Carroll, D. C. (2007). Self-projection and the brain. *Trends in Cognitive Sciences*, 11(2), 49–57.

Cardella, V. (2017). *Language and schizophrenia*. New York: Routledge.

Cermolacce, M., Naudin, J., and Parnas, J. (2007). The "minimal self" in psychopathology: Re-examining the self-disorders in the schizophrenia spectrum. *Consciousness and Cognition*, 16(3), 703–714.

Chen, X. J., Liu, L. L., Cui, J. F., Wang, Y., Chen, A. T., Li, F. H., . . . and Shum, D. H. (2016). Schizophrenia spectrum disorders show reduced specificity and less positive events in mental time travel. *Frontiers in Psychology*, 7, article 1121.

Clayton, N. S., and Dickinson, A. (1998). Episodic-like memory during cache recovery by Scrub Jays. *Nature*, 395(6699), 272–274.

Corballis, M. C. (2017). *The truth about language: What it is and where it came from*. Chicago: University of Chicago Press.

Cosentino, E. (2011). Self in time and language. *Consciousness and Cognition*, 20(3), 777–783.

Cosentino, E., and Ferretti, F. (2015). Cognitive foundations of the narrative self. *Rivista internazionale di Filosofia e Psicologia*, 6(2), 311–324.

Crane, L., and Goddard, L. (2008). Episodic and semantic autobiographical memory in adults with autism spectrum disorders. *Journal of Autism and Developmental Disorders*, 38(3), 498–506.

Cratsley, K., and Samuels, R. (2013). Cognitive science and explanations of psychopathology. In K. W. Fulford, M. Davies, R. Gipps, G. Graham, J. Sadler, G. Stanghellini, and T. Thornton (Eds.), *The Oxford handbook of philosophy and psychiatry* (pp. 413–433). Oxford, UK: Oxford University Press.

Cuervo-Lombard, C., Jovenin, N., Hedelin, G. U. Y., Rizzo-Peter, L., Conway, M. A., and Danion, J. M. (2007). Autobiographical memory of adolescence and early adulthood events: An investigation in schizophrenia. *Journal of the International Neuropsychological Society*, 13(2), 335–343.

Daneš, F. (1974). Functional sentence perspective and the organization of the text. In F. Daneš (Ed.), *Papers on functional sentence perspective* (pp. 106–128). Prague: Academia.

Danion, J. M., Huron, C., Vidailhet, P., and Berna, F. (2007). Functional mechanisms of episodic memory impairment in schizophrenia. *The Canadian Journal of Psychiatry*, 52(11), 693–701.

D'Argembeau, A., Raffard, S., and Van der Linden, M. (2008). Remembering the past and imagining the future in schizophrenia. *Journal of Abnormal Psychology*, 117(1), 247–251.

Dautenhahn, K. (2002). The origins of narrative: In search of the transactional format of narratives in humans and other social animals. *International Journal of Cognition and Technology*, 1, 97–123.

Davidson, L. (2020). Recovering a sense of self in schizophrenia. *Journal of Personality*, 88(1), 122–132.

Dennett, D. C. (1991). *Consciousness explained*. Boston, MA: Little Brown and Company.

Di Francesco, M., Marraffa, M., and Paternoster, A. (2016). *The self and its defenses: From psychodynamics to cognitive science*. London: Palgrave McMillan.

Dimaggio, G., Salvatore, G., Popolo, R., and Lysaker, P. H. (2012). Autobiographical memory and mentalizing impairment in personality disorders and schizophrenia: Clinical and research implications. *Frontiers in Psychology*, 3, 529.

Duff, M. C., Hengst, J. A., Tranel, D., and Cohen, N. J. (2009). Hippocampal amnesia disrupts verbal play and the creative use of language in social interaction. *Aphasiology*, 23(7–8), 926–939.

Elvevåg, B., Kerbs, K. M., Malley, J. D., Seeley, E., and Goldberg, T. E. (2003). Autobiographical memory in schizophrenia: An examination of the distribution of memories. *Neuropsychology*, 17(3), 402–409.

Ferretti, F. (2021). The narrative origins of language. In N. Gontier, A. Lock, and C. Sinha (Eds.), *The Oxford handbook of human symbolic evolution*. Oxford: Oxford University Press.

Ferretti, F., and Adornetti, I. (2020). Why we need a narrative brain to account for the origin of language. *Paradigmi, XXXVIII* (2), 269–292.

Ferretti, F., Adornetti, I., Chiera, A., Nicchiarelli, S., Valeri, G., Magni, R., Vicari, S., and Marini, A. (2018). Time and narrative: An investigation of storytelling abilities in children with Autism Spectrum Disorder. *Frontiers in Psychology*, 9, 944.

Fornara, G. A., Papagno, C., and Berlingeri, M. (2017). A neuroanatomical account of mental time travelling in schizophrenia: A meta-analysis of functional and structural neuroimaging data. *Neuroscience and Biobehavioral Reviews*, 80, 211–222.

Freud, S. (1957). *Neurosis and psychosis* (A. Strachev and J. Strachev, trans.), Collected Papers, Vol. II. London, UK: Hogarth Press.

Frith, C. D. (1992). *The cognitive neuropsychology of schizophrenia*. Hove and New York: Psychology Press.

Frosch, J. (1983). *The psychotic process*. New York: International Universities Press.

Gallagher, S. (2000). Philosophical conceptions of the self: Implications for cognitive science. *Trends in Cognitive Sciences*, 4(1), 14–21.

Gallagher, S. (2003). Self-narrative in schizophrenia. In T. Kircher, A. S. David, and A. David (Eds.), *The self in neuroscience and psychiatry* (pp. 336–357). Cambridge: Cambridge University Press.

Gallagher, S., and Zahavi, D. (2015). Phenomenological approaches to self-consciousness. In E. N. Zalta (Ed.), *The Stanford encyclopedia of philosophy*. http://plato.stanford.edu/archives/spr2015/entries/self-consciousnessphenomenological (accessed 10 July 2020).

Giora, R. (1985). Notes towards a theory of text coherence. *Poetics Today*, 6(4), 699–715.

Glosser, G., and Deser, T. (1990). Patterns of discourse production among neurological patients with fluent language disorders. *Brain and Language*, 40, 67–88.

Habermas, T., and Bluck, S. (2000). Getting a life: The emergence of the life story in adolescence. *Psychological Bulletin*, 126(5), 748–769.

Habermas, T., and de Silveira, C. (2008). The development of global coherence in life narratives across adolescence: Temporal, causal, and thematic aspects. *Developmental Psychology*, 44(3), 707–721.

Habermas, T., and Köber, C. (2014). Autobiographical reasoning is constitutive for narrative identity: The role of the life story for personal continuity. In K. C. McLean and M. U. Syed (Eds.), *The Oxford handbook of identity development* (pp. 1–33). New York: Oxford University Press.

Halliday, M. A. K., and Hasan, R. (1976). *Cohesion in English*. Longman: London.

Hanlon, F. M., Houck, J. M., Pyeatt, C. J., Lundy, S. L., Euler, M. J., Weisend, M. P., . . . and Tesche, C. D. (2011). Bilateral hippocampal dysfunction in schizophrenia. *Neuroimage*, 58(4), 1158–1168.

Hassabis, D., Kumaran, D., and Maguire, E. A. (2007). Using imagination to understand the neural basis of episodic memory. *Journal of Neuroscience*, 27(52), 14365–14374.

Henriksen, M. G., and Nordgaard, J. (2014). Schizophrenia as a disorder of the self. *Journal of Psychopathology*, 20, 435–441.

Hilverman, C., Cook, S. W., and Duff, M. C. (2016). Hippocampal declarative memory supports gesture production: Evidence from amnesia. *Cortex*, 85, 25–36.

Holm, T., Thomsen, D. K., and Bliksted, V. (2016). Life story chapters and narrative self-continuity in patients with schizophrenia. *Consciousness and Cognition*, 45, 60–74.

Hutto, D. (2009). Folk psychology as narrative practice. *Journal of Consciousness Studies*, 16(6–8), 9–39.

Jablensky, A. (2010). The diagnostic concept of schizophrenia: Its history, evolution, and future prospects. *Dialogues in Clinical Neuroscience*, 12(3), 271–287.

James, W. (1950). *The principles of psychology*. New York: Dover. (Original work published 1890.)

Jeannerod, M. (2009). The sense of agency and its disturbances in schizophrenia: A reappraisal. *Experimental Brain Research*, 192, 527–532.

Kalus, P., Buri, C., Slotboom, J., Gralla, J., Remonda, L., Dierks, T., . . . and Kiefer, C. (2004). Volumetry and diffusion tensor imaging of hippocampal subregions in schizophrenia. *Neuroreport*, 15(5), 867–871.

Kano, F., and Hirata, S. (2015). Great apes make anticipatory looks based on longterm memory of single events. *Current Biology*, 25(19), 2513–2517,

Kean, C. (2009). Silencing the self: Schizophrenia as a self-disturbance. *Schizophrenia Bulletin*, 35(6), 1034–1036.

Kensinger, E. A., Ullman, M. T., and Corkin, S. (2001). Bilateral medial temporal lobe damage does not affect lexical or grammatical processing: Evidence from amnesic patient HM. *Hippocampus*, 11(4), 347–360.

Klein, S. B., Loftus, J., and Kihlstrom, J. F. (2002). Memory and temporal experience: The effects of episodic memory loss on an amnesic patient's ability to remember the past and imagine the future. *Social Cognition*, 20(5), 353–379.

Kraepelin, E. (1919). *Dementia praecox and paraphrenia* (M. Barclay, trans.). Bristol, UK: Thoemmes Press, 2002.

Kuperberg, G. R. (2010). Language in schizophrenia part 1: An introduction. *Language and Linguistics Compass*, 4(8), 576–589.

Laing, R. D. (1978). *The divided self*. New York: Pantheon.

Lind, S. E., and Bowler, D. M. (2010). Episodic memory and episodic future thinking in adults with autism. *Journal of Abnormal Psychology*, 119(4), 896.

Lu, H., Zou, Q., Gu, H., Raichle, M. E., Stein, E. A., and Yang, Y. (2012). Rat brains also have a default mode network. *Proceedings of the National Academy of Sciences*, 109(10), 3979–3984.

Lyons, A. D., Henry, J. D., Rendell, P. G., Robinson, G., and Suddendorf, T. (2016). Episodic foresight and schizophrenia. *British Journal of Clinical Psychology*, 55(2), 107–122.

Lysaker, P. H., and Lysaker, J. T. (2002). Narrative structure in psychosis: Schizophrenia and disruptions in the dialogical self. *Theory and Psychology*, 12(2), 207–220.

Lysaker, P. H., and Lysaker, J. T. (2010). Schizophrenia and alterations in self-experience: A comparison of 6 perspectives. *Schizophrenia Bulletin*, 36(2), 331–340.

Maguire, E. A., Intraub, H., and Mullally, S. L. (2016). Scenes, spaces, and memory traces: What does the hippocampus do? *The Neuroscientist*, 22(5), 432–439.

Malek, H. B., D'Argembeau, A., Allé, M. C., Meyer, N., Danion, J. M., and Berna, F. (2019). Temporal processing of past and future autobiographical events in patients with schizophrenia. *Scientific Reports*, 9(1), 1–11.

Marini, A., Ferretti, F., Chiera, A., Magni, R., Adornetti, I., Nicchiarelli, S., Vicari, S., and Valeri, G. (2016). Brief report: Self-based and mechanical-based future thinking in children with autism spectrum disorder. *Journal of Autism and Developmental Disorders*, 46(10), 3353–3360.

Marini, A., Ferretti, F., Chiera, A., Magni, R., Adornetti, I., Nicchiarelli, S., Vicari, S., and Valeri, G. (2019). Episodic future thinking and narrative discourse generation in children with Autism Spectrum Disorders. *Journal of Neurolinguistics*, 49, 178–188.

Marini, A., Spoletini, I., Rubino, I. A., Ciuffa, M., Bria, P., Martinotti, G., . . . and Caltagirone, C. (2008). The language of schizophrenia: An analysis of micro and macrolinguistic abilities and their neuropsychological correlates. *Schizophrenia Research*, 105(1–3), 144–155.

Marraffa, M., and Paternoster, A. (2016). Disentangling the self. A naturalistic approach to narrative self-construction. *New Ideas in Psychology*, 40, 115–122.

McAdams, D. P. (1996). Personality, modernity, and the storied self: A contemporary framework for studying persons. *Psychological Inquiry*, 7(4), 295–321.

McKenna, P. J., Oh, T. M., and Oh, T. (2005). *Schizophrenic speech: Making sense of bathroots and ponds that fall in doorways*. Cambridge: Cambridge University Press.

Mellor, C. S. (1970). First rank symptoms of schizophrenia: I. The frequency in schizophrenics on admission to hospital II. Differences between individual first rank symptoms. *The British Journal of Psychiatry*, 117(536), 15–23.

Minkowski, E. (1987). The essential disorder underlying schizophrenia and schizophrenic thought. In J. Cutting (Ed.), *The clinical roots of the schizophrenic concept*. Cambridge, UK: Cambridge University Press.

Mulcahy, N. J., and Call, J. (2006). Apes save tools for future use. *Science*, 312(5776), 1038–1040.

Musholt, K. (2015). *Thinking about oneself: From nonconceptual content to the concept of a self*. Cambridge, MA: MIT Press.

O'Brien, G., and Opie, J. (2003). The multiplicity of consciousness and the emergence of the self. In T. Kircher and A. David (Eds.), *The self in neuroscience and psychiatry* (pp. 107–120). Cambridge: Cambridge University Press.

Pauselli, L., Halpern, B., Cleary, S. D., Ku, B., Covington, M. A., and Compton, M. T. (2018). Computational linguistic analysis applied to a semantic fluency task to measure derailment and tangentiality in schizophrenia. *Psychiatry Research*, 263, 74–79.

Phillips, J. (2003). Schizophrenia and the narrative self. In T. Kircher and A. David (Eds.), *The self in neuroscience and psychiatry*. Cambridge: Cambridge University Press.

Potheegadoo, J., Berna, F., Cuervo-Lombard, C., and Danion, J. M. (2013). Field visual perspective during autobiographical memory recall is less frequent among patients with schizophrenia. *Schizophrenia Research*, 150(1), 88–92.

Prebble, S. C., Addis, D. R., and Tippett, L. J. (2013). Autobiographical memory and sense of self. *Psychological Bulletin*, 139(4), 815–840.

Race, E., Keane, M. M., and Verfaellie, M. (2015). Sharing mental simulations and stories: Hippocampal contributions to discourse integration. *Cortex*, 63, 271–281.

Raffard, S., D'Argembeau, A., Lardi, C., Bayard, S., Boulenger, J. P., and Van der Linden, M. (2009). Exploring self-defining memories in schizophrenia. *Memory*, 17, 26–38.

Raffard, S., D'Argembeau, A., Lardi, C., Bayard, S., Boulenger, J. P., and Van der Linden, M. (2010). Narrative identity in schizophrenia. *Consciousness and Cognition*, 19(1), 328–340.

Raffard, S., Esposito, F., Boulenger, J. P., and Van der Linden, M. (2013). Impaired ability to imagine future pleasant events is associated with apathy in schizophrenia. *Psychiatry Research*, 209(3), 393–400.

Saks, E. R. (2007). *The center cannot hold: My journey through madness*. London: Hachette UK.

Sass, L. A., and Parnas, J. (2002). Phenomenology of self-disturbances in schizophrenia: Some research findings and directions. *Philosophy, Psychiatry, and Psychology*, 8, 347–356.

Sass, L. A., and Parnas, J. (2003). Schizophrenia, consciousness, and the self. *Schizophrenia Bulletin*, 29(3), 427–444.

Schacter, D. L., and Addis, D. R. (2007). The cognitive neuroscience of constructive memory: Remembering the past and imagining the future. *Philosophical Transactions of the Royal Society B: Biological Sciences*, 362(1481), 773–786.

Singer, J. A., and Salovey, P. (1993). *The remembered self: Emotion and memory in personality*. Old Tappan, NJ: Free Press.

Spalletta, G., Spoletini, I., Cherubini, A., Rubino, I. A., Siracusano, A., Piras, F., . . . and Marini, A. (2010). Cortico-subcortical underpinnings of narrative processing impairment in schizophrenia. *Psychiatry Research: Neuroimaging*, 182(1), 77–80.

Stanghellini, G. (2004). *Disembodied spirits and deanimated bodies: The psychopathology of common sense*. Oxford: Oxford University Press.

Stirling, J. D., Hellewell, J. S., Blakey, A., and Deakin, W. (2006). Thought disorder in schizophrenia is associated with both executive dysfunction and circumscribed impairments in semantic function. *Psychological Medicine*, 36(4), 475–484.

Suddendorf, T., and Corballis, M. C. (2007). The evolution of foresight: What is mental time travel, and is it unique to humans? *Behavioral and Brain Sciences*, 30(3), 299–313.

Tulving, E. (1985). *Elements of episodic memory*. Oxford: Clarendon Press.

Tulving, E. (2005). Episodic memory and autonoesis: Uniquely human? In H. S. Terrace and J. Metcalfe (Eds.), *The missing link in cognition* (pp. 3–56). Oxford: Oxford University Press.

Wang, Y., Wang, Y., Zhao, Q., Cui, J. F., Hong, X. H., and Chan, R. C. (2017). Preliminary study of visual perspective in mental time travel in schizophrenia. *Psychiatry Research*, 256, 225–227.

World Health Organization. *ICD-11 for mortality and morbidity statistics (ICD-11 MMS) 2018 version*. https://icd.who.int/browse11/l-m/en (accessed 27 June 2020).

Yang, Z. Y., Xie, D. J., Zou, Y. M., Wang, Y., Li, Y., Shi, H. S., . . . and Chan, R. C. (2018). Prospection deficits in schizophrenia: Evidence from clinical and subclinical samples. *Journal of Abnormal Psychology*, 127(7), 710.

Zahavi, D. (2005). *Subjectivity and selfhood: Investigating the first-person perspective*. Cambridge, MA: MIT Press.

Zahavi, D. (2010). Minimal self and narrative self. A distinction in need of refinement. In T. Fuchs, H. Sattel, and P. Heningsen (Eds.), *The embodied self: Dimensions, coherence and disorders* (pp. 3–11). Stuttgart: Schattauer.

Zahavi, D. (2014). *Self and other: Exploring subjectivity, empathy, and shame*. Oxford: Oxford University Press.

7

DELUSIONS AND PATHOLOGIES OF BELIEF: MAKING SENSE OF CONSPIRACY BELIEFS VIA THE PSYCHOSIS CONTINUUM

Niall Galbraith

1 Introduction

Delusions are said to fall on a continuum representing the extreme end of a spectrum of psychotic-like traits (Murphy et al., 2010). Consistent with this view is the notion that milder forms of delusional beliefs are observable within the general population, manifesting as unusual ideas which do not cross the thresholds for clinical symptoms, but which might represent a vulnerability for psychotic disorder. In the pre-Internet age, unusual or bizarre beliefs (such as conspiracy theories) would have had fewer opportunities for social acceptance, as the proponents would have less chance to share their ideas with like-minded people. Indeed, part of the DSM-V definition of delusions stipulates that delusions are "not understandable to same-culture peers" (APA, 2013: 90). However, the rise of social media presents new platforms for socially unacceptable beliefs to gain exposure and endorsement from like-minded others, who are no longer limited by geographical constraints (Bell, 2007). Evidence suggests that conspiracy theories and other contentious beliefs have grown in popularity due to the ease with which they are propagated and reinforced through online platforms (Bessi et al., 2015). This chapter reviews the current evidence on the continuity between delusions and conspiracy beliefs. It also explores whether social media and other online platforms make vulnerable individuals more likely to adopt unsound beliefs and consider the effects this might have on mental health as well as the broader social and political implications.

2 Psychosis as a continuum

There is now a considerable body of evidence for the notion that psychosis falls at the extreme end of a spectrum which also includes healthy non-clinical experience. This theory is at odds with Kraepelin (Kraepelin, 1990; see also Bentall, 2003),

TABLE 7.1 Descriptions of the most notable types of delusion

Control	Where feelings, actions, cognitions, or sensations are believed to be under the control of an external source
Grandiose	Where the individual has inflated beliefs about his/her wealth, power, importance, or status in the world
Guilt	Beliefs of unworthiness or shame
Hypochondria	Where the individual falsely believes s/he has a serious disease
Infestation	The belief that one has become infested by small organisms
Jealousy	Where the individual believes that his/her partner is unfaithful
Love	Based upon the false belief that the individual is loved by another person
Misidentification	Where the patient believes that a familiar person has been replaced by an identical impostor (Capgras syndrome), where an unfamiliar person is believed to be someone known to the patient (e.g., their mother; Fregoli syndrome), or where inanimate personal possessions are believed to have been replaced by inferior copies (inanimate doubles)
Persecutory	Where the person believes that they are being pursued, spied on, plotted against, or persecuted
Reference	Where seemingly random events in the person's environment are assumed to have some significance or reference to the self
Religion	Where the person may believe that they have a special relationship with a religious figure or unusual religious powers
Somatic	Delusions relating to the appearance or the functioning of the body

who believed that psychosis (dementia praecox) was utterly distinct from normal behaviour. The traditional Kraepelinian view of psychiatric disorder, still reflected in the DSM-V (APA, 2013), is one where psychiatric symptoms are placed into categories with psychotic disorders falling into either schizophrenia or affective psychoses. However, the validity of such discrete categories has been questioned due to high comorbidity between diagnoses such as schizophrenia and bipolar disorder (Laursen et al., 2009) and the commonality of genetic and environmental risk factors for these diagnoses (e.g., Lichtenstein et al., 2009).

There are two perspectives on the nature of the continuity of psychosis. Firstly, the clinical view put forward by Meehl (1962, 1990) and Lenzenweger (2011) is that certain vulnerable individuals possess an inherited proneness to schizophrenic symptoms. The severity of these symptoms may be measurable along a dimension, but a dimension which is discontinuous with normality (Lenzenweger, 2011; Lenzenweger and Korfine, 1995). Meehl (1990) posits that up to 10% of the population may have such a vulnerability, which is underpinned by a central nervous system anomaly (schizotaxia), and of these, around 50% are expected to develop schizophrenia. Hence, many individuals will carry the latent liability for schizophrenia, but not all of these will develop the disease.

Claridge and Beech (1995) describe Meehl's conceptualization of schizotypy as "quasi-dimensional", in that it represents a disease continuum rather than a full personality dimension. More recently however, large studies of the general population (e.g., Laurens et al., 2012; Mendez et al., 2019; Nuevo et al., 2012) show robust evidence for Claridge and Beech's fully dimensional model of the psychosis continuum. Claridge and Beech view schizophrenia as continuous with normality, a view also referred to as the 'individual differences approach'. The severest forms of the illness exist at the extreme end of the dimension, with healthy experience as its polar opposite. Less severe forms of psychotic behaviour can be found at points along the continuum (see also van Os et al., 2009). Importantly, Claridge and colleagues' argument in favour of the individual differences view incorporates the notion that schizophrenia and the other psychotic disorders are related and represent different points along an illness continuum. The evidence for such a view can be gleaned from three sources: family studies, reports of psychotic-like experiences in healthy individuals, and psychometric data.

a Family studies

Taylor (1992) carried out a review of family studies. He found high incidence of affective disorder in relatives of schizophrenic probands. For example, Tsuang et al. (1980) found that the risk for bipolar affective disorder in first-degree relatives of schizophrenic patients was significantly higher than in first-degree relatives of controls. Similarly, Mendlewicz et al. (1980) reported a high risk for bipolar affective disorder in first-degree relatives of schizophrenic probands. More recent studies support this finding: a higher risk of schizophrenia and schizophrenia spectrum personality disorder among first-degree relatives of recent-onset schizophrenia probands than in first-degree relatives of community control probands (Subotnik et al., 2017). Indeed, large population studies show that a diagnosis of schizophrenia is strongly associated with a range of psychotic disorders in first-degree relatives (Mortensen et al., 2010). Taylor also reviews a number of studies that report a higher occurrence of schizophrenia in relatives of affective disorder patients (e.g., Angst et al., 1980; Scharfetter and Nüsperli, 1980). More recent research concords with this as Vallès et al. (2000) report risk of schizophrenia is higher in relatives of bipolar probands than in relatives of controls. Hochberger et al. (2016) report common neurocognitive dysfunction in probands diagnosed with schizophrenia, schizoaffective disorder, or psychotic bipolar disorder, as well as their first-degree relatives. Facial emotion recognition deficits are found in relatives of probands with schizophrenia, schizoaffective disorder, and bipolar disorder (Ruocco et al., 2014). Consistent with this research is the finding that schizophrenia and bipolar disorder have a common polygenic basis (International Schizophrenia Consortium, 2009).

b Psychotic-like experiences in the general population

Thus, family studies support the continuum model by revealing a genetic basis for a spectrum of psychotic disorder. Further support for the continuum comes from evidence that the spectrum of psychotic-like experience extends into the general population. Numerous studies demonstrate that healthy people can experience milder forms of psychotic-like experience, such as delusions and hallucinations (e.g., Galbraith et al., 2014; Kelleher and Cannon, 2011). For example, Posey and Losch (1983) found that 39% of a student sample reported having previously heard voices. Furthermore, 5% of these claimed to have had conversations with their voices. Tien (1991) reported data collected from approximately 18,000 people as part of a large epidemiological study of psychiatric symptoms in the United States. Between 11% and 13% of the sample reported having hallucinatory experiences at some point. In a later study, van Os et al. (2000) found that nearly 8% of a sample numbering 7076 reported hallucinatory experiences (excluding those attributable to drug use or illness). In addition, van Os et al. (2000) reported that approximately 12% of their sample were found to have delusions of varying intensity (3.3 were adjudged to have had 'true' delusions). In a longitudinal study, Poulton et al. (2000) found that just over 20% of their sample were found to have delusional beliefs. Other types of psychotic symptoms aside from hallucinations and delusions have been reported by healthy people. For example, Poulton et al. (2000) found that nearly 18% of their sample were assessed as having disorganized speech. A meta-analysis of psychosis proneness reports a median prevalence rate of 5% (van Os et al., 2009).

Other characteristics displayed by schizophrenic patients are found in psychometric schizotypes from the normal population. For example, Obiols et al. (1993) found that high schizotypes were poorer on a measure of sustained attention, which is known to be characteristic of people at risk for psychosis (Erlenmeyer-Kimling and Cornblatt, 1987). Cognitive biases (e.g., bias against disconfirmatory evidence or BADE) commonly found in patients with psychosis (Woodward et al., 2006) are also evident in those with subclinical delusional ideation (Zawadzki et al., 2012). People with high schizotypy display schizophrenic phenomenology (Kendler et al., 1985); they show deficits in sustained attention (Lenzenweger et al., 1991; Le Pelley et al., 2010), eye movement dysfunction (Myles et al., 2017; Siever et al., 1990), performance deficits on the Wisconsin Card Sorting Task (Cappe et al., 2012; Lenzenweger and Korfine, 1994), and a data gathering bias on tasks of statistical reasoning (Linney et al., 1998; Ross et al., 2015).

These studies suggest, therefore, that psychotic-like experiences are prevalent in the normal population albeit in a milder form. This implies that the disease continuum proposed by Meehl (1990) extends beyond those who suffer psychiatrically defined psychosis into the healthy section of the population, thus providing support for the individual differences approach advocated by Claridge and Beech (1995).

c Psychometric studies on the structure of psychotic-like experiences

Further support for the notion of a psychosis continuum is provided by psychometric studies. Dissatisfaction with the categorical, Kraepelinian convention has inspired data-driven attempts to map the structure of psychosis in both clinical and non-clinical populations. Psychometric measures have found schizotypal traits to be roughly normally distributed in the general population (Mason et al., 1995; Bentall et al., 1989); furthermore, such measures appear to load onto factors which are consistent with the clusters of symptoms found in psychosis. Typically, the factors on schizotypy measures will reflect positive symptoms, negative symptoms, and disorganization factors (Liddle, 1987; Vollema and Hoijtink, 2000; see also Venables and Bailes, 1994), thus reflecting the major symptom groups of schizophrenia. Other measures have included a fourth factor which appears to reflect impulsive and non-conformist behaviours (e.g., Claridge et al., 1996; Mason et al., 1995) which Mason et al. (1995) suggest is a common feature of schizophrenic spectrum disorders such as bipolar affective disorder. More recently, a five-factor structure – positive symptoms, negative symptoms, cognitive disorganization, affective symptoms, and mania – has been demonstrated both in patients (Stefanovics et al., 2014) and in the general population (Shevlin et al., 2016).

It should be noted, of course, that despite the volume of research evidence available, the continuum model of psychosis is not without criticism. Parnas and Henriksen (2016), for example, argue that psychometric studies of psychotic symptoms reduce such episodes to simplified events, assuming them to be homogeneous and universal. Parnas and Henriksen argue that such a conceptualization of psychosis loses sight of the context or gestalt – the rich, contextual picture of the psychotic experience. When measured psychometrically, subclinical and clinical experiences might superficially appear to represent the same concept, but through careful clinical interview the phenomenology behind apparently similar events can be profoundly distinct (see also David, 2010). Psychometric studies are not suited to capturing the nuanced phenomenology of psychosis. And it has been argued that methodology is crucially important to the way psychopathology is recorded, with different methods accounting for the rather broad incidence rates of psychotic-like experiences reported in the literature (David, 2010). David (2010) goes on to argue that pure quantification of symptoms can be invalid as a measure of severity and that although such measurement is convenient for large statistical surveys, symptoms can only be truly understood when also accounting for their social and phenomenological context.

In defence of the fully dimensional model however, there is evidence that psychometric measures can predict future development of psychosis, which goes some way to support the validity of the continuity model. Chapman et al. (1994) divided a student sample into high and normal scoring groups based on responses to a battery of schizotypy measures. After a ten-year follow-up, 14 of the high scorers had been admitted to hospital with psychosis, whereas in contrast, only one of the normal scorers had been hospitalized with a psychotic episode. Other longitudinal studies have supported these findings showing that risk of developing subsequent psychotic disorder is far higher in those who have reported earlier psychotic-like experiences (Hanssen et al., 2005; Kaymaz et al., 2012; Poulton et al., 2000). Thus, psychometric measures provide evidence that psychotic-like traits are distributed across the general population, and that these traits reflect not just schizophrenic-like behaviours but also the schizophrenia spectrum disorders, including bipolar affective disorder and schizoaffective disorder.

In summary, the literature reviewed here presents an argument for the existence of a psychosis continuum. Research evidence has established that schizophrenia and the schizophrenia spectrum disorders represent a psychosis continuum which extends beyond disease states. There is also evidence that the presence of psychotic-like experiences in the subclinical range represents an elevated risk of subsequent clinical psychosis. This chapter attempts to draw a conceptual link between schizotypy and conspiracy beliefs. We have established that there is evidence for a psychosis continuum, the next step is to consider the continuum of belief, i.e., how beliefs fit into the spectrum of psychosis. To answer this question, we must consider the literature on delusions and attempt to explain how delusions are continuous with other types of belief.

3 Delusions and other implausible beliefs

Delusions have been described as the sine qua non of psychosis (e.g., Kemp et al., 1997) (although the necessity and sufficiency of delusions for the diagnosis of schizophrenia was relaxed in DSM-V [see Bebbington and Freeman, 2017]). Delusions are beliefs which, according to the DSM-V (APA, 2013), are fixed and not amenable to change in the face of conflicting evidence. Delusions are regarded as bizarre if they are clearly implausible or not understandable to same-culture peers. Delusions are also multidimensional and may be assessed in terms of distressed caused, preoccupation, degree of conviction, and action (Garety and Freeman, 1999; Freeman et al., 2016; Gaynor et al., 2013; Sisti et al., 2012). Delusions are most commonly thought of as a symptom of schizophrenia (Tandon and Maj, 2008); however, they are also transdiagnostic and feature in a range of other conditions (e.g., depression; Johnson et al., 1991; see Bebbington and Freeman, 2017). Delusional content can take numerous forms, but certain themes are common (see also Arciniegas, 2015) as can be seen in Table 7.1.

Within the psychosis continuum framework, there has been much research on the relationship between delusional beliefs (or schizotypy more generally) and other types of belief. In the research literature, the beliefs targeted by such research have most commonly been described as magical, superstitious, or paranormal beliefs, anomalous experiences, or fantasy proneness (Brugger and Mohr, 2008; Drinkwater et al., 2020; Eckblad and Chapman, 1983; Hergovich et al., 2008; Swami et al., 2011). These terms are indeed sometimes used interchangeably to refer to the same construct; however, before proceeding we should look at how authors have sought to define these kinds of belief.

In designing the Magical Ideation Scale, Eckblad and Chapman (1983) defined magical thinking as "belief and reported experiences in forms of causation that by conventional standards are invalid" (215). Scores on the magical thinking scale are positively related to Tobacyk and Milford's (1983) Paranormal Belief Scale (PBS;

see Tobacyk and Wilkinson, 1990), who define the paranormal as phenomena which are incompatible with current science and incompatible with "normative perceptions, beliefs, and expectations about reality" (1029). Although the definition of paranormal belief is contentious, paranormal belief is multidimensional: the PBS, for example, and the subsequent revised PBS (RPBS; Tobacyk, 2004) measure belief across seven subscales: religious belief, psi, witchcraft, spiritualism, precognition, superstition, and extraordinary lifeforms. Studies into 'superstitious beliefs' have often employed the superstition subscale of the PBS to measure this construct, but other scales and measures have also been used (see Fluke et al., 2014; Keinan, 2002; Wiseman and Watt, 2004). It should be noted that Wiseman and Watt (2004) note that superstition can often reflect positive beliefs (e.g., charms bringing good luck), whereas the superstition subscale of the PBS tends to focus on superstitions which are negative (e.g., Black cats can bring bad luck).

These definitions have some similarity with Lindeman and Aarnio's (2007) proposal that magical, superstitious, and paranormal thinking are all underpinned by a tendency to make ontological confusions. This is where the core attributes of mental, physical, and biological entities are conflated such that inanimate physical objects are attributed mental ability (e.g., knowledge, desire) or mental phenomena (such as thoughts) are given biological or physical properties.

Based on the foregoing definitions, these types of belief tend to embody a greater willingness to endorse unconventional or unscientific conceptions of phenomena in the world, including the properties of such phenomena and their effects on the environment. For the remainder of this chapter, I shall refer to these types of belief collectively as 'implausible beliefs'. So, what do such beliefs have in common with delusions?

To answer this, let's consider the DSM-V definition of delusions as a reference point. The DSM-V and all the paranormal definitions given previously emphasize beliefs which are held contrary to clear evidence or conventional/scientific knowledge. Both the DSM-V and the foregoing paranormal definitions also emphasize deviation from normal life experiences – which in the case of the DSM-V is a criterion for distinguishing bizarre from non-bizarre delusions. Bizarre delusions are characterized by the DSM as implausible to same-culture peers and not derived from ordinary life experiences, whereas a non bizarre delusion may in theory be plausible (e.g., being under surveillance by the police) but held despite convincing evidence to the contrary. Perhaps the key difference between the DSM-V and paranormal descriptions is the former's emphasis on the conviction and fixedness of the beliefs. Indeed, the DSM-V cites strength of conviction as the index for differentiating delusion from strongly held ideas. Within a continuum framework therefore, we can see that the definitions of delusions and paranormal beliefs have overlap but might be distinguished by degree of conviction.

Thus, the definitions of delusions and other implausible beliefs, such as those relating to the paranormal, have conceptual overlap. Let us now consider the research evidence for how they might coexist on a belief continuum. Firstly, as can be seen in Table 7.1, the paranormal is a common delusional theme and this is supported by empirical studies documenting such delusions (Lange and Houran, 1998, 1999). People reporting more psychotic-like symptoms score higher on the Magical Ideation Scale (Eckblad and Chapman, 1983) and when the MI items were divided into 'paranormal' and 'psychotic' content, both of these subscales correlated with paranormal belief on the Australian Sheep-Goat Scale (Thalbourne and Haraldsson, 1980), hence these relationships were not simply due to similarity between items, but perhaps share a common latent factor (Thalbourne, 1984). The most widely used psychometric measures of delusional ideation, the Community Assessment of Psychic Experiences (CAPE; Wigman et al., 2011), the Peters et al. delusions inventory (PDI; Peters et al., 1999, 2004), and the Schizotypal Personality Questionnaire (SPQ; Raine, 1991), include items on paranormal phenomena. Numerous studies from across the world on the psychometric structure of the CAPE and SPQ group paranormal/magical ideation items with other delusion-like beliefs and positive symptoms (Brenner et al., 2007; Cicero, 2016; Fonseca-Pedrero et al., 2018; Schlier et al., 2015).

Research has revealed that certain cognitive biases associated with delusional beliefs (for a review, see Galbraith and Manktelow, 2014) also co-occur with paranormal beliefs. For example, both delusional and paranormal beliefs are associated with a bias against disconfirmatory evidence (BADE; Woodward et al., 2006), a heightened reluctance to change one's initial hypothesis in the face of new counter-evidence. Both are associated with a liberal acceptance bias (Moritz and Woodward, 2004; Prike et al., 2018) where one is biased to be more accepting of implausible ideas. Both types of belief are associated with a data-gathering bias (Dudley et al., 2016; Fine et al., 2007; Irwin et al., 2014) characterized by a tendency to make hasty decisions based on less evidence. Increased errors in deductive reasoning have been found in both paranormal believers and delusion-prone respondents (Anandakumar et al., 2017; Lawrence and Peters, 2004; Sellen et al., 2005), both types of belief are related to lower reliance on analytic thinking (Freeman et al., 2014; Ross et al., 2017) and both paranormal believers and the delusion-prone respondents show evidence of statistical reasoning errors/biases (Dagnall et al., 2016; Galbraith et al., 2010; Rogers et al., 2017).

Furthermore, both types of belief show neurocognitive similarities. High scores in both magical ideation and schizotypy show reduced left hemisphere dominance for language (Leonhard and Brugger, 1998). This is perhaps due to loose semantic processing and overactivation of the right hemisphere, which Gianotti et al. (2001) argue provide the common factor in paranormal and delusional thinking and which also manifest in higher levels of creativity in both paranormal believers and those with schizotypy (Weinstein and Graves, 2002). Both paranormal believers and those higher in schizotypy show stronger right hemisphere activation (Pizzagalli et al., 2000) and also stronger ambidextrality (Gruzelier, 1994; Nicholls et al., 2005).

Before we move on to consider conspiracy beliefs, we must consider what distinguishes subclinical implausible beliefs from genuine psychotic delusions. Firstly, psychotic delusions are often comorbid with other symptoms such as cognitive disorganization, hallucinations, low mood, mania, negative symptoms, etc. (refs), but this comorbidity is not typical in paranormal beliefs.[1] Secondly, the delusional continuum is indexed by degrees of conviction, preoccupation, and distress (Peters et al., 2004). Similarly, paranormal beliefs are related to negative affect (Dudley, 2000) and, although they are amenable to change (Kane et al., 2010; Wilson, 2018), they can be held with strong conviction (Musch and Ehrenberg, 2002).

Perhaps one of the features of paranormal belief which distinguishes them from delusions is simply how commonplace they are. Unlike psychotic delusions, paranormal beliefs are commonly held within society, with up to 48% of a large UK sample reporting a paranormal experience and with paranormal belief being strongly related to such experience (Pechey and Halligan, 2012). The wide acceptance of such beliefs within society clearly violates another feature of psychotic delusions, i.e., that they should not be shared by same-culture peers. However, the degree to which beliefs are shared by one's culture perhaps represents another dimension to the psychosis continuum, as delusion-like beliefs are also prevalent in the general population: for example, in 39% of a UK general population (Pechey and Halligan, 2011) and ideas of persecution or paranoia can be shared by cultures and communities.

For example, cyber-paranoia and beliefs about online surveillance are widely expressed and are shared by mainly online communities who join in common endorsement of such ideas (Holm, 2009; Mason et al., 2014). It has been argued that these narratives are the product of modern society and are driven by social inequality (Harper, 2011). Indeed, the archetype of paranoia in which an individual believes himself to be persecuted by powerful agencies is no longer solely the domain of the isolated psychotic patient: recent years have seen the emergence of 'targeted' individual' communities, in which members come together online to share their convictions about being the subject of state or agency-driven persecution (Xuan and MacDonald III, 2019).

As we can see, in the decades since the development of the Magical Ideation scale, evidence has mounted in favour of conceptual overlap between delusions and other implausible beliefs, particularly those relating to the paranormal. There is evidence that paranormal or magical beliefs feature in both psychotic delusions and subclinical delusional ideas, thus supporting the notion of a continuum of belief, a dimension of the psychosis continuum which incorporates the varying intensity of delusional beliefs. The question to which we turn next is whether the continuum of delusional belief can be extended to incorporate another type of implausible belief: conspiracies.

4 Do conspiracy beliefs fall on the delusion continuum?

To answer this question, we must consider whether conspiracy beliefs share a conceptual overlap with delusions as other implausible beliefs do (such as those relating to the paranormal). Before that however, let us define what we mean by 'conspiracy theories'.

Conspiracy theories claim that certain events or practices are the doing of omnipotent groups operating in coalition and in secret, often to intentionally control the social order or to achieve malevolent or harmful goals (Fenster, 1999; Sunstein and Vermeule, 2009; Zonis and Joseph, 1994). Conspiracy theories often make claims which are unwarranted or clearly false given the available evidence (Sunstein and Vermeule, 2009), often arguing for patterns or connections between random or coincidental events where mundane explanations are more likely to be true (Ramsay, 2012; van Prooijen, 2018). Sometimes however, conspiracy theories, by their nature, are difficult to falsify (e.g., Newheiser et al., 2011). Although many conspiracy theories have political themes such as the 9/11 attacks, the death of Lady Diana, the Apollo moon landings, or the assassination of John F Kennedy, many others reflect supernatural ideas such as alien abduction or alien impostors (e.g., lizard people) (Banaji and Kihlstrom, 1996; van Den Bulck and Hyzen, 2020).

In line with these features, the definition of conspiracy belief by van Prooijen & van Vugt (2018) summarizes five key characteristics that such beliefs should have: patterns (patterns of events that are not coincidental); agency (events that are caused purposefully not by accident); coalitions (the theory must involve groups working together); hostility (the coalition must be pursuing goals which are selfish and not in the public interest); continued secrecy (coalitions operating in secret, at least until the conspiracy is proven with hard evidence). These characteristics, van Prooijen & van Vugt (2018) argue, are necessary for conspiracy theories. Other types of belief, such as supernatural beliefs, might share some but not all of these features. For example, belief in ghosts might involve detecting patterns and agency but lacks the necessary elements of hostility and coalition (ghosts are not necessarily hostile nor do they *necessarily* co-conspire with others in some hostile plan). These definitions will be useful as we now turn to consider the relation between conspiracy beliefs and delusional beliefs.

4.1 Conspiracy belief and schizotypy

Firstly, the foregoing definitions of conspiracy theory reflect some of the characteristics of delusions and paranormal beliefs, in particular the presence of unwarranted claims and misinterpreted evidence. Hence, grouping conspiracies with other implausible beliefs is justified. Conspiracies also embody some of the paranoia commonly found in delusions, whereby there is suspicion of hostile groups who have malevolent intentions – however, the degree to which the believer is the sole subject of this hostility perhaps distinguishes conspiracy theories from paranoia, an issue we will return to later.

If conspiracy beliefs do fall onto the continuum of delusional belief, then we should see consistent relationships between schizotypy and conspiracist ideation. Such evidence has been mounting over the past decade or so. Darwin et al. (2011) report that both non-clinical paranoid ideation and schizotypy were both strongly related to conspiracy belief. A confirmatory factor analysis modelling the relationships between these variables was stronger when paranormal belief was omitted.

Darwin et al. (2011) suggest this indicates conspiracy beliefs have more in common with paranoia than paranormal beliefs. Conspiracy beliefs reflect milder levels of suspicion towards malevolent others which at more moderate locations on the psychosis continuum are even adaptive and protective. Only if such suspicion reaches an intensity which is maladaptive for mental health and social relationships would it be classed as a clinical delusion warranting clinical care. Numerous other studies have also shown relationships between conspiracy belief and paranoid ideation or other measures of schizotypy (Barron et al., 2018; Bruder et al., 2013; Brotherton and Eser, 2015; Denovan et al., 2020; Georgiou et al., 2019; van der Tempel and Alcock, 2015; see also Imhoff and Lamberty, 2018, for a review).

Also commonly reported in the literature are relationships between conspiracy belief and paranormal belief (Barron et al., 2018; Drinkwater et al., 2012; Lobato et al., 2014). One of the difficulties with such studies however is that the constructs of paranormal belief, magical ideation, and schizotypy can be conflated. As we have already seen, the magical ideation scale is sometimes described as a measure of paranormal belief and sometimes as a measure of schizotypy. Both descriptions have validity. As we have seen, psychometric studies of delusional beliefs incorporate items on magical or paranormal phenomena. This presents a risk of circularity however, where constructs are purported to correlate with one another and yet are measured with the same or very similar instruments.

4.2 Conspiracy belief and cognition

So, there is growing evidence that conspiracy beliefs and schizotypy are related. Let us look next at whether the tendency to believe in conspiracy theories shares some of the underlying psychological factors with delusions or other implausible beliefs. Firstly, there is evidence that certain thinking styles or information processing biases are found in conspiracy belief as they are in delusional or paranormal belief. Belief in conspiracy theories seems to be negatively related to analytical thinking (Barron et al., 2018; Georgiou et al., 2019; Stahl and van Prooijen, 2018; Swami et al., 2014). This suggests that belief in such theories is due in part to a failure or unwillingness to apply rational or critical thought when assessing evidence for one's beliefs and perhaps a greater reliance instead on intuition. This is something which conspiracy beliefs have in common with paranormal belief and delusional ideation (Freeman et al., 2014; Ross et al., 2017; Ward and Garety, 2019). This might be more than simply a correlation too: Swami et al. (2014) found that experimental manipulations to induce better analytical thought also reduced the strength of conspiracist beliefs. Similarly, Orosz et al. (2016) also found that strength of conspiracy belief could be reduced through rational counter-argument. Thus, as with other implausible beliefs, conspiracy beliefs might be more likely in those who are less analytical, less likely to engage in effortful consideration of the evidence, and are more likely to rely on instinctive, intuitive judgements.

The 'need for cognitive closure' (NFCC) construct has also been investigated as a potential factor in conspiracy belief. NFCC is characterized by a desire to gain quick answers to solutions and also a need to preserve the solution, thus maintaining order and structure and avoiding confusion and ambiguity (Webster and Kruglanski, 1994). As NFCC can be both dispositional and situational, it is appealing as an explanation for why strong beliefs are formed and tenaciously held onto – judgements are formed quickly and preserved with little scrutiny of counter-evidence and alternative views, thus avoiding cognitive dissonance (Festinger, 1957). NFCC has been shown to predict political beliefs (Golec de Zavala and van Bergh, 2007) and self-enhancing beliefs about parenting (Taris, 2000) and epistemic beliefs (Rosman et al., 2016).

The evidence for NFCC playing a role in conspiracy belief is reasonably good. Leman and Cinnirella (2013) found that manipulation of NFCC can reduce belief in conspiracy. Other studies show a relation between NFCC and strength of conspiracy belief (Marchlewska et al., 2018; Umam et al., 2018). However, Moulding et al. (2016) found that intolerance of uncertainty did not predict faith in conspiracy theories. van Prooijen and Jostmann (2013) argue though that uncertainty is more likely to influence conspiracy beliefs when there is simultaneously a perception of low morality in authorities. So, there is some support for the idea that NFCC makes one more vulnerable to conspiracy belief. This same cognitive bias has been linked with delusional belief: higher NFCC has been found in delusional patients and delusion-prone non-patients (Bentall and Swarbrick, 2003; Colbert and Peters, 2002; McKay et al., 2006). NFCC has also been proposed as a mechanism for why people with delusions jump to conclusions – hasty decisions are made in order to avoid ambiguity, although the evidence linking NFCC and the JTC bias is mixed (Freeman et al., 2006; McKay et al., 2006).

Delusions, paranormal, and conspiracy beliefs share other cognitive biases too. Teleological bias (seeing intentionality and purpose in naturally occurring events) is related to both conspiracy and paranormal beliefs (Lindeman et al., 2015; Wagner-Egger et al., 2018). Misperception of patterns is evident in paranormal believers and in conspiracist ideators (van Prooijen et al., 2018). Susceptibility to the conjunction fallacy (where one incorrectly judges the conjunction of two events as more likely than either event occurring alone) is higher in conspiracy believers (Brotherton and French, 2014; Dagnall et al., 2017) and proneness for similar statistical reasoning biases is reported in paranormal believers, (e.g., Rogers, 2014) and in delusional/delusion-prone participants (Galbraith and Manktelow, 2014; Galbraith et al., 2010).

The evidence of cognitive bias in conspiracy belief offers encouraging lines of inquiry. However, the number of studies is still quite small and further replications with a broader range of methodologies are needed before strong conclusions can be drawn. A further weakness is the reliance on self-report measures of cognition. The studies on thinking style in conspiracy belief have mostly used only self-report scales such as the Rational Experiential Inventory (REI; Pacini and Epstein, 1999) despite the evidence that the REI does not necessarily correlate with actual thinking performance (Newstead et al., 2004). Similarly, research which relies solely on Webster and Kruglanski's (1994) self-report NFCC scale is questionable for the same reason: self-reporting on one's own cognition is unreliable and stronger conclusions can be drawn from studies which use performance measures or experimental manipulations (e.g., Whiston et al., 2015). When Mikušková (2018) administered both the REI and the cognitive reflection test (CRT; Toplak et al., 2014), as with other studies, self-reported rational thinking on the REI was positively related to strength of conspiracy belief, but actual thinking performance as measured by the CRT was unrelated to it. Stahl and van Prooijen (2018) did however observe a negative relationship between analytic responding on the CRT and conspiracy beliefs. Importantly, Stahl and van Prooijen (1028) also found that scepticism towards conspiracies is predicted not simply by analytic cognitive style, but the combination of this *and* the motivation to think analytically.

Hence, there is mounting evidence that conspiracy beliefs are related to schizotypal traits and the research on cognition shows that conspiracy beliefs share similar cognitive biases with other forms of implausible belief, although this evidence is not without its weaknesses. Like other implausible beliefs, conspiracist ideation is not characterized by system 2 (Evans and Stanovich, 2013) analytical thinking and is instead associated more so with system 1 processing style: a reliance on fast, instinctive, heuristic judgement. What must be stressed however is that cognitive bias is itself continuous much like other traits (Stanovich et al., 2016) and if conspiracy beliefs are characterized by cognitive bias, this should not be taken to mean that conspiracy believers exhibit these biases and non-conspiracy believers do not. No, rather the former might display a stronger tendency for biases which are found to some degree in most individuals.

What other similarities beyond cognitive factors might help to compare or contrast delusional and conspiracy beliefs? The literature on the social and environmental factors underpinning delusions is well developed. There is also growing research evidence for the role that such factors play in conspiracy beliefs.

5 Social and environmental factors in conspiracy beliefs

Conspiracy beliefs have been proposed as serving a psychological function in the face of social threat. When societal perceptions of powerlessness, lack of control, a sense of societal threat, or anomie are prevalent (Abalakina-Paap and Stephan, 1999; Bruder et al., 2013; Jolley et al., 2018; Whitson and Galinsky, 2008), conspiracy beliefs are said to emerge as a way of making sense of and gaining control over these complex social issues (Swami and Coles, 2010). This might lead to mistrust of others and to the externalizing of anger and fear upon perceived enemies within society (Abalakina-Paap et al., 1999; Goertzel, 1994). Indeed, there is experimental evidence that an increase in anxiety can intensify conspiracist thinking towards perceived outgroups (Grzesiak-Feldman, 2013) and the relation between conspiracy and mistrust of authority is well known (Bogart et al., 2016; Freeman et al., 2020). In his existential threat model of conspiracy theories, van Prooijen (2020) proposes that existential threat motivates people to find ways to make sense of their social environment. Such perceived threat exacerbates cognitive processing biases resulting in misinterpretation of information and biased judgements. Conspiracy beliefs then arise if there is a salient and despised outgroup (which can be either low [e.g., ethnic minorities, refugees, etc.] or high in power [political parties, institutions]) onto which negative emotions can be projected. The model incorporates the Adaptive Conspiracism Hypothesis (van Prooijen and van Vugt, 2018), which proposes that conspiracist tendencies have evolved as an adaptive response to intergroup conflict throughout early human history.

According to this view, conspiracy beliefs are a rational reaction to negative societal conditions. van Prooijen's (2020) argument – that emotional (perceived threat), cognitive (epistemic sense-making characterized by cognitive bias), and social factors (perceived ingroups and outgroups) combine in conspiracy beliefs – has similarities with Freeman's threat anticipation model of delusions (Freeman, 2007). Freeman's model proposes that paranoia arises from an interaction between emotion, cognition, experience, and self-concept. Negative schemas (about the self, others, and the world) may prime one to see oneself as vulnerable and inadequate and at the mercy of bad and dangerous people. The anxiety which arises from this makes one hypervigilant for threat, thus biasing the way one processes information, with a reliance on hasty or system 1 thinking. Social and internal experiences will then likely be interpreted through a lens of threat and vulnerability, leading to paranoid hypotheses.

Like van Prooijen, Freeman's model also explains delusions as a rational response to adverse psychosocial conditions, enabling such beliefs to be seen not as pathological but rather as the product of normal belief formation processes. Such a view is implicit in the continuum model of psychosis. Paranoia should only be considered a clinical phenomenon when it becomes incompatible with well-being and reasonable social functioning. In milder form, the ability to feel some paranoia in certain contexts is adaptive, providing the individual with appropriate levels of suspiciousness to be able to detect genuine cheaters, exploiters, and hostiles when they are encountered (see Raihani and Bell, 2019). In van Prooijen's view, the ability to form conspiracy beliefs can serve a similar adaptive function, equipping the individual with the ability to be suspicious when faced with genuine exploitation or threat from hostile groups. As Imhoff and Lamberty (2018) argue, perhaps the principal difference between paranoia and conspiracy is the extent to which perceived threat is projected onto specific outgroups and the degree to which the individual perceives themselves as the specific object of persecution. In paranoia, the hostile others may be less specifically defined than in conspiracy theories (although this is not always the case). In paranoia, the target of the hostility is the self, whereas in conspiracy theories the target is society or communities. If conspiracy beliefs have evolved from adaptive origins, why are they seen as problematic and why have they attracted the interest of so many researchers? In the next section, I will consider this question with particular focus on conspiracy beliefs in the online world.

6 Conspiracy beliefs and social media: causes and effects

Perhaps one of the reasons for the increasing interest from researchers is that conspiracy theories can do significant harm to society. Conspiracy theories about vaccines prevent people from vaccinating themselves or their children placing themselves and society at greater risk of infection (Jolley and Douglas, 2014a). Conspiracy theories about global warming as a hoax prevent people from reducing their carbon footprint (Jolley and Douglas, 2014b). Conspiracy theories often target minority groups putting them in danger (Fekete, 2012). Conspiracy theories are also related to fundamentalism and extremism (van Prooijen et al., 2015) and to mistrust of political parties or of democratic process (Goertzel, 1994; Jolley and Douglas, 2014b). Also, as conspiracies emerge only when there is a perceived hostile outgroup, conspiracies can help to motivate intergroup conflict (van Prooijen et al., 2018). Hence, there are good reasons why conspiracy beliefs might be seen as negative for society.

Another reason for interest in conspiracy beliefs is that modern-day communication, the Internet, and social media, makes conspiracies more accessible and has enabled them to proliferate (Ahmed et al., 2020; Mian and Khan, 2020). So-called echo chambers are characterized by homogeneous clusters of users who assemble online based on common views or attitudes. Such echo chambers have been studied on Facebook (Quattrociocchi et al., 2016) and Twitter (Cossard et al., 2020).

Contrary to conventional belief, humans contribute more to the 'viral' spread of false information online than automated robots, and false information cascades further online than true information does, primarily due to the different emotions that are evoked by false and true material, respectively (Vosoughi et al., 2018). The spread of digital misinformation has been labelled as one of the principal threats to society by the World Economic Forum (Howell, 2013). Facebook, for example, enables the formation of homogeneous communities or echo chambers, clustered around specific narratives (Del Vicario, Bessi et al., 2016). The outcome is that such echo chambers become highly polarized and the narratives within become self-reinforcing, characterized by conformation bias and the cascade of further false narratives, mistrust, and paranoia, with refuting information avoided or ignored (Quattrociocchi et al., 2016). Although it is known that humans are resistant to belief change (Lord et al., 1979), the segregated and homogeneous nature of echo chambers makes this even more difficult to achieve and on Facebook there is evidence that debunking information actually entrenches conspiracy beliefs (Zollo et al., 2017). Evidence also suggests that on Facebook, greater online activity within an echo chamber leads more quickly to more negative sentiments (Del Vicario, Vivaldo et al., 2016). Furthermore, it might be that polarization itself amplifies division: perceiving cohesion in outgroups increases one's sense of social threat from said groups (Greenburgh et al., 2019).

Although acceptance of contradictory information is more likely if it originates from a trusted source (Margolin et al., 2018; Vraga and Bode, 2017), we should recognize that true echo chambers aggressively reject counter-evidence and harbour mistrust of dissenters. They should be distinguished from what Nguyen (2020) calls "epistemic bubbles" where dissenting voices although not visible are not necessarily actively excluded. In this vein, echo chambers exacerbate one of the common features of conspiracy theories whereby contradictory views are seen as further evidence of a hostile conspiracy. Social media also satisfies one of the other functions of a conspiracy theory, namely to offer simplicity in the face of complexity. In echo chambers, the homogeneity of the community is an antidote to confusing social structures, offering togetherness and supporting homophily (Törnberg, 2018).

Furthermore, the nature of echo chambers and social media can exacerbate the cognitive biases that underpin conspiracy beliefs. Conspiracy beliefs are characterized by less analytic thinking. Compared to true news, online political disinformation suppresses analytic responding, particularly extreme forms of disinformation (Barfar, 2019), and susceptibility to fake news is more dependent on such lazy thinking than it is on partisan bias (Pennycook and Rand, 2019). Reliance on the Internet for information begets further use (Storm et al., 2017), and reliance on technology for knowledge increases illusions of knowledge (Hamilton and Yao, 2018). Those who tend to think more intuitively or less analytically are also more likely to cognitively offload onto their device – in other words, to rely on their device to find information (Barr et al., 2015). Conversely, engaging in more analytical thought can reduce people's reliance on smartphones (Pennycook et al., 2015). This suggests that even though conspiracy beliefs are already characterized by lower reliance on analytical thought, the location of conspiracy communities in online social media platforms can exacerbate this kind of lazy thinking even further.

In the pre-Internet age, experiences such as external thought control would have remained idiosyncratic and incompatible with common shared reality. Such experiences are classic first-rank symptoms of psychosis, normally regarded as forming bizarre delusions. A social network analysis of mind control experiences has revealed that online communities, including individuals with apparent signs of psychosis, have formed around common experience or interest in this phenomenon (Bell et al., 2006). This illustrates that the Internet provides a forum for social endorsement of even the most improbable ideas which would be very difficult to re-create in the offline world.

7 Conclusions

Thus, conspiracy beliefs represent significant social challenges, including political extremism, intergroup conflict, environmental protection, faith in democracy, and population health. Although there are likely to be individual differences in one's proneness to conspiracy beliefs, such beliefs likely originate from long-evolved mechanisms which would have been adaptive traits for effective intergroup conflict in early human existence. In the modern day, the shifting and complex social landscape evokes a sense of threat from salient and despised outgroups. This threat drives a need to make meaning out of a confusing social milieu, a desire for sense-making which favours overreliance on cognitive bias and system 1 thinking. The ability of the Internet and in particular social media platforms to accommodate conspiracy networks in ways that the offline world cannot match accentuates the homogeneity and polarization of such groups, the sense of threat posed by opposing outgroups and even the lazy cognitive style which conspiracy believers might have a prior proneness to.

An argument for the existence of a fully dimensional psychosis continuum has been elaborated. Delusional beliefs form an important dimension of this continuum and a question for the chapter was whether conspiracy beliefs can be understood as forming part of the continuum of delusional belief. Many of the characteristics of delusions are found in both paranormal and conspiracy beliefs. Both delusions and conspiracy beliefs emerge from processes which might have been – or remain – adaptive protections against social threat. Whilst delusions and conspiracies might differ with regard to the perceived relevance to the self, this too might represent a further dimension of the belief continuum whereby clinical delusions are characterized by highly personalized sense of threat with the elevated distress and social isolation that such individualized beliefs would present. Suspicion orientated more to the group or to wider society is more (although not always) likely to reflect the definition of conspiracy belief than clinical delusion.

There is perhaps a risk in conceptualizing in psychopathological terms what is after all, a rather common, everyday belief. But the object of this chapter is not to construe conspiracy beliefs as a clinical phenomenon. Conversely, the psychosis continuum is seen as a means of 'normalizing' psychopathological symptoms, of making psychotic behaviours and experiences understandable by referencing them as exaggerated forms of everyday non-clinical existence. Thus, it is important to stress that conspiracy beliefs should not be viewed as psychotic, but rather as a multidimensional belief which can vary in intensity like other types of belief. In this sense, the author hopes that conceptualizing conspiracy belief in relation to the psychosis continuum will be useful for education, intervention, and prevention rather than stigmatization.

Note

1 On the other hand, this is not the case with delusional disorder, where a delusional belief is entrenched but without comorbidities or deficits in social functioning (Marneros et al., 2012); hence, the absence of other symptoms is not sufficient to distinguish regular paranormal beliefs from delusions.

References

Abalakina-Paap, M., Stephan, W., Craig, T., and Gregory, W. L. (1999). Beliefs in conspiracies. *Political Psychology*, 20, 637–647.

Ahmed, W., Vidal-Alaball, J., Downing, J., and Seguí, F. L. (2020). COVID-19 and the 5G conspiracy theory: Social network analysis of Twitter data. *Journal of Medical Internet Research*, 22(5), e19458.

American Psychiatric Association. (2013). *Diagnostic and statistical manual of mental disorders, (DSM V)* (5th ed.). Washington, DC: American Psychiatric Association.

Anandakumar, T., Connaughton, E., Coltheart, M., and Langdon, R. (2017). Belief-bias reasoning in non-clinical delusion-prone individuals. *Journal of Behavior Therapy and Experimental Psychiatry*, 54, 211–218.

Angst, J., Frey, R., Lohmeyer, B., & Zerbin-Rudin, E. (1980). Bipolar manic-depressive psychoses: Results of a genetic investigation. *Human Genetics*, 55, 237–254.

Arciniegas, D. B. (2015). Psychosis. *Continuum: Lifelong Learning in Neurology*, 21, 715–736.

Banaji, M. R., and Kihlstrom, J. F. (1996). The ordinary nature of alien abduction memories. *Psychological Inquiry*, 7(2), 132–135.

Barfar, A. (2019). Cognitive and affective responses to political disinformation in Facebook. *Computers in Human Behavior*, 101, 173–179.

Barr, N., Pennycook, G., Stolz, J. A., and Fugelsang, J. A. (2015). The brain in your pocket: Evidence that smartphones are used to supplant thinking. *Computers in Human Behavior*, 48, 473–480.

Barron, D., Furnham, A., Weis, L., Morgan, K. D., Towell, T., and Swami, V. (2018). The relationship between schizotypal facets and conspiracist beliefs via cognitive processes. *Psychiatry Research*, 259, 15–20.

Bebbington, P., and Freeman, D. (2017). Transdiagnostic extension of delusions: Schizophrenia and beyond. *Schizophrenia Bulletin*, 43(2), 273–282.

Bell, V. (2007). Online information, extreme communities and internet therapy: Is the internet good for our mental health? *Journal of Mental Health*, 16(4), 445–457.

Bell, V., Maiden, C., Muñoz-Solomando, A., and Reddy, V. (2006). 'Mind control' experiences on the internet: Implications for the psychiatric diagnosis of delusions. *Psychopathology*, 39(2), 87–91.

Bentall, R. P., Claridge, G. S., and Slade, P. D. (1989). The multidimensional nature of schizotypal traits: A factor analytic study with normal subjects. *British Journal of Clinical Psychology*, 28, 363–375.

Bentall, R. P., and Swarbrick, R. (2003). The best laid schemas of paranoid patients: Autonomy, sociotropy and need for closure. *Psychology and Psychotherapy: Theory, Research and Practice*, 76(2), 163–171.

Bessi, A., Coletto, M., Davidescu, G. A., Scala, A., Caldarelli, G., and Quattrociocchi, W. (2015). Science vs conspiracy: Collective narratives in the age of misinformation. *PLoS One*, 10(2), e0118093.

Bogart, L. M., Wagner, G. J., Green Jr, H. D., Mutchler, M. G., Klein, D. J., McDavitt, B., . . . and Hilliard, C. L. (2016). Medical mistrust among social network members may contribute to antiretroviral treatment nonadherence in African Americans living with HIV. *Social Science and Medicine*, 164, 133–140.

Brenner, K., Schmitz, N., Pawliuk, N., Fathalli, F., Joober, R., Ciampi, A., and King, S. (2007). Validation of the English and French versions of the Community Assessment of Psychic Experiences (CAPE) with a Montreal community sample. *Schizophrenia Research*, 95(1–3), 86–95.

Brotherton, R., and Eser, S. (2015). Bored to fears: Boredom proneness, paranoia, and conspiracy theories. *Personality and Individual Differences*, 80, 1–5.

Brotherton, R., and French, C. C. (2014). Belief in conspiracy theories and susceptibility to the conjunction fallacy. *Applied Cognitive Psychology*, 28(2), 238–248.

Bruder, M., Haffke, P., Neave, N., Nouripanah, N., and Imhoff, R. (2013). Measuring individual differences in generic beliefs in conspiracy theories across cultures: Conspiracy Mentality Questionnaire. *Frontiers in Psychology*, 4, 225.

Brugger, P., and Mohr, C. (2008). The paranormal mind: How the study of anomalous experiences and beliefs may inform cognitive neuroscience. *Cortex*, 44(10), 1291.

Cappe, C., Herzog, M. H., Herzig, D. A., Brand, A., and Mohr, C. (2012). Cognitive disorganisation in schizotypy is associated with deterioration in visual backward masking. *Psychiatry Research*, 200(2–3), 652–659.

Chapman, L. J., Chapman, J. P., Kwapil, T. R., Eckblad, M., and Zinser, M. C. (1994). Putatively psychosis-prone subjects 10 years later. *Journal of Abnormal Psychology*, 103(2), 171–183.

Cicero, D. C. (2016). Measurement invariance of the Schizotypal Personality Questionnaire in Asian, Pacific Islander, White, and multiethnic populations. *Psychological Assessment*, 28(4), 351.

Claridge, G. S., and Beech, T. (1995). Fully and quasi-dimensional constructions of schizotypy. In A. Rain, T. Lencz & S.A. Mednick (Eds.). *Schizotypal Personality*. New York: Cambridge University Press.

Claridge, G., McCreery, C., Mason, O., Bentall, R., Boyle, G., Slade, P., and Popplewell, D. (1996). The factor structure of "schizotypal" traits: A large replication study. *British Journal of Clinical Psychology*, 35(1), 103–115.

Colbert, S. M., and Peters, E. R. (2002). Need for closure and jumping-to-conclusions in delusion-prone individuals. *The Journal of Nervous and Mental Disease*, 190(1), 27–31.

Cossard, A., Morales, G. D. F., Kalimeri, K., Mejova, Y., Paolotti, D., and Starnini, M. (2020, May). Falling into the echo chamber: The Italian vaccination debate on twitter. *Proceedings of the International AAAI Conference on Web and Social Media*, 14(1), 130–140. Retrieved from https://ojs.aaai.org/index.php/ICWSM/article/view/7285:

Dagnall, N., Denovan, A., Drinkwater, K., Parker, A., and Clough, P. (2016). Toward a better understanding of the relationship between belief in the paranormal and statistical bias: The potential role of schizotypy. *Frontiers in Psychology*, 7, 1045.

Dagnall, N., Denovan, A., Drinkwater, K., Parker, A., and Clough, P. (2017). Statistical bias and endorsement of conspiracy theories. *Applied Cognitive Psychology*, 31(4), 368–378.

Darwin, H., Neave, N., and Holmes, J. (2011). Belief in conspiracy theories. The role of paranormal belief, paranoid ideation and schizotypy. *Personality and Individual Differences*, 50(8), 1289–1293.

David, A. S. (2010). Why we need more debate on whether psychotic symptoms lie on a continuum with normality. *Psychological Medicine*, 40(12), 1935–1942.

Del Vicario, M., Bessi, A., Zollo, F., Petroni, F., Scala, A., Caldarelli, G., . . . and Quattrociocchi, W. (2016). The spreading of misinformation online. *Proceedings of the National Academy of Sciences*, 113(3), 554–559.

Del Vicario, M., Vivaldo, G., Bessi, A., Zollo, F., Scala, A., Caldarelli, G., and Quattrociocchi, W. (2016). Echo chambers: Emotional contagion and group polarization on facebook. *Scientific Reports*, 6, 37825.

Denovan, A., Dagnall, N., Drinkwater, K., Parker, A., and Neave, N. (2020). Conspiracist beliefs, intuitive thinking, and schizotypal facets: A further evaluation. *Applied Cognitive Psychology*, 34(6), 1394–1405.

Drinkwater, K., Dagnall, N., and Parker, A. (2012). Reality testing, conspiracy theories, and paranormal beliefs. *Journal of Parapsychology*, 76(1), 57–77.

Drinkwater, K., Denovan, A., Dagnall, N., and Parker, A. (2020). Predictors of hearing electronic voice phenomena in random noise: Schizotypy, fantasy proneness, and paranormal beliefs. *Journal of Parapsychology*, 84(1), 96–113.

Dudley, R. T. (2000). The relationship between negative affect and paranormal belief. *Personality and Individual Differences*, 28(2), 315–321.

Dudley, R., Taylor, P., Wickham, S., and Hutton, P. (2016). Psychosis, delusions and the "jumping to conclusions" reasoning bias: A systematic review and meta-analysis. *Schizophrenia Bulletin*, 42(3), 652–665.

Eckblad, M., and Chapman, L. J. (1983). Magical ideation as an indicator of schizotypy. *Journal of Consulting and Clinical Psychology*, 51(2), 215.

Erlenmeyer-Kimling, L., Golden, R. R., and Cornblatt, B. A. (1987). A taxometric analysis of cognitive and neuromotor variables in children at risk for schizophrenia. *Journal of Abnormal Psychology*, 98, 203–208.

Evans, J. S. B., and Stanovich, K. E. (2013). Dual-process theories of higher cognition: Advancing the debate. *Perspectives on Psychological Science*, 8(3), 223–241.

Fekete, L. (2012). The Muslim conspiracy theory and the Oslo massacre. *Race and Class*, 53(3), 30–47.

Fenster, M. (1999). *Conspiracy theories: Secrecy and power in American culture*. University of Minnesota Press: Minnesota, USA.

Festinger, L. (1957). *A theory of cognitive dissonance* (Vol. 2). Stanford University Press; California, USA.

Fine, C., Gardner, M., Craigie, J., and Gold, I. (2007). Hopping, skipping or jumping to conclusions? Clarifying the role of the JTC bias in delusions. *Cognitive Neuropsychiatry*, 12(1), 46–77.

Fluke, S. M., Webster, R. J., and Saucier, D. A. (2014). Methodological and theoretical improvements in the study of superstitious beliefs and behaviour. *British Journal of Psychology*, 105(1), 102–126.

Fonseca-Pedrero, E., Chan, R. C., Debbané, M., Cicero, D., Zhang, L. C., Brenner, C., . . . and Cohen, A. (2018). Comparisons of schizotypal traits across 12 countries: Results from the International Consortium for Schizotypy Research. *Schizophrenia Research*, 199, 128–134.

Freeman, D. (2007). Suspicious minds: The psychology of persecutory delusions. *Clinical Psychology Review*, 27, 425−457.

Freeman, D., Bradley, J., Antley, A., Bourke, E., DeWeever, N., Evans, N., . . . and Slater, M. (2016). Virtual reality in the treatment of persecutory delusions: Randomised controlled experimental study testing how to reduce delusional conviction. *The British Journal of Psychiatry*, 209(1), 62–67.

Freeman, D., Garety, P., Kuipers, E., Colbert, S., Jolley, S., Fowler, D., . . . and Bebbington, P. E. (2006). Delusions and decision-making style: Use of the Need for Closure Scale. *Behaviour Research and Therapy*, 44(8), 1147–1158.

Freeman, D., Lister, R., and Evans, N. (2014). The use of intuitive and analytic reasoning styles by patients with persecutory delusions. *Journal of Behavior Therapy and Experimental Psychiatry*, 45(4), 454–458.

Freeman, D., Waite, F., Rosebrock, L., Petit, A., Causier, C., East, A., . . . and Bold, E. (2020). Coronavirus conspiracy beliefs, mistrust, and compliance with government guidelines in England. *Psychological Medicine*, 1–30.

Galbraith, N. D., and Manktelow, K. I. (2014). A psychological model of delusional belief: Integrating reasoning biases with perceptual, self-concept and emotional factors. In N. D. Galbraith (Ed.), *Aberrant beliefs and reasoning*. Hove, UK: Psychology Press.

Galbraith, N. D., Manktelow, K. I., and Morris, N. G. (2010). Subclinical delusional ideation and appreciation of sample size and heterogeneity in statistical judgement. *British Journal of Psychology*, 10(4), 621–635.

Galbraith, N. D., Manktelow, K. I., Chen-Wilson, C. H., Harris, R. A., and Nevill, A. (2014). Different combinations of perceptual, emotional, and cognitive factors predict three different types of delusional ideation during adolescence. *The Journal of Nervous and Mental Disease*, 202(9), 668–676.

Garety, P. A., and Freeman, D. (1999). Cognitive approaches to delusions: A critical review of theories and evidence. *British Journal of Clinical Psychology*, 38, 113–154.

Gaynor, K., Ward, T., Garety, P., and Peters, E. (2013). The role of safety-seeking behaviours in maintaining threat appraisals in psychosis. *Behaviour research and therapy*, 51(2), 75–81.

Georgiou, N., Delfabbro, P., and Balzan, R. (2019). Conspiracy beliefs in the general population: The importance of psychopathology, cognitive style and educational attainment. *Personality and Individual Differences*, 151, 109521.

Gianotti, L. R., Mohr, C., Pizzagalli, D., Lehmann, D., and Brugger, P. (2001). Associative processing and paranormal belief. *Psychiatry and Clinical Neurosciences*, 55(6), 595–603.

Goertzel, T. (1994). Belief in conspiracy theories. *Political Psychology*, 15, 731–742.

Golec de Zavala, A., and van Bergh, A. (2007). Need for cognitive closure and conservative political beliefs: Differential mediation by personal worldviews. *Political Psychology*, 28(5), 587–608.

Greenburgh, A., Bell, V., and Raihani, N. (2019). Paranoia and conspiracy: Group cohesion increases harmful intent attribution in the Trust Game. *PeerJ*, 7, e7403.

Gruzelier, J. H. (1994). Syndromes of schizophrenia and schizotypy, hemispheric imbalance and sex differences: Implications for developmental psychopathology. *International Journal of Psychophysiology*, 18(3), 167–178.

Grzesiak-Feldman, M. (2013). The effect of high-anxiety situations on conspiracy thinking. *Current Psychology*, 32(1), 100–118.

Hamilton, K. A., and Yao, M. Z. (2018). Blurring boundaries: Effects of device features on metacognitive evaluations. *Computers in Human Behavior*, 89, 213–220.

Hanssen, M., Bak, M., Bijl, R., Vollebergh, W., and van Os, J. (2005). The incidence and outcome of subclinical psychotic experiences in the general population. *British Journal of Clinical Psychology*, 44(2), 181–191.

Harper, D. J. (2011). Social inequality and the diagnosis of paranoia. *Health Sociology Review*, 20(4), 423–436.

Hergovich, A., Schott, R., and Arendasy, M. (2008). On the relationship between paranormal belief and schizotypy among adolescents. *Personality and Individual Differences*, 45(2), 119–125.

Hochberger, W. C., Hill, S. K., Nelson, C. L., Reilly, J. L., Keefe, R. S., Pearlson, G. D., . . . Sweeney, J. A. (2016). Unitary construct of generalized cognitive ability underlying BACS performance across psychotic disorders and in their first-degree relatives. *Schizophrenia Research*, 170(1),156–161.

Holm, N. (2009). Conspiracy theorizing surveillance: Considering modalities of paranoia and conspiracy in surveillance studies. *Surveillance and Society*, 7(1), 36–48.

Howell, L. (2013). Digital wildfires in a hyperconnected world. *WEF Report 2013*. reports.weforum.org/global-risks-2013/risk-case-1/digital-wildfires-in-a-hyperconnected-world (accessed 17 July 2020).

Imhoff, R., and Lamberty, P. (2018). How paranoid are conspiracy believers? Toward a more fine-grained understanding of the connect and disconnect between paranoia and belief in conspiracy theories. *European Journal of Social Psychology*, 48(7), 909–926.

International Schizophrenia Consortium. (2009). Common polygenic variation contributes to risk of schizophrenia that overlaps with bipolar disorder. *Nature*, 460(7256), 748.

Irwin, H. J., Drinkwater, K., and Dagnall, N. (2014). Are believers in the paranormal inclined to jump to conclusions? *Australian Journal of Parapsychology*, 14(1), 69.

Johnson, J., Horwath, E., and Weissman, M. M. (1991). The validity of major depression with psychotic features based on a community study. *Archives of General Psychiatry*, 48(12), 1075–1081.

Jolley, D., and Douglas, K. M. (2014a). The effects of anti-vaccine conspiracy theories on vaccination intentions. *PLoS One*, 9(2), e89177.

Jolley, D., and Douglas, K. M. (2014b). The social consequences of conspiracism: Exposure to conspiracy theories decreases intentions to engage in politics and to reduce one's carbon footprint. *British Journal of Psychology*, 105(1), 35–56.

Jolley, D., Douglas, K. M., and Sutton, R. M. (2018). Blaming a few bad apples to save a threatened barrel: The system-justifying function of conspiracy theories. *Political Psychology*, 39(2), 465–478.

Kane, M. J., Core, T. J., and Hunt, R. R. (2010). Bias versus bias: Harnessing hindsight to reveal paranormal belief change beyond demand characteristics. *Psychonomic Bulletin and Review*, 17(2), 206–212.

Kaymaz, N., Drukker, M., Lieb, R., Wittchen, H. U., Werbeloff, N., Weiser, M., . . . and van Os, J. (2012). Do subthreshold psychotic experiences predict clinical outcomes in unselected non-help-seeking population-based samples? A systematic review and meta-analysis, enriched with new results. *Psychological Medicine*, 42(11), 2239–2253.

Keinan, G. (2002). The effects of stress and desire for control on superstitious behavior. *Personality and Social Psychology Bulletin*, 28(1), 102–108.

Kelleher, I., and Cannon, M. (2011). Psychotic-like experiences in the general population: Characterizing a high-risk group for psychosis. *Psychological Medicine*, 41(1), 1–6.

Kemp, R., Chua, S., McKenna, P., and David, A. (1997). Reasoning and delusions. *British Journal of Psychiatry*, 170, 398–405.

Kendler, K. S., Masterson, C. C., and Davis, K. L. (1985). Psychiatric illness in first-degree relatives of patients with paranoid psychosis, schizophrenia and medical illness. *British Journal of Psychiatry*, 147, 524–531.

Kraepelin, E. (1899/1990). *Psychiatry: A textbook for students and physicians. Volume 1: General psychiatry*. Watson Publishing International: Massachusetts, USA.

Lange, R., and Houran, J. (1998). Delusions of the paranormal: A haunting question of perception. *The Journal of Nervous and Mental Disease*, 186(10), 637–645.

Lange, R., and Houran, J. (1999). The role of fear in delusions of the paranormal. *The Journal of Nervous and Mental Disease*, 187(3), 159–166.

Laurens, K., Hobbs, M., Sunderland, M., Green, M., and Mould, G. (2012). Psychotic-like experiences in a community sample of 8000 children aged 9 to 11 years: An item response theory analysis. *Psychological Medicine*, 42(7), 1495–1506.

Laursen, T. M., Agerbo, E., and Pedersen, C. B. (2009). Bipolar disorder, schizoaffective disorder, and schizophrenia overlap: A new comorbidity index. *The Journal of Clinical Psychiatry*, 70(10), 1432–1438.

Lawrence, E., and Peters, E. (2004). Reasoning in believers in the paranormal. *The Journal of Nervous and Mental Disease*, 192(11), 727–733.

Le Pelley, M. E., Schmidt-Hansen, M., Harris, N. J., Lunter, C. M., and Morris, C. S. (2010). Disentangling the attentional deficit in schizophrenia: Pointers from schizotypy. *Psychiatry Research*, 176(2–3), 143–149.

Leman, P. J., and Cinnirella, M. (2013). Beliefs in conspiracy theories and the need for cognitive closure. *Frontiers in Psychology*, 4, 378. https://doi.org/10.3389/fpsyg.2013.00378

Lenzenweger, M. F., Cornblatt, B. A., and Putnick, M. (1991). Schizotypy and sustained attention. *Journal of Abnormal Psychology*, 100, 84–89.

Lenzenweger, M. F., and Korfine, L. (1992). Confirming the latent structure and base rate of schizotypy: A taxometric analysis. *Journal of Abnormal Psychology*, 101, 567–571.

Lenzenweger, M. F., and Korfine, L. (1994). Perceptual aberrations, schizotypy, and the Wisconsin Card Sorting Test. *Schizophrenia Bulletin*, 20(2), 345–357.

Lenzenweger, M.F. and Korfine, L. (1995). Tracking the taxon: On the latent structure and base rate of schizotypy. In A. Raine, T. Lencz & S. A. Mednick (Eds.), *Schizotypal Personality*. New York: Cambridge University Press.

Leonhard, D., and Brugger, P. (1998). Creative, paranormal, and delusional thought: A consequence of right hemisphere semantic activation? *Neuropsychiatry, Neuropsychology, and Behavioral Neurology*, 11(4), 177–183.

Lichtenstein, P., Yip, B. H., Björk, C., Pawitan, Y., Cannon, T. D., Sullivan, P. F., and Hultman, C. M. (2009). Common genetic determinants of schizophrenia and bipolar disorder in Swedish families: A population-based study. *The Lancet*, 373(9659), 234–239.

Liddle, P. F. (1987). The symptoms of chronic schizophrenia: A re-examination of the positive-negative dichotomy. *The British Journal of Psychiatry*, 151, 145–151.

Lindeman, M., and Aarnio, K. (2007). Superstitious, magical, and paranormal beliefs: An integrative model. *Journal of Research in Personality*, 41(4), 731–744.

Lindeman, M., Svedholm-Häkkinen, A. M., and Lipsanen, J. (2015). Ontological confusions but not mentalizing abilities predict religious belief, paranormal belief, and belief in supernatural purpose. *Cognition*, 134, 63–76.

Linney, Y. M., Peters, E. R., and Ayton, P. (1998). Reasoning biases in delusion-prone individuals. *British Journal of Clinical Psychology*, 37, 285–302.

Lobato, E., Mendoza, J., Sims, V., and Chin, M. (2014). Examining the relationship between conspiracy theories, paranormal beliefs, and pseudoscience acceptance among a university population. *Applied Cognitive Psychology*, 28(5), 617–625.

Lord, C. G., Ross, L., and Lepper, M. R. (1979). Biased assimilation and attitude polarization: The effects of prior theories on subsequently considered evidence. *Journal of Personality and Social Psychology*, 37(11), 2098.

Marchlewska, M., Cichocka, A., and Kossowska, M. (2018). Addicted to answers: Need for cognitive closure and the endorsement of conspiracy beliefs. *European Journal of Social Psychology*, 48(2), 109–117.

Margolin, D. B., Hannak, A., and Weber, I. (2018). Political fact-checking on Twitter: When do corrections have an effect? *Political Communication*, 35(2), 196–219.

Marneros, A., Pillmann, F., and Wustmann, T. (2012). Delusional disorders: Are they simply paranoid schizophrenia? *Schizophrenia Bulletin*, 38(3), 561–568.

Mason, O., Claridge, G., and Jackson, M. (1995). New scales for the assessment of schizotypy. *Personality and Individual Differences*, 18(1), n7–13.

Mason, O. J., Stevenson, C., and Freedman, F. (2014). Ever-present threats from information technology: The Cyber-Paranoia and Fear Scale. *Frontiers in Psychology*, 5, 1298.

McKay, R., Langdon, R., and Coltheart, M. (2006). The persecutory ideation questionnaire. *The Journal of Nervous and Mental Disease*, 194(8), 628–631.

Meehl, P. E. (1962). Schizotaxia, schizotypy, schizophrenia. *American Psychologist*, 17, 827–838.

Meehl, P. E. (1990). Toward an integrated theory of schizotaxia, schizotypy, and schizophrenia. *Journal of Personality Disorders*, 4, 1–99.

Mendez, I., Axelson, D., Castro-Fornieles, J., Hafeman, D., Goldstein, T. R., Goldstein, B. I., . . . and Hickey, M. B. (2019). Psychotic-like experiences in offspring of parents with bipolar disorder and community controls: A longitudinal study. *Journal of the American Academy of Child and Adolescent Psychiatry*, 58(5), 534–543.

Mendlewicz, J., Linkowski, P., and Wilmotte, J. (1980). Relationship between schizoaffective illness and affective disorder or schizophrenia: Morbidity risk and genetic transmission. *Journal of Affective Disorders, 2*, 289–302.

Mian, A., and Khan, S. (2020). Coronavirus: The spread of misinformation. *BMC Medicine*, 18(1), 1–2.

Mikušková, E. B. (2018). Conspiracy beliefs of future teachers. *Current Psychology*, 37(3), 692–701.

Moritz, S., and Woodward, T. S. (2004). Plausibility judgment in schizophrenic patients: Evidence for a liberal acceptance bias. *German Journal of Psychiatry*, 7(4), 66–74.

Mortensen, P. B., Pedersen, M. G., and Pedersen, C. B. (2010). Psychiatric family history and schizophrenia risk in Denmark: Which mental disorders are relevant? *Psychological Medicine*, 40(2), 201.

Moulding, R., Nix-Carnell, S., Schnabel, A., Nedeljkovic, M., Burnside, E. E., Lentini, A. F., and Mehzabin, N. (2016). Better the devil you know than a world you don't? Intolerance of uncertainty and worldview explanations for belief in conspiracy theories. *Personality and Individual Differences*, 98, 345–354.

Murphy, J., Shevlin, M., Adamson, G., and Houston, J. E. (2010). Positive psychosis symptom structure in the general population: Assessing dimensional consistency and continuity from "pathology" to "normality". *Psychosis*, 2(3), 199–209.

Musch, J., and Ehrenberg, K. (2002). Probability misjudgement, cognitive ability, and belief in the paranormal. *British Journal of Psychology*, 93(2), 169–177.

Myles, J. B., Rossell, S. L., Phillipou, A., Thomas, E., and Gurvich, C. (2017). Insights to the schizophrenia continuum: A systematic review of saccadic eye movements in schizotypy and biological relatives of schizophrenia patients. *Neuroscience and Biobehavioral Reviews*, 72, 278–300.

Newheiser, A. K., Farias, M., and Tausch, N. (2011). The functional nature of conspiracy beliefs: Examining the underpinnings of belief in the Da Vinci Code conspiracy. *Personality and Individual Differences*, 51(8), 1007–1011.

Newstead, S. E., Handley, S. J., Harley, C., Wright, H., and Farrelly, D. (2004). Individual differences in deductive reasoning. The Quarterly Journal of Experimental Psychology Section A, 57(1), 33–60.

Nguyen, C. T. (2020). Echo chambers and epistemic bubbles. *Episteme*, 17(2), 141–161.

Nicholls, M., Orr, C., and Lindell, A. (2005). Magical ideation and its relation to lateral preference. *Laterality: Asymmetries of Body, Brain, and Cognition*, 10(6), 503–515.

Nuevo, R., Chatterji, S., Verdes, E., Naidoo, N., Arango, C., and Ayuso-Mateos, J. L. (2012). The continuum of psychotic symptoms in the general population: A cross-national study. *Schizophrenia Bulletin*, 38(3), 475–485.

Obiols, J. E., García-Domingo, M., de Trinchería, I., and Doménech, E. (1993). Psychometric schizotypy and sustained attention in young males. *Personality and Individual Differences*, 14(2), 381–384.

Orosz, G., Krekó, P., Paskuj, B., Tóth-Király, I., Bőthe, B., and Roland-Lévy, C. (2016). Changing conspiracy beliefs through rationality and ridiculing. *Frontiers in Psychology*, 7, 1525.

Pacini, R., and Epstein, S. (1999). The relation of rational and experiential information processing styles to personality, basic beliefs, and the ratio-bias phenomenon. *Journal of Personality and Social Psychology*, 76(6), 972.

Parnas, J., and Henriksen, M. G. (2016). Epistemological error and the illusion of phenomenological continuity. *World Psychiatry*, 15(2), 126.

Pechey, R., and Halligan, P. (2011). The prevalence of delusion-like beliefs relative to sociocultural beliefs in the general population. *Psychopathology*, 44(2), 106–115.

Pechey, R., and Halligan, P. (2012). Prevalence and correlates of anomalous experiences in a large non-clinical sample. *Psychology and Psychotherapy: Theory, Research and Practice*, 85(2), 150–162.

Pennycook, G., Fugelsang, J. A., and Koehler, D. J. (2015). Everyday consequences of analytic thinking. *Current Directions in Psychological Science*, 24(6), 425–432.

Pennycook, G., and Rand, D. G. (2019). Lazy, not biased: Susceptibility to partisan fake news is better explained by lack of reasoning than by motivated reasoning. *Cognition*, 188, 39–50.

Peters, E. R., Joseph, S. A., Day, S., and Garety, P. (2004). Measuring delusional ideation: The 21-item Peters et al. Delusions Inventory (PDI). *Schizophrenia Bulletin*, 30(4), 1005–1022.

Peters, E. R., Joseph, S. A., and Garety, P. A. (1999). Measurement of delusional ideation in the normal population: Introducing the PDI (Peters et al. Delusions Inventory). *Schizophrenia Bulletin*, 25(3), 553–576.

Pizzagalli, D., Lehmann, D., Gianotti, L., Koenig, T., Tanaka, H., Wackermann, J., and Brugger, P. (2000). Brain electric correlates of strong belief in paranormal phenomena: Intracerebral EEG source and regional Omega complexity analyses. *Psychiatry Research: Neuroimaging*, 100(3), 139–154.

Posey, T. B., and Losch, M. E. (1983). Auditory hallucinations of hearing voices in 375 normal subjects. *Imagination, Cognition and Personality*, 2, 99–113.

Poulton, R., Caspi, A., Moffitt, T. E., Cannon, M., Murray, R., and Harrington, H. (2000). Children's self-reported psychotic symptoms and adult schizophreniform disorder: A 15-year longitudinal study. *Archives of General Psychiatry*, 57(11), 1053–1058.

Prike, T., Arnold, M. M., and Williamson, P. (2018). The relationship between anomalistic belief and biases of evidence integration and jumping to conclusions. *Acta Psychologica*, 190, 217–227.

Quattrociocchi, W., Scala, A., and Sunstein, C. R. (2016). *Echo chambers on Facebook*. SSRN 2795110.

Raihani, N. J., and Bell, V. (2019). An evolutionary perspective on paranoia. *Nature Human Behaviour*, 3(2), 114–121.

Raine, A. (1991). The SPQ: A scale for the assessment of schizotypal personality based on *DSM – III – R* criteria. *Schizophrenia Bulletin*, 17, 555–564. http://doi.org/10.1093/schbul/17.4.555

Ramsay, R. (2012). Conspiracy theories. Oldcastle Books: Hertfordshire, UK.

Rogers, P. (2014). Paranormal believers' proneness to probabilistic reasoning biases. In N. Galbraith (Ed.) *Aberrant beliefs and reasoning*. Psychology Press: Sussex, UK.

Rogers, P., Fisk, J., and Lowrie, E. (2017). Paranormal belief and errors of probabilistic reasoning: The role of constituent conditional relatedness in believers' susceptibility to the conjunction fallacy. *Consciousness and Cognition*, 56, 13–29.

Rosman, T., Mayer, A. K., Peter, J., and Krampen, G. (2016). Need for cognitive closure may impede the effectiveness of epistemic belief instruction. *Learning and Individual Differences*, 49, 406–413.

Ross, R. M., Hartig, B., and McKay, R. (2017). Analytic cognitive style predicts paranormal explanations of anomalous experiences but not the experiences themselves: Implications for cognitive theories of delusions. *Journal of Behavior Therapy and Experimental Psychiatry*, 56, 90–96.

Ross, R. M., McKay, R., Coltheart, M., and Langdon, R. (2015). Jumping to conclusions about the beads task? A meta-analysis of delusional ideation and data-gathering. *Schizophrenia Bulletin*, 41(5), 1183–1191.

Ruocco, A. C., Reilly, J. L., Rubin, L. H., Daros, A. R., Gershon, E. S., Tamminga, C. A., . . . and Sweeney, J. A. (2014). Emotion recognition deficits in schizophrenia-spectrum disorders and psychotic bipolar disorder: Findings from the Bipolar-Schizophrenia Network on Intermediate Phenotypes (B-SNIP) study. *Schizophrenia Research*, 158(1–3), 105–112.

Scharfetter, C., and Nüsperli, M. (1980). The group of schizophrenia, schizoaffective psychoses and affective disorders. *Schizophrenia Bulletin*, 6(4), 586–591.

Schlier, B., Jaya, E. S., Moritz, S., and Lincoln, T. M. (2015). The community assessment of psychic experiences measures nine clusters of psychosis-like experiences: A validation of the German version of the CAPE. *Schizophrenia Research*, 169(1–3), 274–279.

Sellen, J. L., Oaksford, M., and Gray, N. S. (2005). Schizotypy and conditional reasoning. *Schizophrenia Bulletin*, 31(1), 105–116.

Shevlin, M., McElroy, E., Bentall, R. P., Reininghaus, U., and Murphy, J. (2016). The psychosis continuum: Testing a bifactor model of psychosis in a general population sample. *Schizophrenia Bulletin*, 43(1), 133–141.

Sisti, D., Rocchi, M. B., Siddi, S., Mura, T., Manca, S., Preti, A., and Petretto, D. R. (2012). Preoccupation and distress are relevant dimensions in delusional beliefs. *Comprehensive Psychiatry*, 53(7), 1039–1043.

Ståhl, T., and van Prooijen, J. W. (2018). Epistemic rationality: Skepticism toward unfounded beliefs requires sufficient cognitive ability and motivation to be rational. *Personality and Individual Differences*, 122, 155–163.

Stanovich, K. E., West, R. F., and Toplak, M. E. (2016). *The rationality quotient: Toward a test of rational thinking*. Cambridge, MA: MIT Press.

Stefanovics, E. A., Elkis, H., Zhening, L., Zhang, X. Y., and Rosenheck, R. A. (2014). A cross-national factor analytic comparison of three models of PANSS symptoms in schizophrenia. *Psychiatry Research*, 219(2), 283–289.

Storm, B. C., Stone, S. M., and Benjamin, A. S. (2017). Using the Internet to access information inflates future use of the Internet to access other information. *Memory*, 25(6), 717–723.

Subotnik, K., Asarnow, R., Fogelson, D., Kendler, K., Heidi, K., Woo, S., . . . and Nuechterlein, K. (2017). SA96. Schizophrenia and schizophrenia-spectrum disorders in the first-degree relatives of children and adults with schizophrenia: The UCLA family study. *Schizophrenia Bulletin*, 43(suppl. 1), S147–S147.

Sunstein, C. R., and Vermeule, A. (2009). Conspiracy theories: Causes and cures. *Journal of Political Philosophy*, 17(2), 202–227.

Swami, V., and Coles, R. (2010). The truth is out there. *The Psychologist*, 23, 560–563.

Swami, V., Pietschnig, J., Stieger, S., and Voracek, M. (2011). Alien psychology: Associations between extraterrestrial beliefs and paranormal ideation, superstitious beliefs, schizotypy, and the Big Five personality factors. *Applied Cognitive Psychology*, 25(4), 647–653.

Swami, V., Voracek, M., Stieger, S., Tran, U. S., and Furnham, A. (2014). Analytic thinking reduces belief in conspiracy theories. *Cognition*, 133(3), 572–585.

Tandon, R., and Maj, M. (2008). Nosological status and definition of schizophrenia: Some considerations for DSM-V and ICD-11. *Asian journal of psychiatry*, 1(2), 22.

Taris, T. W. (2000). Dispositional need for cognitive closure and self-enhancing beliefs. *The Journal of Social Psychology*, 140(1), 35–50.

Taylor, M. A. (1992). Are schizophrenia and affective disorder related? A selective literature review. *The American Journal of Psychiatry*, 149(1), 22–32.

Thalbourne, M. A. (1984). Are believers in psi more prone to schizophrenia? *Research in Parapsychology*, 85–88.

Thalbourne, M. A., and Haraldsson, E. (1980). Personality characteristics of sheep and goats. *Personality and Individual Differences*, 1, 180–185.

Tien, A. (1991). Distribution of hallucinations in the population. *Social Psychiatry and Psychiatric Epidemiology*, 26, 287–292.

Tobacyk, J. J. (2004). A revised paranormal belief scale. *The International Journal of Transpersonal Studies*, 23(23), 94–98.

Tobacyk, J. J., and Milford, G. (1983). Belief in paranormal phenomena: Assessment instrument development and implications for personality functioning. *Journal of Personality and Social Psychology*, 44, 1029–1037.

Tobacyk, J. J., and Wilkinson, L. V. (1990). Magical thinking and paranormal beliefs. *Journal of Social Behavior and Personality*, 5, 255–264.

Toplak, M. E., West, R. F., and Stanovich, K. E. (2014). Assessing miserly information processing: An expansion of the Cognitive Reflection Test. *Thinking & Reasoning*, 20, 147 168.

Törnberg, P. (2018). Echo chambers and viral misinformation: Modeling fake news as complex contagion. *PLoS One*, 13(9), e0203958.

Tsuang, M. T., Winokur, G., and Crowe, R. R. (1980). Morbidity risks of schizophrenia and affective disorders among first-degree relatives of patients with schizophrenia, mania, depression and surgical conditions. *British Journal of Psychiatry*, 137, 497–504.

Umam, A. N., Muluk, H., and Milla, M. N. (2018). The need for cognitive closure and belief in conspiracy theories: An exploration of the role of religious fundamentalism in cognition. In A. Ariyanto, H. Muluk, P. Newcombe, F. Piercy, E. Poerwandari, and S. Suradijono (Eds.), *Diversity in unity: Perspectives from psychology and behavioral sciences*. London and New York: Taylor and Francis.

Vallès, V., van Os, J., Guillamat, R., Gutiérrez, B., Campillo, M., Gento, P., and Fañanás, L. (2000). Increased morbid risk for schizophrenia in families of in-patients with bipolar illness. *Schizophrenia Research*, 42(2), 83–90.

van den Bulck, H., and Hyzen, A. (2020). Of lizards and ideological entrepreneurs: Alex Jones and Infowars in the relationship between populist nationalism and the post-global media ecology. *International Communication Gazette*, 82(1), 42–59.

van der Tempel, J., and Alcock, J. E. (2015). Relationships between conspiracy mentality, hyperactive agency detection, and schizotypy: Supernatural forces at work? *Personality and Individual Differences*, 82, 136–141.

van Os, J., Hansen, M., Bijl, R. V., and Ravelli A. (2000). Strauss (1969). Revisited: A psychosis continuum in the general population? *Schizophrenia Research*, 45, 11–20.

van Os, J., Linscott, R. J., Myin-Germeys, I., Delespaul, P., and Krabbendam, L. J. P. M. (2009). A systematic review and meta-analysis of the psychosis continuum: Evidence for a psychosis proneness-persistence-impairment model of psychotic disorder. *Psychological Medicine*, 39(2), 179.

van Prooijen, J.-W. (2020). An existential threat model of conspiracy theories. *European Psychologist*, 25(1), 16–25.

van Prooijen, J.-W., and Douglas, K. M. (2018). Belief in conspiracy theories: Basic principles of an emerging research domain. *European Journal of Social Psychology*, 48(7), 897–908.

van Prooijen, J.-W., Douglas, K. M., and De Inocencio, C. (2018). Connecting the dots: Illusory pattern perception predicts belief in conspiracies and the supernatural. *European Journal of Social Psychology*, 48(3), 320–335.

van Prooijen, J.-W., and Jostmann, N. B. (2013). Belief in conspiracy theories: The influence of uncertainty and perceived morality. *European Journal of Social Psychology*, 43(1), 109–115.

van Prooijen, J.-W., Krouwel, A. P., and Pollet, T. V. (2015). Political extremism predicts belief in conspiracy theories. *Social Psychological and Personality Science*, 6(5), 570–578.

van Prooijen, J.-W., and van Vugt, M. (2018). Conspiracy theories: Evolved functions and psychological mechanisms. *Perspectives on Psychological Science*, 13(6), 770–788.

Venables, P. H., and Bailes, K. (1994). The structure of schizotypy, its relation to subdiagnoses of schizophrenia and to sex and age. *British Journal of Clinical Psychology*, 33(3), 277–294.

Vollema, M. G., and Hoijtink, H. (2000). The multidimensionality of self-report schizotypy in a psychiatric population: An analysis using multidimensional Rasch models. *Schizophrenia Bulletin*, 26(3), 565–575.

Vosoughi, S., Roy, D., and Aral, S. (2018). The spread of true and false news online. *Science*, 359(6380), 1146–1151.

Vraga, E. K., and Bode, L. (2017). Using expert sources to correct health misinformation in social media. *Science Communication*, 39(5), 621–645.

Wagner-Egger, P., Delouvée, S., Gauvrit, N., and Dieguez, S. (2018). Creationism and conspiracism share a common teleological bias. *Current Biology*, 28(16), R867–R868.

Ward, T., and Garety, P. A. (2019). Fast and slow thinking in distressing delusions: A review of the literature and implications for targeted therapy. *Schizophrenia Research*, 203, 80–87.

Webster, D. M., and Kruglanski, A. W. (1994). Individual differences in need for cognitive closure. *Journal of Personality and Social Psychology*, 67(6), 1049.

Weinstein, S., and Graves, R. E. (2002). Are creativity and schizotypy products of a right hemisphere bias? *Brain and Cognition*, 49(1), 138–151.

Whitson, J. A., and Galinsky, A. D. (2008). Lacking control increases illusory pattern perception. *Science*, 322(5898), 115–117.

Whiston, J. A., Galinsky, A. D., and Kay, A. (2015). The emotional roots of conspiratorial perceptions, system justification, and belief in the paranormal. *Journal of Experimental Social Psychology*, 56, 89–95.

Wigman, J. T., Vollebergh, W. A., Raaijmakers, Q. A., Iedema, J., van Dorsselaer, S., Ormel, J., . . . and van Os, J. (2011). The structure of the extended psychosis phenotype in early adolescence: A cross-sample replication. *Schizophrenia Bulletin*, 37(4), 850–860.

Wilson, J. A. (2018). Reducing pseudoscientific and paranormal beliefs in university students through a course in science and critical thinking. *Science and Education*, 27(1–2), 183–210.

Wiseman, R., and Watt, C. (2004). Measuring superstitious belief: Why lucky charms matter. *Personality and Individual Differences*, 37(8), 1533–1541.

Woodward, T. S., Moritz, S., Cuttler, C., and Whitman, J. C. (2006). The contribution of a cognitive bias against disconfirmatory evidence (BADE) to delusions in schizophrenia. *Journal of Clinical and Experimental Neuropsychology*, 28(4), 605–617.

Xuan, L., and MacDonald III, A. (2019). T120. Examining psychosis in social media: The targeted individuals movement and the potential of pathological echo-chambers. *Schizophrenia Bulletin*, 45(Suppl 2), S250.

Zawadzki, J. A., Woodward, T. S., Sokolowski, H. M., Boon, H. S., Wong, A. H. C., and Menon, M. (2012). Cognitive factors associated with subclinical delusional ideation in the general population. *Psychiatry Research*, 197(3), 345–349.

Zollo, F., Bessi, A., Del Vicario, M., Scala, A., Caldarelli, G., Shekhtman, L., . . . and Quattrociocchi, W. (2017). Debunking in a world of tribes. *PLoS One*, 12(7), e0181821.

Zonis, M., and Joseph, C. M. (1994). Conspiracy thinking in the Middle East. *Political Psychology*, 443–459.

PART 2

Psychopathology and human nature

8

NORMALITY AT THE MIRROR OF MADNESS: HISTORICAL CONSIDERATIONS ON A CHIMERIC BOUNDARY[1]

Francesco Paolo Tocco

1 Preliminary warnings

It should be useful to start this chapter with some preliminary warnings. The first one – probably the most important one – is that the chapter is elaborated by a historian, which means that for the author, it is not only possible but also essential to analyse the arguments concerning medical and psychological aspects of mental diseases – or better, as it was mainly named until not so many years ago, mental insanity – not only from a psychiatric or a psychological or a philosophical perspective, but especially from cultural history perspective. Historical perspective could give a dynamic vision on items primarily studied through structuralist methodologies, from scholars that are often more interested about the recognition and classification of symptoms rather than their outset, evolution, and permutation or, sometimes, disappearance.

Another warning, which depends strictly on the historical point of view that I've just highlighted, must concern the fact that – opposite to an often not explicit but usually passively accepted hypothesis – conceptions and mentalities towards mental disease are not even the same all over the world: not only during the past centuries, but also in present times. It is a fact, this one, that has been recently efficaciously demonstrated among others by Alan Ehrenberg's studies (Ehrenberg, 2010), that enforces our awareness of the differences existing between the American and the French approach to psychological problems, despite the cultural uniformity caused by globalization that leads us to erroneously think that the psychological dimension should be uniform all over the world.

The third, but not less important, warning consists in the fact that in comparison to an enormous number of scientific ponderings on mental insanity, it is – apparently incredibly – less easy to find well-founded reflections about normality. So, we are almost compelled to try to reach normality moving necessarily from madness or, more generally, from the so-called (but today unmentionable – at least officially) abnormality.

2 Normality: a self-evident concept?

If we meditate on the evanescence of commonly accepted definitions of normality (especially in the psychological field), we have to admit that this is the basic problem of all the DSMs (*Diagnostic and Statistical Manual of Mental Disorders*). It is a problem getting more and more serious from the birth of the manual in the middle of the twentieth century until its most recent edition. Nikolas Rose summarizing the history of DSM writes:

> The first Diagnostic and Statistical Manual of Mental Disorders, published in 1952, was prepared by a Committee on Nomenclature and Statistics of the American Psychiatric Association in the wake of psychiatry's wartime experience and conceived mental disorders as reactions of the personality to psychological, social, and biological factors . . . . DSM II, published in 1968, was 134 pages and had 180 categories framed in the interpretative language of psychoanalysis. DSM III, published in 1980, ran to almost 500 pages and is often seen as a response to the crisis in legitimacy of psychiatry over the 1970s (American Psychiatric Association, 1980). The revised version of 1987 had 292 categories, each defined by a set of objective "visible" criteria. Ideally, each of these categories was a distinct disorder, with a unique aetiology and prognosis, amenable to a specific kind of treatment. DSM IV, published in 1994, runs to 886 pages and classifies some 350 distinct disorders, from Acute Stress Disorder to Voyeurism. DSM IV cautions that individuals within any diagnostic group are heterogeneous: its categories are only intended as aids to clinical judgment. But it promotes an idea of specificity in diagnosis that is linked to a conception of specificity in underlying pathology.
>
> *(Rose, 2007: 199)*

In light of this concise summary, it should be evident that the reason why DSM-V avoids to define what exactly should be considered a mental disorder is strictly related to the problem that it is impossible to assert with absolute certainty what constitutes normal behaviour. A problem which is well pointed out by Wakefield in his reflections about the most appropriate terms to efficiently describe mental disease (Wakefield, 1992, 1999, 2006). Wakefield avoids, more or less consciously, to define normality, but he does not renounce to define "abnormality" from a psychiatric point of view. Wakefield's definition of abnormality is well known, but it is important to mention it, because we will return on some of the terms used in this definition:

> I argue that a disorder is a harmful dysfunction, wherein harmful is a value term based on social norms, and dysfunction is a scientific term referring to

> the failure of a mental mechanism to perform a natural function for which it was designed by evolution.
>
> *(Wakefield, 1992: 373)*

This definition and the problem raised by the absence of a definition of normality has been debated by many scholars, and has been well highlighted by Massimiliano Aragona in his studies (Aragona, 2009, 2013) about mental disorder and the debate on its denomination during the elaboration of the DSM-V:

> [I]t would be very difficult to find clear and consensual definition/description of what is exactly to be intended as *normal reaction proportional and appropriate response* and so on. . . . Who must decide what should be intended for disproportionate? When should a response to a living situation be considered exaggerated, and who decides what is exaggerated? Who knows when stimuli are appropriated? How many specific circumstances are known that in normal conditions invariably elicit has given response? Are rational decisions synonymous of normal decisions? . . . [T]he question that implicitly underlies the overinclusion problem, that is "what (who) is normal and what (who) is mentally disordered?" should be reconsidered, being significantly influenced by what is conceived as normal and what is thought to be a mental pathology in our society and our era.
>
> *(Aragona, 2009: 8)*

The majority of the insider beneficiaries of the recent DSM-V, whose purpose was to give an order to the knowledge, diagnosis, and potentially to the cure of mental diseases, admits that this ambitious volume has not clarified the problems that it wanted to resolve, making the *status quaestionis* more uncertain than before. Moreover, this latest version of the DSM has produced a sort of explosion of new pathologies, which can hardly be considered as an aid to the diagnosis.

Moreover, there is a minority of professionals who not only find the new DSM impractical, but who also criticize it strongly from a point of view which is, at least at a first glance, diametrically opposite to the authors of the manual.

Indeed, Lennard J. Davis, the author of *The End of Normal. Identity in a Biocultural Era*, a well-constructed hymn to the cultural integration of the diverse, writes in his book:

> The *Diagnostic and Statistical Manual-V* (*DSM-V*) has elaborated a dizzying display of lifestyle illnesses that demand medical treatments to cure and normalize people. Sadness, shyness, obsession, sexual desire, anger, adolescent rebellion, and the like now fall under a bell curve whose extremes become pathologies. Surgical and pharmaceutical interventions are designed to return normalcy or the appearance of normalcy to aberrant bodies.
>
> *(Davis, 2014: 7–8)*

And, as we will see up ahead, to aberrant minds.

On the other side, the current psychiatric perspective, that we can consider the most popular in the last 30 years, and that is well represented by the recent studies of many scholars like the psychiatrist Oleguer Plana Ripoll and the public health specialist Benjamin Lahey, criticizing the chaos generated by the DSM-V, supposes that behind this multiplicity of illnesses, there must be a unique biological – or better, genetic – cause of all mental diseases.

In a very recent article, Michael Marshall writes:

> Some psychiatrists have put forward a radical hypothesis that they hope will allow them to make sense of the chaos. If disorders share symptoms, or co-occur, and if many genes are implicated in multiple disorders, then maybe there is a single factor that predisposes people to psychopathology.
>
> *(Marshall, 2020: 21)*

In both theories (of Davis and Lahey) normality comes into play, in a way that is explicit in Davis' words and implicit in the recent researches of neuropsychiatry. At first glance, it seems we are in front of two different, and apparently, opposite kind of normalities.

According to Lahey, we can divide people into two distinct categories: the normal ones, and the 'abnormal' ones, genetically predisposed to mental illness, although on different levels. It is important to observe that the abnormal ones, if looked after, could belong to the world of normal people. But only if they recognize that their behaviour is constitutively damaged, which medical therapies and treatments aim to control or, better, eliminate.

The first theory is more sophisticated. Let Davis speak for himself:

> We are all humans, diverse as we may be. In that sense, although our diversity is a sign of our difference, it is also a sign of our sameness, the sameness of being human. This is a proposition with which few will disagree. There is a built-in contradiction to the idea of diversity in neoliberal ideology, which holds first and foremost each person to be a unique individual. Individualism does not meld easily into the idea of group identity. And yet for neoliberalism it must be part of a "different" group – ethnic, gendered, raced, sexual. It is considered boring if not limiting, under the diversity aegis, to be part of the nondiverse (usually dominant) group. So diversity demands difference so it can claim sameness. In effect, the paradoxical logic is: we are all different; therefore we are all the same.
>
> *(Davis, 2014: 13)*

Davies then highlights the dark side of the neoliberal ideology with a series of observations:

> What is suppressed from the imaginary of diversity, a suppression that actually puts neoliberal diversity into play, are various forms of inequality,

> notably economic inequality. . . . But what is also suppressed . . . is disability – particularly a notion of disability without cure. In this sense disability (along with poverty) represents that which must be suppressed for diversity to survive as a concept. . . . Thus "we are all different; therefore we are all the same" becomes "we are all the same because we aren't that kind of different." "*that* kind of different" would refer to that which cannot be chosen – the intractable, stubborn, resistant, and yet constitutive part of neoliberal capitalism – *zoe*, bare life, the ethnic order, the abject, the disabled – that which cannot be transmuted into the neoliberal subject of postmodernity.
>
> (*Davis, 2014: 13*)

This cogent reflection ends with a very incisive sentence regarding the contemporary notion of normality that – let's bear it in mind – is substantially accepted by Davis himself:

> Disability is an identity that is unlike all the others in that it resists change and cure. It is not chosen, and therefore it is outside of the dominant ethic of choice. It is an atavism representing the remainder of normal at the end of normal. But such it isn't an anomaly, but rather the capstone that upholds the arch of the neoliberal notions of diversity. It is the difference that creates the fantasy of a world in which we are all so diverse that we become the same. As such, paradoxically, it upholds meaning and significance because without difference there can be no meaning. Thus disability is the ultimate modifier of identity, holding identity to its original meaning of being one with oneself. Which after all is the foundation of difference.
>
> (*Davis, 2014: 14*)

3 Can the history of words help us?

At this point, it seems to be clear that scholars considerably debate about abnormality, difference, and mental disease, but at the same time and with the same determination they accurately avoid to explain what normality should be for them. Let us try to see if a historical analysis based on linguistic landmarks can help us to reach this elusive concept, starting from the basic question whether the couple 'madness-normality' has been characterized during the centuries by the same kind of relation, and even whether this pair has always existed.

First of all, it will be useful to debunk the myth of the scarceness of scientific researches about madness in Greek, Roman, and Medieval societies. Conversely, we have a very rich stream of high-level works, especially regarding the first two cultures. This myth has been promoted by some opening observations in the classic Foucaultian work about madness in Classical age – we must remember that 'classic' in Foucault means 'Early Modern', and that the American translation of the original locution is 'Age of Reason' – and this commonplace was acceptable at the time when Foucault wrote his book. But from the 1970s, scholars have abundantly provided for this lack in research.

So, we can affirm with a high degree of certainty that in the ancient Greek culture – from its beginning until the first centuries of the Christian Era – the disorder of the mind was a phenomenon which did not have a univocal definition. There were different words to indicate mental disease, each investing in different kinds of behaviour and emotions. To indicate the furious madness, the Greeks used the word μελαγχολία – from which derives the word melancholy, which has however acquired a different semantic meaning. But the most probably used and known word to generically suggest madness was μανία, a term documented since fifth century B.C. and ascribable to irrationality and furious passion more than exclusively to pathology. Ancient Greeks believed that mental diseases were originated from the possession of the person by many Gods. Moreover, it is important to underline that lunacy and prophetic inspiration were strictly associated. Indeed, the words μαντική, meaning 'prophetic art', and μανική, meaning 'madness', are etymologically connected. In this culture, madness doesn't represent uniquely the obnubilation or, worse, the vanishing of reason, but also a different and superior kind of knowledge. This higher knowledge could be reached by the ἐνθουσιασμός, inspiring energy that permits to earn a real awareness, supported by a God (Guidorizzi, 2010: 11; 94). For this reason, probably, crazy people had to be differentiated from other people by wearing headgear and it is quite certain that there did not exist any form of repression of people who suffered from mental illnesses. To the demented, it was only forbidden to bring weapons, to serve in the military, and to make a will.

The situation in the ancient Roman world was richer and more articulated than in the Greek one, but it was nonetheless homogeneous to the other one. The Latin vocabulary is more accurate than the Greek one, and it makes a distinction between *insania* and *furor*. Cicero wrote that this second term was more precise than the generic μελαγχολία of the Greeks, because it showed better physical and moral causes of madness. *Furor* is a very severe form of mental disease and it is more dangerous than *insania*, but it is a kind of more noble madness (Diliberto, 1984: 27) that can strike the sapient too – differently from *insania*, which is nothing more than a kind of *stultitia*, that is to say foolishness. According to the philosophy of the Stoics, Cicero asserts that people in good health are those whose mind is not disturbed by passions: all the other people, the majority, suffer from that disease that can be named *insania*.

It is important to observe that to be *furiosus* does not imply the loss of role and dignity. These prerogatives must be maintained, as there is always the possibility to leave this condition. But if the condition persists, the *furious* cannot practice the office of judge, even if it will be in his power if he returns to normality. Moreover, the *furious* does not lose the *patria potestas* (Rizzelli, 2014: 157–158).

At this point, it should be clear that in classical Western cultures madness was a component of human life: an unfortunate, problematic, also painful one, like in our Western contemporary culture. However, differently from our beliefs, it was not a state directly related to the abnormality, at least in the sense we now give to this word, as we will see beyond. Also, it is important to observe that the terms used in these two ancient languages to indicate normality are in Greek κανονικός, which has to do with the word that means 'rule'; and in Latin *rectus*, *iustus*, *solitus*, *medius*. The Latin words enrich the Greek semantic field related to the rule, adding notions connected to the idea of normality as 'most likely frequency'. What we must focus on is the linguistic component that suggests the concept of rule, or better, of the law (*iustus*), because we will find it again in the final paragraphs of this work.

4 An imperceptible but radical transition

During the Middle Ages, things imperceptibly start to change, especially during the last centuries of the period (Horn and Frohne, 2013). Concepts linked to mental illness – aside from the representation of literature, that we intentionally will not consider, as, after all, we have already done for Greek and Roman cultures – are analysed and reported almost uniquely in juridical environments (Metzler, 2010): with the flourishing of written texts starting from the thirteenth century, it emerges a certain number of very important juridical lexicographies, in which a specific space is dedicated to illness and madness (Mayali, 1987).

One of the first of this kind of *lexicons* was the one written by Alberico da Rosciate of Bergamo at the middle of fourteenth century entitled *Alphabetum*, trivially known as *Dictionarium iuris tam civilis quam canonicis* (*Dictionary of Civil and Canonic law*) (Silanos, 2015: 31)

In Alberico da Rosciate's *Alphabetum*, the headword *infirmity* is divided into three basic groups: physical debility (*infirmitas corporis*), mental disability (*dementia*), and spiritual weakness, which we could call sin (*infirmitas animi*). It is important to highlight that physical and mental disabilities, in substantial continuity with the Roman tradition, are considered conditions that exempt from penalties and exonerate from guilt. In the specific case of mental disease, there is a distinction between two kinds of illnesses: the actual madness, *amentia*, a condition in which the person is not imputable of a crime, and *dementia*, that is the inability to express self-will, which is contemplated only for issues pertinent to canonic law, like weddings or sacred orders (Silanos, 2015: 33–35). Regardless, we can affirm that late Medieval civil right is not particularly interested in any kind of invalidities, neither physical nor mental, as in ancient Rome. This is another fact that attests that mental disease in Medieval world was considered one of the multiple aspects of "normal" human life (Turner, 2010).

But there was a special case where madness put men out of humanity: the *Furor Hereticorum*, that is, the 'madness' of the heretics. This exception appeared very soon, at the beginning of the institutionalization of Christianity in the late Roman Empire (Zuccotti, 1992: 48–57). This kind of *furor* during the thirteenth century will be connected to the crime of lese-majesty against the Emperor and later the Kings, but – especially from the time of Pope Innocence IV – against the popes, the vertex of the social world of that time. Only in this case we can say that madness was a form of shocking damage of the social and consequently universal order, punishable with the death penalty.

Medieval civilization did not know any difference between invalidity (the physical/mental problem in the strict sense) and handicap (that is to say, the sociocultural image regarding the subject affected by an invaliding sickness). All infirmed people, especially since the last centuries of the Middle Ages, were simply 'useless' (*inutiles personae*), even if terminology related to mental illnesses was a bit richer, with terms like *furiosus*, *mentecaptus* (stupid), *non sanae mentis* (insane). They are all *pauperes* and *miserabiles* (poor and miserable), because, as Mollat has efficaciously observed: "The poor is one who lived – permanently or temporarily – in a condition of weakness, reliance or humiliation, characterized by the lack of tools of power and of social respect" (Mollat, 2001: 7). Mollat identified morbidity as one of the causes that transformed a state of precariousness in a state of need.

During the end of the Middle Ages, the social aspects of the mental disease start to change compared to the past centuries and, in general, compared to non-Christian Mediterranean civilizations. We will return to this observation, but first of all, we must focus on the aspects of this change. We have to recognize that the behaviour that urban Italian legislators implemented to regulate the social problem of disabled can be efficaciously represented by the sociological couple inclusion/exclusion. The first one, inclusion, suggests the juridical protection of people affected by physical or psychical infirmity; the second one consists in the 'social exclusion' of particular sick persons whose presence in the town could be dangerous for the whole community. It is a process that starts during the thirteenth century and that at the beginning concerns only the leprous, with a degree of expulsion that will increase with time. With this notice about the marginalization of the leprous, we have reached the first chapter of Foucault's masterpiece, *Madness and Civilization: A History of Insanity in the Age of Reason* (this is the American translation of the title), in which the French philosopher underlines the switch of marginalization from the leprous to those who suffered from mental diseases. We will return to examine several observations of Foucault's book. However, before doing so we must focus on some other aspects of the Middle Ages' culture and society.

First of all, it is essential to underline that the word 'normal' appears for the first time exactly during the Middle Ages. And that its semantic field is unequivocally tied to the dimension of rule and law. If we read the lemmas related to the word 'normal' in the richest vocabulary of Medieval Latin (Du Cange, 1883–87), we can find many meanings of the word. The first meaning is enlightening, because it is *Regula monastica* (Monastic Rule) and it is quite old, tracing back to the year 770. The second one is the earliest word, from which all the other meanings develop: *Norma*, a Latin word of unknown origin that indicates "carpenter's square, rule, pattern". The derivatives of *Norma* are quite interesting too: *Normatrix*, that is abbess; *Normales limites*, a word used by the land surveyors to signify the line traced from the border of a land to another one; *Normalis honor*, that is the proper deference to religious authorities. To have a clear perspective of the evolution of this word from its birth to modernity, we will report the meanings of the voice 'normal' from the *Oxford Online Dictionary*, which gives us its first attestation in the English language:

> c. 1500, "typical, common"; 1640s, in geometry, "standing at a right angle, perpendicular," from Late Latin *normalis* "in conformity with rule, normal," in classical Latin "made according to a carpenter's square," from norma "rule, pattern," literally "carpenter's square," a word of unknown origin (see norm). Meaning "conforming to common standards or established order or usage, regular, usual" is attested from 1828 but probably is older than the record [Barnhart]. Meaning "heterosexual" is by 1914. As a noun meaning "usual state or condition," from 1890 (in geometry as "a perpendicular" from 1727). Sense of "a normal person or thing" is attested by 1894. Normal school "training college for teachers" (1835) is a translation of French école normale (1794), a creation of the French Republic; the notion is of "serving to set a standard".

To end our reconstruction, we will report the adverb derived from normal, 'normally':

> 1590s, "regularly, according to general custom" (a sense now archaic or obsolete), from normal + ly. Meaning "under ordinary conditions" is by 1838.

Through the reading of this simple quotes from dictionaries – although it may be a bit boring – we can adequately understand how a word that formerly had to do with the establishment of rules and the administration of people, unambiguously – only a well-used carpenter's square allows erecting flawless buildings – transformed itself in a word that should be meaning 'being within certain limits that define the range of normal functioning'.

An equivalent process happens when analysing the linguistic history of 'rationality', whose loss is still considered by many people and a certain number of physicians as automatically associated with mental disorders. Recent studies, on the contrary, have abundantly demonstrated that people affected by mental disorders have more logical abilities as compared to the so-called normal people (Cardella, 2018). There is probably a historical reason behind this commonplace. If we read on the Du Cange the voice *Ratio* and all the correlated voices, we understand that they mainly concern the semantic field that has to do with juridical trials and accounts. The first item for *Ratio* gives *Jus, causa, judicium* (Law, trial); then we have *Rationis Consules* (Judges); *Rationis exercere* (to issue laws); *Mittere/Ponere ad rationem* (to summon); *Rationator, Ratiocinator* (attorney); *Ratiocinare* (*Litigare, in jure agere, jus suum disceptare, ad rationem ponere, causam suam coram judice rationibus probare, rem quampiam, rationibus ad id adductis, sibi asserere, crimen rationibus in judicio a se amoliri*). The other items for *Ratio* are "goods", "ration", "descendants", "measure", and "straight line" according to the agricultural writers.

This long list of terms can be reconnected to the ancient Latin meanings of the word and to its etymological origin. The word *ratio* comes from *ratus*, the past participle of the verb *reor*, whose original meaning is sum, count, calculation. Ancient people knew very well that people with mental diseases usually had a working *ratio*, as it is demonstrated by the fact that the terms used to define crazy people very rarely concerns rationality. Insanity, in the Greek and Roman cultures, was principally to be furious, not to be irrational. Things started partially to change during the end of the Middle Ages (Murray, 1978), with an important semantic relocation in many vernaculars that facilitated the present misconception about the irrationality of people with mental diseases. Alexander Murray reminds us:

> In this period [towards the end of the XII century] a wider audience had given the verb *rationare* the plain meaning "to talk" (the first known example of this usage in Italy dates back to 1228). This connotation, too, perhaps had its antecedent in ancient vulgar Latin, but in the Middle Ages it undoubtedly developed partially in symbiosis with the equivalence *ratio* "courthouse", as *rationare* had taken on the meaning "to press charges". However, the correlation "to reason/to talk" became so deeply rooted in vulgar languages that it gave birth to new acceptations. A French saying – paradoxical only on a surface level – that is around 1260 stated: "Keep your tongue or else *resun* [speaking] will make you feel embarrassed".
>
> *(Murray, 2011: 933)*

5 From 'God-signed' to dangerous marginalized

So far, we have tried to show how, during the long centuries of the evolution of Greek, Latin and, for the most part, Medieval civilizations, the room of madness was a 'piece' of the social world. A certainly troubled and suffering piece (Pfau, 2010), that could be nevertheless become noble, a voice of God, able to force humanity to meditate on its meaningless ambitions. This conception received its most relevant celebration, thanks to Erasmus Roterodamus with his *The Praise of Folly*, ironically written at the turning point of the social conception of the mental disease: a panegyric which exactly behind its humanistic and highbrow weaving seems to hide the symptoms of a tragic change under the sign of the banishment of the lunatics from the humanity. Foucault's work shows clearly how during Renaissance and until the beginning of the sixteenth century, insanity, in a way that is ironic and tragic at the same time, can help us to reflect about the sense of life and the real consistence of reason:

> Finally, at the centre of all these serious games, the great humanist texts: the *Moria rediviva* of Flayder and Erasmus's *Praise of Folly*. And confronting all these discussions, with their tireless dialectic, confronting these discourses constantly reworded and reworked, a long dynasty of images, from Hieronymus Bosch with *The Cure of Madness* and *The Ship of Fools*, down to Brueghel

> and his Dulle Griet; woodcuts and engravings transcribe what the theatre, what literature and art have already taken up: the intermingled themes of the Feast and the Dance of Fools. Indeed, from the fifteenth century on, the face of madness has haunted the imagination of Western man. A sequence of dates speaks for itself: the *Dance of Death* in the *Cimetiere des Innocents* doubtless dates from the first years of the fifteenth century, the one in the Chaise-Dieu was probably composed around 1460; and it was in 1485 that Guyot Marchant published his *Danse macabre*. These sixty years, certainly, were dominated by all this grinning imagery of Death. And it was in 1494 that Brant wrote the *Narrenschiff*; in 1497 it was translated into Latin. In the very last years of the century Hieronymus Bosch painted his *Ship of Fools*. The Praise of Folly dates from 1509. The order of succession is clear. Up to the second half of the fifteenth century, or even a little beyond, the theme of death reigns alone. The end of man, the end of time bears the face of pestilence and war. What overhangs human existence is this conclusion and this order from which nothing escapes. The presence that threatens even within this world is a fleshless one. Then in the last years of the century this enormous uneasiness turns on itself, the mockery of madness replaces death and its solemnity. From the discovery of that necessity which inevitably reduces man to nothing, we have shifted to the scornful contemplation of that nothing which is existence itself.
>
> *(Foucault, 1963: 15–16)*

But with the seventeenth century, the destiny of the fouls is marked by the triumph of modern Rationalism: the insane must be closed, forever far from society. Insanity gives to us no more kind of benefit. Reason does not need the self-critical role of madness anymore:

> Since delirium is the dream of waking persons, those who are delirious must be torn from this quasi-sleep, recalled from their waking dream and its images to an authentic awakening, where the dream disappears before the images of perception. Descartes sought this absolute awakening, which dismisses one by one all the forms of illusion, at the beginning of his Meditations, and found it, paradoxically, in the very awareness of the dream, in the consciousness of deluded consciousness. But in madmen, it is the medicine which must effect the awakening, transforming the solitude of Cartesian courage into an authoritarian intervention, by the man awake and certain of his wakefulness, into the illusion of the man who sleeps waking: a short cut that dogmatically reduces Descartes's long road. What Descartes discovers at the end of his resolution and in the doubling of a consciousness that never separate from itself and does not split, medicine imposes from outside, and in the dissociation of doctor and patient. The physician, in relation to the madman, reproduces the moment of the Cogito in relation to the time of the dream, of illusion, and madness. A completely exterior Cogito, alien to

> cogitation itself, and which can be imposed upon it only in the form of an invasion.
>
> *(Foucault, 1963: 184–185)*

With Descartes, with the triumph of a new Rationality, never seen in the past centuries, there is only a place for the insane ones and their reiterated dangerous uselessness: the hospital.

> It is common knowledge that the seventeenth century created enormous houses of confinement; it is less commonly known that more than one out of every hundred inhabitants of the city of Paris found themselves confined there, within several months. It is common knowledge that absolute power made use of *lettres de cachet* and arbitrary measures of imprisonment; what is less familiar is the judicial conscience that could inspire such practices. Since Pinel, Tuke, Wagnitz, we know that madmen were subjected to the regime of this confinement for a century and a half, and that they would one day be discovered in the wards of the Hospital General, in the cells of prisons; they would be found mingled with the population of the workhouses or Zuchthäusern. But it has rarely been made clear what their status was there, what the meaning was of this proximity which seemed to assign the same homeland to the poor, to the unemployed, to prisoners, and the insane. It is within the walls of confinement that Pinel and nineteenth-century psychiatry would come upon madmen; it is there – let us remember – that they would leave them, not without boasting of having "delivered" them. From the middle of the seventeenth century, madness was linked with this country of confinement, and with the act which designated confinement as its natural abode. A date can serve as a landmark: 1656, the decree that founded, in Paris, the Hopital General.
>
> *(Foucault, 1963: 38)*

6 What Foucault has neglected

At this point we have to return to the end of the Middle Ages. There were some places in the South of Europe and in the Mediterranean area where the attitude towards illness and crazy people was characterized – even if based on the same social and cultural atmosphere of the fifteenth and sixteenth centuries – by care and inclusion, most probably, thanks to ideas and strategies originated in the Islamic culture.

On 24th February 1409, friar Joan Gilabert Jofré was headed to the cathedral of Valencia. As he was walking, he chanced upon a group of young people abusing and insulting a madman, as they believed the poor man to be possessed. After defending the insane man, the friar brought him into his convent and two days later, during his sermon at the Cathedral, he exhorted believers to put an end to the cruel persecution of innocent and powerless people like the mad ones. A few months later, a group of artisans and merchants gathered some funds to build a hospital for people with mental diseases. After an official authorization by the King of Aragon Martin the Humane and by Pope, Benedict XIII, on 1st June 1410, the hospital started its life under the protection of the 'Holy innocent Martyrs' – the children killed by King Herod – the only canonized saints that lacked reason. It was a clear sign that there was a place in heavens for lunatics, too.

Then, other hospitals aimed to recover all kind of innocent and troubled people (e.g., castaways, disabled, and prostitutes), which were built. The hospital of Valencia encouraged the spring of many other foundations of this kind, starting from the one founded in Zaragoza by Alfons V of Aragon '*the Magnanimous*' in 1425. All these hospitals applied to insane people the treatment that many centuries later became known as 'moral treatment', a well-known practice in the history of psychiatry. The hospitalized spent their time doing physical exercise, group games, working, attending ludic performances, and following specific diets and hygiene programs. It is most important to highlight that the rules of the hospital of Valencia, which were authorized by King Martin, provided the *Clavarius* or *Hospitaler* (*Hospital Manager*) to gather the insane tramps wandering into the town and to bring them to the hospital willingly or unwillingly. There, the manager was responsible for them and with time he was vulgarly named 'Father of Insanes', a locution denoting a protective connection between him and the lunatics (López-Ibor, 2009).

Many scholars believe that the role model of the Hospital of Valencia was the *Maristán* of Granada, a hospital for insane people founded in the Islamic Emirate of Granada from emir Muhammad V during the years 1365–1367 (Fernández Vázquez and Mañá Ares, 2016). This building had surely been created to put into practice Islamic beliefs on madness, which can be considered an evolution of the ancient Greek and Roman attitudes towards crazy people. Muslim society generally considered madness as the possession by spirits or magical creatures such as genies (*djinn or jinn*), intelligent beings with great knowledge, who control the actions of those innocents that they possess. The most used word to define lunatics is *majnun*, which is directly translatable as "possessed by a *jinn*". The connection between madness and possession is the basis of a great number of beliefs and practices linked to religion and magic, and it was generally accepted by Medieval Islamic society. Together with this widespread belief, Islamic medicine – developed from the theories of Hippocrates and Galenus (Pérez et al., 2012) – supposes that mental illnesses can be treated with a certain degree of success and that, in any case, crazy people must be helped and respected. the mentally ill must not be excluded from society because they are proof of human diversity. This attitude was certainly driven and reinforced by religious prescriptions. Indeed, a verse of the Qur'an (IV, 4) delivers "And do not give the weak-minded your property, which Allah has made a means of sustenance for you, but provide for them with it and clothe them and speak to them words of appropriate kindness". This attitude was different from that of Christian charity – that we have seen abundantly applied to the lunatics – and it can be considered an aspect of Islamic *ihsan*, that means "to do beautiful things", one of the three basilar dimensions of the Islamic religion, which encourages social responsibility and a mutual exchange of good deeds.

For all of these reasons, *bimaristans* were scattered all over the Islamic world. These were both helpful centres, for people affected by mental or physical invalidity, and educational centres, for those who took up healthcare careers. Towards the end of the Middle Ages, the majority of *bimaristanes* received insane people almost exclusively. At the end of thirteenth century, *bimaristanes* were well attested in the oriental area of the Islamic world, in Damascus, Baghdad, Antioch, Aleppo, Jerusalem, and Cairo, whereas the diffusion in the West Islamic countries was tardive, starting from Morocco (Issa, 1928). It is very likely that the *Maristán* of Granada was the first and probably the only one in Islamic Europe.

We must not emphasize the nobleness of Spanish catholic mental institutions, because insane were not always treated as their statutes prescribed. This is especially true over time as attested by the life and initiatives of Juan Ciudad Duarte, canonized as Saint John of God, who was sectioned for a short time exactly in the hospital of Granada where he saw the tortures inflicted to insane patients. For this reason, when he returned to free life in 1535, he founded another hospital in Granada: this one based on humanitarian practices whose success will be unquestionable, playing a crucial role in the foundation of the hospitaller order commonly known as 'Brothers of Mercy'. This order supervises hundreds of hospitals all over the world still now.

7 From marginalization to declassification

Now we can return to the time of the decree of the foundation of the Hopital General in Paris, at the half of the seventeenth century, but not before having explained the purpose of the previous paragraph. It is not an erudite critique of Foucault's quotes. The *History of Insanity* remains a masterpiece, and his silence on the Spanish hospitals and the Islamic concept of insanity has its reasons: the winning worlds are the French, the English, and later the German and the American one: the Western world. But it does not mean that there were no other contemporary approaches to the cure of lunatics and above all, contemporary conceptions of the social role of madness which differed drastically from the one described by Foucault. To give a further example, it is enough to remember that precisely during the 'infamous' seventeenth century, in many towns of the Ottoman Empire crazy people could walk freely along the streets without being confined or abused or ridiculed as it was observed by many astonished Western observers and by some grateful Islamic travellers. This last one was the case of Evliya Çelebi: in 1648, while he was in Damascus, he was

> invited by ten Turkish officers to join them for a night of revelry in a house of ill repute . . . . En route to the establishment, Evliya suddenly came face to face with a local *majdhub* (holy fool) by the name of Shaykh Bakkar.
>
> *(Scalenghe, 2014: 102)*

Shaykh Bakkar acted foolishly and embarrassingly towards him. However, these are the words that Çelebi employs in recounting his experience:

> I was on my way with these men to the den of vice. But because I am one of those who bear God's holy word, having memorized the Koran, his holiness Shayk Bekkar received divine inspiration and seized me from the midst of those doomed men. He paraded me round about, crying: "One sinner!" and so rescued me – may his secret be sanctified. Owing to that saintly man I was saved from that abyss.
>
> *(Scalenghe, 2014: 103)*

It cannot be denied that during those years in Europe, some people could ponder on the meaning of life after witnessing embarrassing behaviours of madmen. However, these attitudes towards madness became more and more an exception rather than the norm, which was, if anything, internment. Insane people were locked up together with syphilitics, lascivious men, homosexuals, and blasphemers, and in this way madness was inexorably enchained to the sin.

At the same time, the sign that during the seventeenth and eighteenth centuries will identify the madmen is the absence of reason. This fact is well explicated by Foucault:

> We no longer understand unreason today, except in its epithetic form: the *Unreasonable*, a sign attached to conduct or speech, and betraying to the layman's eyes the presence of madness and all its pathological train; for us the unreasonable is only one of the madness's modes of appearance. On the contrary, unreason, for classicism, had a nominal value; it constituted a kind of substantial function. It was in relation to unreason and to it alone that madness could be understood. Unreason was its support; or let us say that unreason defined the locus of madness's possibility. For classical man, madness was not the natural condition, the human and psychological root of unreason; it was only unreason's empirical form; and the madman, tracing the course of human degradation to the frenzied nadir of animality, disclosed that underlying realm of unreason which threatens man and envelops – at a tremendous distance – all the forms of his natural existence.
>
> *(Foucault, 1963: 83)*

So, we can say that also Shayk Bekkar, for the 'classical man', should be only a dangerous beast to chain up and enclose.

8 The last step: from degradation to abnormality

At the end of eighteenth century and the beginning of nineteenth century, things seem to change. A revolutionary swing appears to take place, thanks to Tuke, Pinel, Esquirol, and all the representants of the 'moral treatment'. But it's a short spring, which turns out to be unable to truly modify the tendency towards the degradation of insane people. And, after all, this change would have been unfeasible in the society of the industrial revolutions; a society which aspires to the reification of man, to the exploitation of the *utilitas* that we have seen mentioned for the first time in late Middle Ages in Italian towns. A society, therefore, which cannot give dignity or freedom to all kinds of *inutiles personae*, and which – thanks to the development of science and its application to technology, and in our case to medicine – classifies all deviants under a new mark (Knepper and Ystehede, 2013). The mark of mental insanity, the mark of an abnormal biological and chronic condition for some failed humans: the degenerates.

> On the basis of the constitution of the degenerate, set in place in the tree of heredity and bearing a condition that is not a condition of illness but one of abnormality, we can see that the theory of *degeneratio* enables psychiatry, with its divergent power relation and object relation, to function. Even better, the degenerate gives a considerable boost to psychiatric power. In fact, you can see that when it became possible for psychiatry to link any deviance, difference, and backwardness whatsoever to a condition of degeneration, it thereby gained a possibility of indefinite intervention in human behaviour. However, by giving itself the power to dispense with illness, by giving itself the power with the ill or the pathological and to connect a deviation of conduct directly with a definitive and hereditary condition, psychiatry gave itself the power of dispensing with the need to find a cure. Certainly, at the beginning of the century mental medicine had made a great deal of incurability, but incurability was defined as such precisely in virtue of what was the necessary major role of mental medicine, namely, to cure. Moreover, incurability was only the current limit of the essential curability of madness.
>
> *(Foucault, 1999: 315–316)*

As it is well known, Foucault identifies three historical characters who prepare the way to the creation of the 'abnormal' and his dangerous significance inside the institution: the 'human monster', the 'man to correct', and the 'masturbating child'. The latter is the origin of all sickness according to certain successful nineteenth-century medicine theories. This genealogy is effective in describing most of the prejudices that are even now ascribed to the abnormal.

To prevent the risk constituted by the abnormals, from the half of the nineteenth century, psychiatric power moves its first, incessant steps towards the control of all lives (Foucault, 2003) in perfect harmony with a society in which work and accumulation of wealth are, always more frequently, the only aim of human life. Foucault explains very efficaciously how psychiatry is first of all the watchdog of any dominant social system, even when it seems to be opposed to Capitalism. This is true also for the historical actualization of Communism, which has substantially resulted in a mere deviation from Capitalism instead of an overcoming of the latter.

Presently, the political embodiment of this assertion can be found in the Popular Republic of China.

As highlighted by Foucault:

> Psychiatry no longer seeks to cure, or in its essence no longer seeks to cure. It can offer merely to protect society from being the victim of the definitive dangers represented by people in abnormal condition. . . . With the medicalization of the abnormal and by dispensing with the ill and the therapeutic, psychiatry can claim for itself the simple function of protection and order. It claims the role of generalized social defence and, at the same time, through the notion of heredity, it claims the right to intervene in familial sexuality.
>
> *(Foucault, 1999: 316)*

Consequently, the political, medical, and psychiatric control of sexuality and reproduction becomes one of the most efficacious ways of social regimentation: a man who is not part of the biological coordinate of this new, apparently scientific kind of normality is not only an abnormal but also a degenerate that can only reproduce other degenerates and that must be shut in, inspected, subdued, and in many cases erased, in the name of normality:

> With this notion of degeneration and these analyses of heredity, you can see how psychiatry could plug into, or rather give rise to, a racism that was very different in this period from what could be called traditional, historical racism, from ethnic racism. The racism that psychiatry gave birth to in this period is racism against the abnormal, against individuals who, as carriers of a condition, a stigma, or any defect whatsoever, may more or less randomly transmit to their heirs the unpredictable consequences of the evil, or rather the non-normal, that they carry within them. . . . It is internal racism that permits the screening of every individual within a given society.
>
> *(Foucault, 1999: 316–317)*

9 Has abnormality been defeated at last?

To put an end to this chapter, let's make a conceptual experiment. Let's imagine a 16-year-old guy surviving a shipwreck in the Ocean. He reaches a desert island very far from other inhabited places where he is the only survivor. At the age of 25, he starts hearing voices and experiencing several delusions. Therefore, he experiences the symptoms of schizophrenia, a psychosis of which he has never heard a word of before the shipwreck. Would he consider himself sick – especially, insane? Anybody who has been reading the paper up to this point can imagine that my answer would be negative. That is, for the simple reason that there would be nobody to tell him that what he senses is not real. On the contrary, if he suffered from some other illness – even one never heard before his shipwreck – he most probably would be able to understand that he is sick, or more optimistically that he is feeling unwell. He would never guess to be insane for the simple reason that there would not be any society around him to govern his concept of normality and reality.

Through this conceptual experiment I have tried to explain, although in a quite trivial way, what Georges Canguilhem had already written several years ago, especially in his *The Normal and the Pathological*, published in 1943 and then enriched in 1966. Canguilhem's theory can be immediately recognized behind these words of Foucault (1954):

> [B]ut with that we came perhaps to one of the paradoxes of mental illness, which forces us to look for new analysis forms: if subjectivity of what is senseless is, at the same time, a plea and a way to lose oneself to the world, isn't it perhaps to the world itself that we must ask for the secret of its enigmatic statute? Does not illness perhaps implicate a nucleus of meanings derived from the environment where it arose – and, in the first place, the plain fact of being defined by it for the reason of being an illness?[2]
>
> *(Foucault, 1954: 65)*

After all, the pathological process is, as Binswanger puts it, a *Verweltlichung*, a "*Mundanization*", or "total affinity to the world" (Binswanger, [1949] 1968: 284). But in the case of mental illness, the world is split into two parts: while the first one defines a specific ordinance for mental illness, the second one creates a stigma against the mental illness through the creation of new significance and truths. These two components brilliantly outline how modern subjectivity is constantly forced between subjectification and subjugation and how individual self-determination and self-recognition in the modern world is made possible precisely because of this strain. Foucault argues that analysing the history of psychiatry through an epistemological and political lens allows an understanding of a historical-genealogical mechanism whose functioning is essential in determining modern power relations and discursive regimes.

We are not only in front of a simple repressive attitude, but in front of something more complex and oppressive: the positive imposition of normality, the only one possible in our society. And this is true for our contemporary society too, despite the elaborate and cogent Foucault's critical work. Furthermore, despite the enormous efforts of a homogeneous coalition of scholars active in several regions of the Western world, like Erich Fromm, the members of the school of Palo Alto, Franco Basaglia, and many others, are part, everybody with his specificity, of the so-called Antipsychiatry:

> Foucault's reflection has often been compared to the one of Antipsychiatry, although the French philosopher himself outlines the differences of method, especially on the issue of "political ontology": anti-psychiatric readings – such as the one of Italian Franco Basaglia – were focused especially on a criticism of the repressive form acquired by institutions – in other words, power

> was interpreted as something which "deprives", while the "psychiatrized" subject was considered an object of "deprivation". In the same period Foucault was moving towards a different idea on how power relations operate in capitalistic western modernity: these relations may not be only "repressive" and, if anything, they may not produce "deprivation" dynamics. Rather, they might be "productive" in so far as the "psychiatrized subject" is found in the condition to have to cause a process of subjectification on himself. This process determines and shapes the subject through feedback from objective to subjective in a productive accent.
>
> *(Salottolo, 2015: 88)*

It is the norm more than the law that operates in those new power devices associated with the bourgeois ascent. Law, which establishes what must not be done, is by nature a repressive force, whereas norm, which dictates what must be done, produces truth, institutions, and subjectivity. For this reason

> [n]ormalization can be nearly total, in so far as any subject must adjust to it to feel "normal" and to be part of organized social life's "normalcy". The passage from the dimension of "law" and "taxation" to that of "norm" and "production" – a passage which complicates instead of excluding – sets forth the birth of the capitalistic social organization. In a few words, the question on normality and abnormality – together with how easily one can move from one to the other – is what defines the fundamental problem.
>
> *(Salottolo, 2015: 91)*

As an operational reaction to psychiatric normalization, Antipsychiatry has undoubtedly been successful for two decades (the 1960s and the 1970s):

> A certain number of professionals soon understands that psychiatric rehabilitation is filtered through society's awareness. . . . In other words, the concern is not with patients' rehabilitation, as in orthopaedics, but with rehabilitating communities to welcome insane people. [But] nowadays, this democratic break is subject to alarming countertrends: classic coercive systems are reactivated in different shapes from the past. . . . When dominant psychiatry becomes aware of this mental revolution, it looks for shelter, finding it in an official present trend; that is to say, in the DSM.
>
> *(Barbetta, 2014: 115)*

The relentlessly rising number of mental illnesses for each new DSM, and especially for the most recent version, gives us evidence of the permanence and paradoxical growth of the psychiatric power as denounced, even if against different targets, by Foucault (Still and Velody, 1992) and by Antipsychiatry at the same time. Most of the present psychiatry avoid accurately of speaking of abnormals, at least ostensibly, but always seems to be tempted to find exclusively biological causes of mental illnesses and, if possible, only one cause. In doing so, contemporary psychiatry rebirths the misconceptions of the recent past. At the moment, psychiatry is contented with the creation of new forms of mental diseases for which it offers to supposedly new patients two desired interdependent gifts: an official pathological label for what in the past would have simply been considered an oddity or a distress (e.g., premenstrual dysphoric disorder, caffeine withdrawal, rapid eye movement sleep behaviour disorder, restless legs syndrome, or apotemnophilia, an attraction to the idea of being an amputee) (Wieczner, 2013) and, at the same time – in the context of the same procedure – to remove the social stigma against these new mental pathologies, obviously by dosing these patients with an appropriate psychiatric drug.

All of that can be shown simply by reading Bruce A. Thyer's cutting off of the nosological criteria of the most recent DSM. Firstly, however, let's read the DSM-V definition of mental disorder:

> A mental disorder is a syndrome characterized by clinically significant disturbance in an individual's cognition, emotion regulation or behavior that reflects a dysfunction in the psychological, biological or developmental processes underlying mental functioning. Mental disorders are usually associated with significant distress or disability in social, occupational or other important activities.
>
> *(APA, 2013: 20)*

Thyer rightly highlights that:

> The beginning and the ending of this definitional sentence reads: "A mental disorder is a syndrome characterized by clinically significant disturbance in . . . processes underlying mental functioning." By itself this is tautological, repeating the same sense in different words, and hence is unsatisfactory from a scientific standpoint. . . . [T]he DSM-V definition of mental disorder significantly expands beyond the definition found in the four previous versions of this manual. . . . The DSM-V greatly expands upon that of its predecessors by creating nine different pathways for mental disorder, with three potential sources of disturbance or aetiology (psychological processes, biological processes, and developmental processes) causing dysfunctions in three domains (cognition, emotional regulation, and behavior).
>
> *(Thyer, 2015: 47)*

10 Conclusions

To sketch a very synthetic conclusion to this chapter, I would like to remind the readers of a sentence which is very often repeated by Vittorino Andreoli, a well-known Italian psychiatrist: "Nowadays, if you want to be considered 'normal' you have to state that you are a bit 'abnormal'" (2018, audio of a public lecture in Rovigo).

I believe that this paradoxical assertion can tell us much more than we can suppose at a first glance. To do it, we must return to Davis when he writes:

> What is suppressed from the imaginary of diversity, a suppression that actually puts neoliberal diversity into play, are various forms of inequality, notably economic inequality. . . . But what is also suppressed . . . is the disability – particularly a notion of disability without a cure. In this sense disability (along with poverty) represents that which must be suppressed for diversity to survive as a concept.
>
> *(Davis, 2014: 13)*

Therefore, Andreoli's aphorism shows efficaciously how – since capitalism has reinforced its cultural hegemony all over the world – by admitting and often asking for recognition of each diversity, everybody proves to be an efficient consumer. By demonstrating this, each one of us attests that he is not a poor, nor a fool unwilling to acknowledge his insanity or to ask for medications to cure illnesses whose number is ever more increasing, as is the case for depression, the most common mental disease of our times which increases more and more every day. This illness, as emphasized already in 1990 in a famous *The Lancet* article, could be erased simply by taking a pill: *Take a pill and be happy!* In this way, when everybody takes his 'personal' pill, we can all live in an enormous, coloured, happy asylum, even if in an uneasy society, as Alain Ehrenberg reminds us (Ehrenberg, 1998, 2010). Everybody, freely imprisoned and inevitably protected by institutions that ground their authority on scientific and algorithmic certainties (Medeghini, 2015), performs his desirably long biopolitical life and believes to be able to sustain the unsustainable effort to be at the same time always efficient and capable of continuously taking decisions and pragmatic actions, as the dominant ideology wants, although it is not explicitly imposed (Frances, 2013). In exchange, he receives an online echo chamber where he can meet the 'different ones' who all live in a state of identical diversity and who reinforce each other's repetitive identity (Dardot – Laval, 2009). Quite a very efficaciously normed normality. Normality has died, long live normality!

Notes

1 I wish to thank my daughter Francesca Maria for her precious support, both linguistic and critical, during my composition of the chapter.

2 Text translated from the Italian edition.

References

American Psychiatric Association (APA). (1980). *Diagnostic and statistical manual of mental disorders* (3rd ed.). Washington, DC: American Psychiatric Association.

American Psychiatric Association (APA). (2013). *Diagnostic and statistic manual of mental disorders* (5th ed.). Washington, DC: American Psychiatric Association.

Andreoli, V. (2018). *La normalità perduta* (Audio of a public lecture in Rovigo). www.vittorinoandreoli.it/conferenze/audio/tag/Normalit%C3%A0%20e%20Follia.html

Aragona, M. (2009). The concept of mental disorder and the DSM-V. *Dialogues in Philosophy, Mental and Neuro Sciences*, 2(1), 1–14.

Aragona, M. (2013). Neopositivism and the DSM psychiatric classification. An epistemological history. Part 1: Theoretical comparison. *History of Psychiatry*, 24(2), 166–179.

Barbetta, P. (2014). *La follia rivisitata*. Milano: Mimesis.

Binswanger, L. (1949). Studien zum Schizophrenieproblem. 3. Studie. Der Fall Lola Voss. *Schweizer Archiv fuer Neurologie und Psychiatrie*, (63), 29–57. (Engl. Transl.) Teedleman, J. (1968). The case of Lola Voss. In *Being-in-the world: Selected Papers of Ludwig Binswanger*. New York: Harper Torchbooks, pp. 266–341, 284.

Cardella, V. (2018). Premessa ad ogni possibile psichiatria: riflessioni sul concetto di normalità. In V. Cardella and A. Gangemi (Eds.), *La logica della follia. Razionalità e irrazionalità nella psicopatologia*. Messina: Corisco.

Dardot, P., and Laval, C. (2009). *La nouvelle raison du monde: Essai sur la société néolibérale*. Paris: La Découverte. (2014). *The new way of the world: On neoliberal society*. English trans. by Elliot, G. New York and London: Verso.

Davis, J. L. (2014). *The end of normal: Identity in a biocultural era*. Chicago: The University of Michigan Press.

Diliberto, O. (1984). *Studi sulle origini della 'Cura furiosi'*. Napoli: Jovene.

Du Cange, C. (1883–87). *Glossarium mediae et infimae latinitatis* (Ed. augm). Niort: L. Favre. Online version. ducange.enc.sorbonne.fr

Ehrenberg, A. (1998). *La fatigue d'être soi: dépression et société*. Paris: Éditions Odile Jacob. English trans. by Caouette, E., Homel, J., Homel, D., and Winkler, D. (2010). *The weariness of the self: Diagnosing the history of depression in the contemporary age*. Montreal: McGill-Queen's University Press.

Ehrenberg, A. (2010). *La société du malaise. Le mental et le social*. Paris: Éditions Odile Jacob.

Fernández Vázquez, A., and Mañá Ares, R. (2016). El legado islámico en los cuidados psiquiátricos. El Maristán de Granada. *Cultura de los Cuidados*, 20(45) (digital edition). http://doi.org/10.14198/cuid.2016.45.06

Foucault, M. (1954). *Maladie mentale et Personnalité*. Paris: PUF. Italian trans. (1997) *Malattia mentale e psicologia*. Milano: Raffaello Cortina Editore.

Foucault, M. (1963). *Folie et déraison: histoire de la folie à l'age classique*. Paris: Gallimard. English trans. by Howard, R. (1973). *Madness and civilization: A history of insanity in the age of reason*. New York: Vintage. Latest english translation by Murphy, J., and Khalfa, J. (2006). *History of madness*. London: Routledge.

Foucault, M. (1999). *Les anormaux. Cours au Collège de France. 1974–75*. Paris: Seuil/Gallimard. English trans. by Burchell, G. (2004). *Abnormal: Lectures at the Collège of France. 1974–75*. London and New York: Verso.

Foucault, M. (2003). *Le pouvoir psychiatrique. Cours au Collège de France. 1973–74*. Paris: Seuil/Gallimard.

Frances, A. (2013). *Primo, non curare chi è normale. Contro l'invenzione delle malattie*. Torino: Bollati Boringhieri.

Guidorizzi, G. (2010). *Ai confini dell'anima. I Greci e la follia*. Milano: Raffaello Cortina editore.

Horn, K.-P., and Frohne, B. (2013). On the fluidity of "disability" in medieval and early modern studies. Opportunities and strategies in a new field of research. In S. Barsch, S., Klein, A., and Verstraete, P. (Eds.), *The imperfect historian: Disability histories in Europe* (pp. 17–40). Frankfurt am Main: Peter Lang.

Issa, A. (1928). *Histoire des Bimaristans (hopitaux) a l'époque islamique*. El Cairo: Paul Barbey.

Knepper, P., and Ystehede, P. J. (Eds.). (2013). *The Cesare Lombroso handbook*. London: Routledge.

López-Ibor, J. J. (2009). La fundación en Valencia del primer hospital psiquiátrico del mundo. *Actas Españolas de Psiquiatría*, 36(1), 23–31.

Marshall, M. (2020). Roots of mental illness. *Science*, 581, 19–21.

Mayali, L. (1987). La folie et la norme dans la science juridique au Moyen Age. *Rechtshistorisches Journal*, 6, 211–229.

Medeghini, R. (Ed.). (2015). *Norma e normalità nei Disability Studies. Riflessioni e analisi critica per ripensare la disabilità* (pp. 11–38). Milano: Erickson Editore.

Metzler, I. (2010). What's in a name? Considering the onomastics of disability in the middle ages. In Turner, W. J., Vandeventer Pearman, T. (Eds.), *The treatment of disabled persons in Medieval Europe* (pp. 15–50). Lewiston, UK: Edwin Mellen Press.

Mollat, M. (1974). *Etudes sur l'histoire de la pauvreté (Moyen Âge – XVIe siècle)*. Paris: Publications de la Sorbonne. Italian trans. (2001) *I poveri nel Medioevo*. Roma-Bari: Laterza.

Murray, A. (1978). *Reason and society in the Middle Ages*. Oxford: Oxford University Press.

Murray, A. (2011). *Ragione. Dizionario dell'Occidente medievale* (Le Goff, J., Schmitt J.-C. Eds., pp. 928–943). Torino: Einaudi.

Pérez, J., Baldessarini, R. J., Undurraga, J., and Sánchez-Moreno J. (2012). Origins of psychiatric hospitalization in Medieval Spain. *The Psychiatric Quarterly*, 83, 419–430. https://doi.org/10.1007/s11126-012-9212-8

Pfau, A. (2010). Protecting or restraining? Madness as a disability in late medieval France. In Eyler, J. (Ed.), *Disability in the middle ages: Reconsiderations and reverberations*. Farnham: Ashgate Publishing Limited.

Rizzelli, G. (2014). *Modelli di "follia" nella cultura dei giuristi romani*. Lecce: Grifo.

Rose, N. (2007). *The politics of life itself: Biomedicine, power, and subjectivity in the twenty-first century*. Princeton: Princeton University Press.

Salottolo, D. (2015). L'impasse epistemologica, le relazioni di potere e lo stigma. Alcuni appunti sulla storia della psichiatria. *Scienza & Filosofia*, 13, 75–99.

Scalenghe, S. (2014). *Disability in the Ottoman Arab World, 1500–1800*. Cambridge: Cambridge University Press.

Silanos, P. (2015). *Homo debilis in civitate*. Infermità fisiche e mentali nello spettro della legislazione statutaria dei comuni cittadini italiani. In Varanini, G. M. (Ed.), *Deformità fisica e identità della persona tra medioevo ed Età Moderna*. Firenze: Firenze University Press.

Still, A., and Velody, I. (Eds.). (1992). *Rewriting the history of madness*. London: Routledge.

Thyer, B. A. (2015). The DSM-5 definition of mental disorder: Critique and alternatives. In *Critical thinking in clinical assessment and diagnosis* (pp. 45–68). Berlin and New York: Springer.

Turner, W. J. (2010). *Madness in medieval law and custom*. Leiden and Boston: Brill.

Wakefield, J. C. (1992). The concept of mental disorder. On the boundary between biological facts and social values. *American Psychologist*, 47(3), 373–388.

Wakefield, J. C. (1999). Evolutionary versus prototype analyses of the concept of disorder. *Journal of Abnormal Psychology*, 108, 374–399.

Wakefield, J. C. (2006). Personality disorder as harmful dysfunction: DSM's cultural deviance criterion reconsidered. *Journal of Personality Disorders*, 20(2), 157–169.

Wieczner, J. (2013). 15 new mental illnesses in DSM-5. *MarketWatch*. www.marketwatch.com/story/15-new-mental-illnesses-in-the-dsm-5-2013-05-22

Zuccotti, F. (1992). *"Furor haereticorum". Studi sul trattamento giuridico della follia e sulla persecuzione della eterodossia religiosa nella legislazione del tardo impero romano*. Milano: Giuffré.

9

"THERE IS A SYSTEM IN LUNACY": MORALITY AND NORMATIVITY IN MENTAL DISORDERS

Leonarda Vaiana

1 Normativity/normality in health mental sciences

The general question to be addressed involves primarily the "normativity", which is not so much – or simply – a great philosophical theme: it is, rather, the essence of philosophy from Plato to contemporary philosophy until W.V. Quine (1969) gave rise to the naturalistic turn. Yet, it is curious that, in the last years, platonic normality has been taken into account within the philosophy of medicine (Chadwick, 2017: 19). On the other hand, Ian Hacking (1990: 160), while reporting that in the early 1820s the word "normality" was coined to signify "a way to be 'objective' about human beings", also underlines that "it uses a power as old as Aristotle to bridge the fact/value distinction, whispering in your ear that what is normal is also right".

Understandably so, within the sciences of mental health, which are the starting point of this study, after the influential Hempel's (1965) paper recommending the use of a scientific language supported by observational terms, the core concept became that of "normality". Adopting this term, psychiatrists and other mental health professionals generally aim to define the mental disorders by an alleged free-value concept. Yet, it is argued by some authors (Wachbroit, 1994; Catita et al., 2020) that sciences as biology and medicine treat the concept of normality as a supposed ideal to which refer the standard accounts of biological or physiological functions. Still it should be reminded that this ideal and its normative function applying to psychiatry were criticized not only by an eccentric historian of thought as M. Foucault (1961), but also by an influential psychiatrist as T. Szasz (1960), both protesting the 'normalizing' function of psychiatric practices and their grounding on the social construction and stigmatization of mental illness.

Perhaps, as a consequence of these strong philosophical and sociological trends of 'antipsychiatry', the word 'normality' is not expressly mentioned in DSM-5 definition of mental disorders: we read, rather, that "mental disorders are usually associated with significant distress or disability in social, occupational, or other important activities" (American Psychiatric Association, 2013: 20).

Yet, there is no author who, although questioning the definition of 'mental disorder' (Bolton, 2008; Stein et al., 2010), does not use the term 'normal' positing it on the side of mental health, and the term 'abnormal' on the side of mental disorders, so that the latter can be explained, as a consequence, since they differ from 'normal' mental functions. Allan V. Horowitz (2015: 340), for example, comments the DSM-5 definition of mental disorder stating that it stresses "the difference between a painful but normal emotion and a mental disorder". In scientific studies, hence, it is generally taken for granted what is the normal functioning of the mind (Regier et al., 2013), whereas it is obvious, on the other hand, that some "abnormal" behaviours or capacities, such as high level of intelligence, or high level of artistic performances are not considered examples of mental disorder.

The question, however, arises as problematic mental conditions such as adolescent antisocial behaviour, intense sadness, intense worry, intense shyness, failure to learn to read, and other types of behaviour are "not merely a form of normal, albeit undesirable and painful, human functioning, but indicative of psychiatric disorder" (Wakefield, 2007: 149). More generally, it is admitted a "normal pain" or "normal grief", as a standard way in which "normal brains respond to such adverse circumstances with negative feelings". So, within the mental health science, although that there is little or no consensus about the meaning of "mental disorder" (Graham, 2002; Wakefield, 2007; Bolton and Gillett, 2019), it seems that there is a large consensus on what is a 'normal' mental functioning, so that "the normal-disordered boundary" is accepted as an unquestioned ground for diagnosis (Wakefield, 2013: 604–605).

Alternatively, "statistically normal" is generally accepted as an explanation of what is normal, and as a value-free concept (Wilkinson, 2000: 290). There are some reservations about the fact that a science such as statistics may be value free. The concept of 'normal distribution' itself is not the representation of merely raw data, but depends on chosen independent variables such as blood pressure and cholesterol measurement, sex, age, pre-existing morbidity, genetic predisposition, nutrition, and similar variable. Therefore, even if Lennard Davis' (1995: 30) stigmatization of the eugenic trend of earlier statistics may refer to an obsolete problem, the fact remains that statistics is born as and is still a normative science. Furthermore, on the side of common people's view on normality, recent studies have also suggested that it involves representations of both statistical norms and prescriptive norms (Bear and Knobe, 2016).

Another way to reduce normality to a scientific concept is to take normality as a biological function (Wakefield, 1999, 2000; Horowitz and Wakefield, 2007), but this approach also meets objections. One of them is that function and dysfunction, being both natural phenomena, should be governed and explained by the same system of natural law. So it is questioned how to mark their difference, if the same biological system can obey to natural rules and can also disobey to them. An answer seems to be that function and dysfunction are two qualitative faces of the same trait that differ in the value associated with this variable (Roux, 2018). Thus, we are back again to value and the question of whether disease and illness are normative concepts or value-free scientific terms (Kendell et al., 1986).

A more general objection to the classic Wakefield's definition of 'mental disorder' as 'harmful dysfunction' was put forward from the evolutionary conceptual framework, which explains mental disorder as "an inability of some internal mechanism to perform its natural function" (Wakefield, 1992: 373). But Laurence J. Kirmayer and Allan Young (1999: 449) refuted this view as a form of biological reductionism, arguing that "cognitive theories of psychopathology suggest that there are disorders that are due to bad programming, not flawed hardware design or damage". In this connection, they mention Daniel Dennett, as a champion of evolutionary theory and cognitive neuroscience who, on his turn, claimed that "whereas animals are rigidly controlled by their biology, human behaviour is largely determined by culture, a largely autonomous system of symbols and values, growing from a biological base, but growing indefinitely away from it" (Dennett, 1995: 491).

Besides, it is worth reminding that almost in the same years, Hilary Putnam (1992: 20) noticed: "evolutionists are extremely cautious about saying which capacities and organs, and so on, were specifically selected for (were 'adaptations') in the evolutionary history of a species and which ones arose serendipitously. Philosophers, however, are not so cautious". It might be added that psychiatrists are not too, since despite the notion of normal function is controversial, they still use it.

Today the distinction between normality and abnormality, although its questionability is no more denied (Singh and Sinnott-Armstrong, 2015), seems to be working for the diagnostic purposes of the sciences of mental health, since normal and abnormal are taken as different points of a continuous distribution (Rössler, 2013; Nuevo et al., 2012; Manwell et al., 2015; Clark et al., 2017), underlying symptomatology compatible with both categorical and dimensional classifications (Watson, 2005: 533).

A general conclusion about the question of normality is therefore that psychiatric diagnoses do not constitute mental illness entities, since "categorical classification systems constitute agreed-upon definitions for pragmatically assigning mental illnesses" (Rössler, 2013: 2).

Within this view, the notion of normality plays only a pragmatically necessary role to distinguish patients in need of clinical treatment from sane people, without carrying any moral or social stigma (Clark et al., 2017).

2 Normality and normativity in law

The problem of normality, which can be overlooked in mental health sciences contexts, becomes stringent when we move to consider the perspective of criminal law. Within this context, the scenery changes, since the main topic is the notion of culpability and responsibility, and it must be analysed in relation to the normal/abnormal mental condition of the defendant.

A general point of view, which is the starting point for the alleged not guilty of an agent due to mental disorders, is the notion of 'mental impairment', according to which a person should not be held criminally responsible if, at the time of the criminal act, the agent lacked the mental capacity to know the nature and quality of her actions or, if she knew the nature and quality of her actions, she did not know, however, that her actions were wrong or she was unable to control her actions.

This is a long-standing rule within the legal tradition and, at the same time, a long-discussed rule: in the legal system, the definition of what constitutes 'mental impairment' is a matter of law, though it refers to an underlying pathological infirmity of the mind that can be ascertained only by a clinical diagnosis. It seems important, therefore, to take into account the debate about the legal and scientific definitions of mental disorder trying to understand also the difference between the law and the mental system's approaches.

Stephen J. Morse (2011: 888) highlighted this difference stating that "the former is primarily concerned with justice and social safety; the latter is primarily concerned with the prevention and treatment of mental disorders". More specifically, as regards the "insanity defence", which is a crucial field of law and psychiatry, law aims to find if the defendant is innocent because of his mental impairment. Innocence and guilt, however, are not a matter of psychiatric diagnosis, but of moral and legal judgements.

Therefore, in the field of criminal law and justice, a largely shared view includes that (1) "insanity", or its recent replacement with the term of "mental impairment", aiming to avoid the "stigma" related to the word "insanity" (CMIA, 4.13), is a legal concept; (2) law is not bound by extra-legal scientific or professional criteria; (3) psychiatry is not an exact science and its allowed concept of "mental disorder" is broad, vague, and questionable; (4) law also belongs to folk psychology, and (5) it has a wider and stronger social impact than psychiatry.

In principle, therefore, not only the Anglo-American legal system but also many other legal systems (Math et al., 2015; Kooijmans and Meynen, 2017; Baiguera Altieri, 2017) limit the influence of forensic psychiatry to the extent that it can only give suggestions for the court's decision that, ultimately, determines what mental behaviour can be accepted for the insanity defence, according to normative standards (Allnutt et al., 2007).

On the other hand, the difference between clinical and legal assumptions concerning mental disorders is underlined by forensic psychiatrists who admit that

> clinicians entering the forensic arena, however, for the most part, do not immerse themselves in thinking about the current social definition or understanding of mental illness. Because of their training and experience, clinicians most often resort to explaining mental illness through the lens of the most widely accepted classification system.
>
> *(Johnson and Elbogen, 2013: 204)*

This explains why they think, in turn, that "legal definitions of mental disorders are often quite vague across statutes and can at times be inconsistent with the psychiatric definitions" (Johnson and Elbogen, 2013: 207).

To understand the deep reason of this divergence, it is necessary, however, to address a notion that is often related to that of 'insanity', namely 'the lack of the capacity for rationality'. The latter introduces a broader topic, on which the legal and clinical definition of insanity itself depends, that is the philosophical and common view of rationality. On this issue, it is worth to emphasize two further differences between law and mental health science: (1) law assumes a normative concept of rationality, while mental health sciences refer to an empirically based understanding of rationality, so that, on this point, the law is more suited to both philosophy and common view; (2) not only law but also philosophy (strange as it may seem) is more related to people's language and understanding than mental health sciences, so scientific objections to the notion of the rationality of psychology of common sense are uninfluential for law and philosophy (Morse, 2011; Sifferd, 2006).

In this connection, it seems interesting to me to take into account the interrelated concepts whose meaning is not univocally understood within the aforementioned perspectives, namely the concepts of evidence and causation.

As regards the evidence, scientists know of course that its relation to data depends on a complex set of interrelated theoretical premises, hypotheses, and observations that do not prevent them from relying, ultimately, on evidence. In the legal system, however, the main question is concerned with the reliability of identifying witnesses, who are often compromised by voluntary or involuntary perception biases. In the US and UK legal systems (Edmond, 2012; Roberts, 2012), it was accepted that the jurors, being alerted by the court about the unreliability of identification evidence, are capable of assessing the credibility and reliability of a witness without expert assistance since "each juror brings to bear on that judgement his experience of life and human affairs"(*Gage v HM Advocate [2011]* HCAJC 40, para 28 see also Roberts, 2012; Nicolson and Auchie, 2017; Kirgis, 2002). Yet, according to a long-standing tradition, expert's opinion is admissible with some caveats: (1) expert's competence is to be recognized by the scientific community; (2) the court must be furnished with scientific information which is likely outside its experience; (3) it is required, however, that experts did not trouble juror's understanding by using scientific jargon or by offering complex and conflicting opinions; finally, (4) it is refuted any pretence to override the role of a jury in the trial (Nicolson and Auchie, 2017).

So again, we can notice that the essential intent of the legal system is to contrast common knowledge and common mind to specialized knowledge and scientific mind. Actually, it has been admitted the necessity to refer to expert testimony, to understand matters related to specialized knowledge such as ballistic analysis, physical matching, and similar topics, as well as genetic science, psychology, and psychiatry (Nicolson and Auchie, 2017). Yet, Gary Edmond (2012: 32) referring to the Law's Commission report, complained that in England and Wales' jurisdiction, "expert opinion evidence has been admitted in criminal proceedings too readily and with insufficient scrutiny". And Andrew Roberts (2012: 105), analysing the Gage's case, concluded that "the question of the admissibility of expert evidence might boil down to a question of risk allocation".

On the other hand, legal system, accepting the contribution of expert testimony, on its turn must depend on the general assumptions and constraints governing the method and criteria of the scientific practice. Forensic psychiatry, as any other science, is characterized by intrinsic limits (Stone, 2008), and evidence sometimes is judged "surprisingly equivocal", for example, when child sexual abuse is considered an evident cause of later violent behaviour (Kennedy, 2005: 4). It is well known that scientific evidence has been debated for decades, from Rudolf Carnap's (1947: 138–139) requirement of "total evidence", which in recent times has been criticized for its implicit grounding on "ideally epistemically rational agents" (Santana, 2017: 4), to current theories of scientific evidence (Scheiner, 2004), where evidence is rather formulated as an interrelated set of elements, including empirical observation and its cognitive biases, background information and its selection, and logical relations between hypothesis and expected evidence. Besides, this setting is embedded in a framework where, as Putnam (2002) showed years ago, it is difficult to maintain the dichotomy fact/value. Of course, many epistemologists still claim a real realism (Kitcher, 2001), which is not, however, ingenuously refuting the idea that both scientific and everyday judgements have a broadly normative content.

The same question can be put forward about the related concept of causation. Is it to be treated as the complex concept as it is used by science or as it is understood in everyday life and law system, that is, as a normative concept? Micheal S. Moore (2009), in his influential work on legal causation, aims to explain how it is possible to reconcile normative uses of the concept, which do not involve the technical or special definition, with causal ordinary and scientific uses of the concept. At the same time, we find again that legal system wants to distinguish its field from those scientific and philosophical approaches that interfere with a plain understanding of these central concepts of the decision-making process of juries and courts. Morse has recently pointed out that the most important thing to recognize for lawyers and policymakers is that mental disorders, which play a causal role, do not turn the person into an automaton:

> People with mental disorders act for reasons just like people without such disorders. . . . Their criminal acts should not be understood mechanistically, like a fever that spikes as the result of an underlying infection. Causation should be understood in this context in terms of assessing the defendant's reasons for action.
>
> *(Morse, 2018: 259)*

One could be tempted to think that mental disorders can be compared to physiological or physical phenomena and, consequently, that they are governed by the same causal mechanism and determinism that are at work in nature. Yet, this sort of reasoning is designated by Morse (2011: 899) as "the fundamental psycho-legal error", which consists in assuming that, if the behaviour of an agent is caused by mental disorder, is excused. However, physical causation is not to be meant as a legal or moral or excusing condition because, if all behaviour depended only on physical causes, then no behaviour would involve any responsibility, and could ever be appreciated, blamed, or justifiably punished (Berman, 2008). This consequence would be, of course, at odd with the legal point of view, but also with common sense, both sharing the assumption that people can act for and respond to reason, that is the general requirement for law's concern on "the lack of rational capacity" (Morse, 2011: 934), the only condition diminishing responsibility. Furthermore, science has not yet shown that the folk psychology's laws fail to explain human behaviour in daily contexts (Dennett, 1987; Dennett, 1998; Lyre, 2018), which are the same that law is concerned with (Morse, 2009, 2011).

These plain reflections would be sufficient to show that the capacity of understanding and using a moral and legal rule for acting has nothing to do with the metaphysical problem of the contrast between causal determinism and free will (Morse, 2007). Yet, also theoretical tenets supported the determinist's perspective in law (Julian, 1970), and a shared solution to this problem was the so-called compatibilism, a philosophical view according to which responsibility – the capacity for free decisions and actions – is independent from the causal mechanism which determines the neurological processes of the brain (Morse, 2000; Dworkin, 2011; Vincent, 2015). Besides, it is shown, however, that mental disorders, like other mental states, are not to be considered a deterministic cause of the behaviour. Morse's example of an agent affected by hypomania is persuasive. According to DSM-5, hypomania is "a distinct period of abnormally and persistently elevated, expansive, or irritable mood and abnormally and persistently increased activity or energy, lasting at least four consecutive days" that includes some symptoms such as "inflated self-esteem or grandiosity", "decreased need for sleep", and "increase in goal-directed activity (at work, at school, or sexually) or psychomotor agitation" (American Psychiatric Association, 2013: 124). Morse's argument is the following:

> [I]magine a "career" armed robber who suffers from clinical hypomania. Suppose our robber never robs except when he is in a hypomanic state because only then does he feel sufficiently confident and energetic to rob. If he is charged with an armed robbery committed while he is hypomanic, his clinical condition played a causal role in explaining his criminal conduct, but no excusing condition necessarily obtains.
>
> *(Morse, 2011: 899)*

In this case, the agent's behaviour seems to be intentionally caused and rational, but just for this reason it is not excusable: even if there is a clinical condition explaining his behaviour, it is not sufficient to show that it is lacking of rationality, and consequently involuntary or unintentional.

An antimechanicistic view of causation is widely spread among legal scholars. Indeed, several studies show that people who are alcohol or drugs addicted, or mentally impaired, may be considered responsible for their conditions. For example, although many people are likely advantaged by an alcohol intolerance in avoiding alcohol use, nevertheless alcohol addicts seem responsible of their condition to the extent that "biological variation is not behavioural imperative" (Mitchell, 1986: 277). Therefore, other types of causes, namely non-physical, like having alcoholic parents, living in adverse circumstances, and complying personal desires may be taken into account as resulting in alcohol abuse. Moreover, a "purposive meta-responsibility" is assigned to people mentally impaired, in as much "mental disorder represents strategic and willful behaviour on the part of the patient in an attempt to influence his personal and social situation" (Mitchell, 1999: 599). If this is the case, psychiatric evidence is provided as a mitigatory rather than an excusatory factor. Finally, "where a crime has been a product of a mental disorder, and that disorder has been culpably caused, then the defendant should not be eligible for a full acquittal (whether due to automatism, insanity or otherwise)" (Mitchell, 1999: 614).

Also, recent findings in cognitive neuroscience, aiming to fulfil the gap between mechanistic and neurological explanations of voluntary actions on the one hand, and commonsensical explanations on the other hand, are promising but still uncertain about date interpretation (Schurger et al., 2016; Schultze-Kraft et al., 2016). These results seem to give reason to Morse's previsions, dating back to some years ago, that he expressed in the following way:

> Although I predict that we will see far more numerous attempts to use neuroscience in the future as evidence in criminal cases and to affect criminal justice policy, I have elsewhere argued (Morse, 2008) that for conceptual and scientific reasons, there is no reason at present to believe that we are not agents. . . . What is the nature of the "agent" that is discovering the laws governing how incentives shape behaviour? Could understanding and providing incentives via social norms and legal rules simply be epiphenomenal interpretations of what the brain has already done? How do "we" "decide" which behaviours to reward or punish? What role does "reason" – a property of thoughts and agents, not a property of brains – play in this "decision"? . . . Normativity depends on reason and thus the radical view is normatively inert. Neurons and neural networks do not have reasons. Only people do. If reasons do not matter, then we have no genuine, non-illusory reason to adopt any morals or politics, any legal rule, or to do anything at all.
>
> *(Morse, 2011: 966)*

3 Normativity and moral philosophy

Interestingly, Morse applies to the legal question of responsibility the long-standing normative view of intentionality and rationality in philosophy. Yet, there is a point in his argument from which it is possible to take a cue for developing a view of mental disorders not yet developed enough. It is 'the lack of rationality', that is the main law's concern for insanity or mental impairment. Philosophy's concern may be different, however, in as much as it may invert the question to be put forward. It will be no more whether mentally impaired people, failing to recognize the normative aspects of the social world, may be excused. The questions will be instead, for example: are psychiatric patients immoral? In breaking the alleged moral rules, do they think to act morally? If this is the case, what can mental disorders teach us about the normative character of moral choices? Can mental disorders shed light on the complex nature of morality? It will be stressed that, putting these questions, the philosophical perspective may propose a new approach to the problem of mental disorders. Unlike mental health sciences and criminal law, whose aim is to certain – clinically or legally – the lack of rationality of people, philosophy can rather address the question of the rationality of patients and their models of morality.

Before proposing this issue, however, it is necessary to try to summarize the main trends of extensive literature on delusional beliefs for two main reasons. The first is because the mainstream philosophical approaches to moral responsibility have been centred on the topic of 'doxastic responsibility', which includes both 'normal' beliefs and delusional beliefs. The second is because, after reporting the main points of a still ongoing debate, I will focus on this 'dominance of belief', as I would call it, to defend an approach on the morality of impaired patients which seems to be more open to new developments.

This topic is characterized by a great division between doxasticism, a view that – unlike the question previously considered about the insanity defence – psychiatrists and other professionals share with common people, and anti-doxasticism, a more sophisticated view introducing some alternatives to the notion of belief. DSM-5's definition of delusion is grounded on the notion of belief:

> A false belief based on incorrect inference about external reality that is firmly held despite what almost everyone else believes and despite what constitutes incontrovertible and obvious proof or evidence to the contrary.
>
> *(American Psychiatric Association, 2013: 819)*

In line with this definition, defenders of doxasticism (Bayne and Pacherie, 2005; Bortolotti, 2010, 2018; Bortolotti and Miyazono, 2015; McCormick, 2011) maintain that, although in a defective sense, delusions must be regarded as beliefs. Marga Reimer (2010: 317) even argues that they are anomalous or unusual beliefs, whose refutation implies a "fallacy of ignoring anomalies", since "if something is unusual for an x, even highly unusual for an x, we cannot conclude without further argument that it is not an x", and parallels them to philosophers' bizarre nihilist claims.

On the contrary, defenders of anti-doxasticism aim to show that delusions' failures, or irrationality, or weakness are just what makes them different from beliefs. So, ironically, the same defeating features are the object of contrasting rating by the two trends. Let us take some exemplar properties of the standard view of beliefs: they are contentful, evidence responsible, consistent, they have a functional role and are context-sensitive. Both doxasticists and anti-doxasticists find arguments to take the presence or absence of certain features as a support of their account and as a refutation of the opposite account. Although scholars have minutely examined each of the aforementioned features, only some key points of the ascription of contentful beliefs to delusional patients will be discussed, in as much as it includes, in some measure, all the others.

A recent study aims to show that Capgras, Fregoli, or Cotard delusions, from folk psychology, are readily classified as stereotypical beliefs. The authors (Rose et al., 2014: 3) present evidence that "people view these delusions as beliefs because frequent assertion is a powerful cue to belief ascription", even if the same participants also notice that patients maintain contradictory beliefs. It seems strange, however, that the experimenters may drive a robust conclusion from such evidence, grounding more on the frequency of patients' assertions rather than on the consistency of their beliefs, which is notoriously a major constraint of common sense psychology (Dennett, 1979, 1987), and a canonical way of beliefs' attribution. On the contrary, arguments supporting the opinion that delusions are contentful but not stereotypical – because they stem from "non-standard perceptual and affective conditions" of patients – have been pointed out (Bayne and Pacherie, 2005: 184) to refute anti-doxasticist objections against delusions' content, while other objections such as irrationality, absence of evidence (indeed counter-evidence), and lack of commitment of delusions are overcome in that the latter are not exclusive features of delusions.

Another line of reasoning, dating back to K. Jaspers (1963: 59), finds that several mental disorders, despite their diversity, share the relation to content, so that "hypochondriacal contents, whether provided by voices, compulsive ideas, overvalued ideas or delusional ideas, remain identifiable as content". Still Jaspers, explaining the concept of delusions, states that "their content is impossible" (Jaspers, 1963: 96) and "un-understandable". It is therefore not surprising to find many scholars referring to Jaspers with the aim of focusing on the opposite view, according to which delusions are not beliefs. Delusions are rather seen as mere "empty speech acts" and "so unlike 'normal beliefs' that it must be asked why we persist in calling them beliefs at all" (Berrios, 1991: 7–8). As a consequence, delusions are taken as "non-assertoric" verbal expression. For example, when a patient says: "I am Napoleon", his words are not to be meant as expressing a literary content (Sass, 1994). Indeed, they may be meaningful if they are understood as metaphors, as in a case of unilateral somatoparaphrenia where the patient said that his foot was like a cow's foot (Halligan et al., 1995). Yet, such arguments are refuted by Andrew W. Young, who defends, on his turn, the content of delusions: although admitting that generally delusions do not result neither in consequential nor in violent actions, he stresses nevertheless that delusions are not "invariably metaphors, empty speech acts, or solipsistic reflections" (Young: 581), just because Capgras delusion, for example, sometimes caused violent behaviour – as in the famous case of a patient decapitating his father (misidentified by him as a robot), in search of his hardware.

As the last-mentioned case shows, content's question is far from being unconnected with other features as lack of evidence, of coherence, of control and functional role. Still many studies could be examined that lead, in my opinion, to the same conclusion: any feature of belief is attributed to delusions in a quite idiosyncratic way and, on the other hand, it is admitted that also beliefs reveal many failures. On the contrary, anti-doxasticists, while questioning the content of delusions, do not deny that beliefs are also imputable, in some measure, of the same failing features. Finally, Bortolotti (2010, 2018) offers a general frame of the whole question of belief ascription that seems to me to end in a *cul de sac*, not promising for future developments of the topic. In particular, Bortolotti challenges the content of delusions by three constraints: procedural rationality, epistemic rationality, and agency rationality. She argues persuasively that all these constraints-having to do with the following subjects' capacities: (1) to make consistently logical inferences, (2) to form new beliefs or to update existing beliefs supported by available evidence, (3) to form beliefs that are interpretable as reasons guiding action-reveal several and meaningful failures regarding not only delusional, but also "normal" beliefs. She rightly concludes therefore that "there is considerable continuity between delusions and beliefs" (Bortolotti, 2010: 57). Yet, in my opinion this is not a reason "to take seriously the doxastic conception of delusions" because even if it is true that also common beliefs are affected by several limitations to rationality, it is nevertheless true that these limitations are easily understood and managed within the common contexts of communication. However, this does not happen in the context of delusional language where there is no level of shared communication. So, in the case of delusional patient's verbal behaviour, it does not seem to me that "words speak louder than actions", as Rose et al. (2014) maintain, while I understand Quine, a master of the criticism of intentional language, when he said: "Actions, behaviour teaches, speak louder than words" Quine (1987: 19).

This is not to say that I will follow Quine thinking that beliefs are just dispositions, since this is just another issue that has been discussed at length by doxasticists. To report the aforementioned opposite opinions is just a way to take a distance from the philosophical debate on the concept of belief which, besides being controversial, is so extensive and dominant as to overshadow other sides of morality that is worth, for me, to address.

4 Kant's view of mental disorder: a different kind of rationality

In particular, in my opinion, Kant's perspective on morality is particularly interesting, just because it is the most rigorous view of practical rationality. Some philosophical studies, centred on the relation between Kant's moral philosophy and mental disorders, are still concerned with the question of doxastic and moral responsibility and thereby with the area of interest of law and mental health sciences

(White, 2012; Cohen, 2013; Scolten, 2016; Golob, 2017). Few studies (Frierson, 2009a, 2009b) aim to suggest cues of reflections that go beyond the boundaries of the question of responsibility, addressing the relation between Kant's principle of 'the sovereignty of reason', which is the keystone of his philosophy, and its interest in the broad concept of 'human nature' including also its irrational sides flowing into mental illness. This relation is considered important for both its implications for Kant's philosophy and today's reflections about the discipline of psychiatry. Interestingly, in these studies, Kant's concern for rationality is highlighted against the background of 'anthropology', which Kant himself overtly considers as a secondary and irrelevant disciplinary approach to the question of morality. Yet, despite this notorious Kantian claim, his three major works on the critique of reason were preceded by a minor text like *Essay on the Maladies of the Head* (1764), and followed by the more important *Anthropology from a Pragmatic Point of View* (1798), and by other essays and lectures also referring to the problem of mental illness. So, in a recent study (Sisti, 2012), the blindness of Kant's scholars with regard to the proximity between thought and madness as a constant dimension of Kant's philosophical reflection has been complained.

My reading of this proximity, as it appears in Kant's *Anthropology*, however, aims to emphasize not the importance of Kant's reflections for current psychiatry, although it is also appreciable for me, but the originality of Kant's moral findings on mental disorder. Contrary to what one would think, the philosopher of unfailing practical rationality admits a different form of rationality experienced by mentally impaired persons. Describing the 'inconceivable' content, made famous by Jaspers, of *Vesania*, Kant states: "this fourth kind of derangement could be called systematic". In a marginal note he also writes: "There is a system in lunacy". So this state of mind of "a deranged *reason*" is not to be meant, unlike *Insania*, as a lack of reason or as a cognitive deficit. It rather shows a different type of cognitive capacity that is far from being irrational. In Kant's words:

> For in this last kind of mental derangement there is not merely disorder and deviation from the rule of the use of reason, but also *positive unreason*; that is, *another* rule, a totally different standpoint into which the soul is transferred, so to speak, and from which it sees all objects differently. And from the *Sensorio communi* that is required for the unity of *life* (of the animal), it finds itself transferred to a faraway placed (hence the word "derangement") [in marginal note Verrückung – which can also mean "displacement"] – just as a mountainous landscape sketched from a bird's eye view prompts a completely different judgment about the region than when it is viewed from level ground. . . . It is astonishing, however, that the powers of the unhinged mind still arrange themselves in a system, and that nature even strives to bring a principle of unity into unreason, so that the faculty of thought does not remain idle. Although it is not working objectively toward true cognition of things, it is still at work subjectively, for the purpose of animal life.
>
> *(Kant, 2007: 321)*

This, then, is a subjective state of 'unreason' of a subject experiencing the unity and division of his mind, when he "flies over the entire guidance of experience and chases after principles that can be completely exempted from its touchstone" (Kant, 2007: 321). Some contemporary psychiatrists, criticizing the concept of delusions, find that Kant's understanding of this mental disorder is more accurate than current understanding in terms of 'delusions' and, following Jaspers, prefer to turn back to the concept of '*Ichstörungen*', namely 'disorders of the experiencing I' (Spitzer, 1990).

What is more relevant from my point of view, which is not concerned with replacing diagnostic criteria with philosophical intuitions, is to underline other sides of this radical subjectivism. Kant (2007: 324) insists that "the only universal characteristic of madness is the loss of common sense (*sensus communis*) and its replacement with logical private sense (*sensus privatus*)" that is self-deceptive and illusory. A few pages later, he describes passion as a chronic and severe illness such as *dementia* (Kant, 2007: 355) and stresses again the rationality (now focusing on moral rationality) of these states of mind and their implying an act of choice:

> Inclination that prevents reason from comparing it with the sum of all inclinations in respect to a certain choice is *passion* (*passio animi*). Since passions can be paired with the calmest reflection, it is easy to see that they are not thoughtless, like affects, nor stormy and transitory; rather, they take root and can even co-exist with rationalizing. . . . Passion always presupposes a maxim on the part of the subject, to act according to an end prescribed to him by his inclination. Passion is therefore always connected with his reason, and one can no more attribute passion to mere animals than to pure rational beings. The manias for honor, revenge, and so forth, just because they are never completely satisfied, are therefore counted among the passions as illnesses for which there is only a palliative remedy.
>
> *(Kant, 2007: 367)*

Finally, the connection with moral egoism can be highlighted, since it is the crucial point which may suggest that a radical egoism may be connected to pathological states such as passions. Of course, Kant's description of this topic shows a steady will to judge morally wrong egoism and passions. Putting in brackets the long-standing question of Kantian moral rigorism, which is not part of my argument, it is remarkable that Kant described egoism as a mental state which stems from an unlimited sense of "I" and maintained that moral egoism is opposite to pluralism, "the way of thinking in which one is not concerned with oneself as the whole world, but rather regards and conducts oneself as a mere citizen of the world" (Kant, 2007: 240–242). For Kant, of course, this was the accomplishment of his theory of mental illness: to suggest how to overcome a moral evil such as egoism means to open the way to overcome mental damage.

Yet, from Kant's approach, questions not yet discussed may arise: what suggestions can result from empirical studies about this particular "derangement" of the reason that has been compared by many psychiatrists to schizophrenia? Do we have any confirmation that Kantian equation between morality and health and between moral egoism and mental disorder is well outlined?

A glimpse into recent literature does not allow to give certain and unambiguous answers, for a reason which needs to be underlined to prospect the questions addressed in the right way. The reason can be expressed referring to a couple of terms, such as 'normative' and 'natural', that is matching to the couple normative/normal opening this study. Philosophical approaches to morality, both rationalistic and empiricist, are normative or, in other words, are governed by the famous Hume's law. On the contrary, mental health sciences, discovering in recent times the question of morality, of course have treated it from a naturalistic, namely descriptive, perspective (Edwards, 2009). So, when the concept of moral reasoning is analysed, from both rationalistic or intuitionistic perspectives, reasons and intuitions lose their normative role and are reduced to motives. Indeed, if this difference were meant as an insuperable divide, it would imply negative consequences both for philosophers – which in my opinion are always in need of relation to empirical grounds – and for mental scientists, in need of conceptual clarification for drawing good experimental designs.

This difference is clearly visible in the case in question: to find empirical support or counter-evidence to Kant's approach on the anomaly of moral rationality is a questionable goal, because experimental researches on moral psychology lie outside Kant's philosophical perspective. Mostly studies are designed to test moral judgement with five psychological systems, that Jonathan Haidt and Jesse Graham (2007) described as the most general concepts on which all the culture, in a different way, ground their forms of life. Later the same authors and others (Glenn et al., 2009) took these five couples of values, harm/care, fairness/reciprocity, ingroup/loyalty, authority/respect, and purity/sanctity, as standards to which relate empirical findings about psychopaths' moral judgement. The most meaningful result of their study was low 'Perspective Taking' and 'Empathic Concern' by psychopaths that were interpreted as primarily responsible for moral judgements violating both harm and fairness value. Mostly experimenters shared this assumed lack of concern for others, arriving indeed to unexpected results in studies concerned with utilitarianism and altruism. For example, in a study into economic decision-making (Wischniewski and Brüne, 2011), patients with schizophrenia seemed to be less sensitive towards unfairness to their disadvantage but, contrary to experiment ers' prediction, they were punished more than healthy controls, depending on the degree of unfairness shown by the virtual proposer in the Dictator Game. An opposite interpretation of similar results was given by Gábor Csukly et al. (2011), according to whom the higher acceptance rate at unfair proposal and the lower acceptance rate at fair proposal suggested higher ratio of inconsistent decisions, a behaviour that was related to a failing ability to perform altruistic punishment. Again, similar findings are reported by Jonathan McGuire et al. (2014), who underline that fairness and harm are different moral domains and recommends caution as to generalize from economic decision-making to harm-related moral cognition.

Indeed, their results seem to show that people with schizophrenia take a meaningful utilitarian and consequentialist stance as regards moral dilemmas. Moreover, they assume that these subjects are more concerned with outcomes rather than intentions, when making moral judgements and blaming others' harmful actions. One could object that this utilitarianism is at odd with the impaired abilities as rational maximizers that the authors also noticed, but a further rejoinder could be that we should not expect an overall coherence of moral reasoning from schizophrenics, but only specific-domain moral judgements.

Finally, other studies may significantly be compared with the previous ones in order to propose a different comment which will bring to Kant' moral philosophy. In my opinion, some studies are very interesting for showing a close relation between moral cognition, firm moral convictions, religious fanaticism, and violent behaviour, to the extent that actions like killings, feuds, crimes of passion, punishments, and honour killings are all associated with specific moral foundation (Glenn et al., 2009; O'Reilly et al., 2019). Intimate partner violence has been also analysed (Vecina et al., 2015) in connection with an autoreferential moral conception, including the utmost certainty of the subject about his moral principles and about what is right, a high moral self-concept, and high level of self-deception whereby he believes to be acting morally while acting selfishly. Curiously, the authors assert that "intimate partner violence is not a disease" (Vecina et al., 2015: 121), presumably to avoid any excusing condition. However, this overvaluation of self, shown by the violent subjects, reminds Kant's moral egoism and its lack of concern with a shared point of view. The authors, after mentioning several studies ascertaining the presence of antisocial, borderline, and narcissistic characteristics, report their results from two studies conducted on men convicted of domestic violence during their court-mandated psychological treatment, confirming their strong self-concern, and even a sense of moral superiority towards the psychologists who treated them, besides a high level of self-deception.

Another type of moral violence that can be framed into a form of Kantian deontology goes beyond punishment tied to moral egoism. It was analysed to distinguish moral violence, seen as morally justified, obligatory, and even praise, from instrumental violence, experienced as morally objectionable but desirable for instrumental reasons. The authors (Rai et al., 2017) present case studies showing that whereas the latter is supported by a process of dehumanization of the victims nullifying the need of moral desert, the former does need that the victims are perceived by perpetrators as morally deserved, as it happens in police violence act, kingpins' protecting acts, terrorist bombing, and honour killings.

Going back from these serious cases of righteous violence to the previous studies inspired by the harm/care foundation, by utilitarian and altruist approaches, we can reflect upon the incongruences that we previously detected. The main perplexing problem which received contrasting comments by experimenters is the acceptance of unfairness by patients with schizophrenia, accompanied by a strong wish of punishment. Interpreting this attitude as indifference towards others, the experimenters find support to maintain a low sensitivity of these subject to harm/care foundation but this conclusion is odd with altruistic punishment, which shows, on the contrary, a strong concern for others. Indeed, the pioneering study of Johnson (1960) on the moral judgement of schizofrenics, grounding on Baruk's (1947) classification of moral models, reported as 'deviant' the judgements that justified the punishment in as much as for these patients "social relations are judged in terms of efficiency and orderliness instead of sympathy and compassion. People are viewed and judged as mere object, hardly different from inanimate objects" (Johnson, 1960: 283). The lack of concern for harm/care values, which Johnson called "humanitarian" values, was already determinant in order to consider immoral the punishment. However, it would not be judged immoral from a rigorous Kantian perspective. To support this claim, I will refer to one of the case studies reported by Johnson: a frail and sick woman uses an electrical heater to warm herself violating the restrictions of the use of electricity imposed during a war. She is accused of stealing electricity and imprisoned. While from a humanitarian, harm/care, or empathic perspective, this act is unequivocally immoral; from the rigorous perspective ruled by the Kantian categorical imperative, it should not be. In fact, the rationale of this principle, also known as the Formula of Universal Law, is just that a maxim is permissible because its opposite is logically and practically contradictory, regardless of any other concern that would reduce its applicability. This golden rule seems to be applied in the previous case: if during wartime all people used electricity, the consequence would be a universal damage.

In my opinion, patients with schizophrenia may be considered as unaware Kantian agents, as it is also indirectly revealed from their failures as utilitarian agents in economic decision-making games. Studies designed to investigate this topic could be promising for new findings.

References

Allnutt, S. et al. (2007). The insanity defence: From wild beasts to M'Naghten. *Australasian Psychiatry*, 15(4), 292–298.

American Psychiatric Association (APA). (2013). *Diagnostic and statistical manual of mental disorders* (5th ed.). Washington, DC: American Psychiatric Association.

Baiguera Altieri, A. (2017). Le turbe mentali nel Diritto Penale italiano. *Diritto & Diritti*, 1–10.

Baruk, H., and Ribière, M. (1947). Présentation d'un test tsedek. *Annales médico- psychologiques*, 19(4).

Bayne, T., and Pacherie, E. (2005). In defence of the doxastic conception of delusions. *Mind & Language*, 20(2), 163–188.

Bear, A., and Knobe, J. (2016). Normality: Part descriptive, part prescriptive. *Cognition*, 167, 25–37.

Berman, M. N. (2008). Punishment and justification. *Ethics*, 118(2), 258–290.

Berrios, G. E. (1991). Delusions as "wrong beliefs": A conceptual history. *British Journal of Psychiatry*, 159, 6–13.

Bertolotti, L., and Miyazono, K. (2015). Recent work on the nature and development of delusions. *Philosophy Compass*, 10(9), 636–645.

Bolton, D. (2008). *What is a mental disorder? An essay in philosophy, science, and values*. New York: Oxford University Press.

Bolton, D., and Gillett, G. (2019). *The biopsychosocial model of health and disease. New philosophical and scientific developments*. Cham, Switzerland: Palgrave Macmillan.

Bortolotti, L. (2010). *Delusions and other irrational beliefs*. Oxford, UK: Oxford University Press.

Bortolotti, L. (2018). Delusions and three myths of irrational belief. In L. Bertolotti (Ed.), *Delusions in context*. Birmingham, UK: Palgrave Macmillan.

Carnap, R. (1947). On the application of inductive logic. *Philosophy and Phenomenological Research*, 8(1), 133–148.

Catita, M., Águas, A., and Morgado, P. (2020). Normality in medicine: A critical review. *Philosophy, Ethics, and Humanities in Medicine*, 15(3), 1–6.

Chadwick, R. (2017). Normality as convention and as scientific fact. In Th. Schramme and S. Edwards (Eds.), *Handbook of the philosophy of medicine*. Dordrecht: Springer.

Clark, L. A. et al. (2017). Three approaches to understanding and classifying mental disorder: ICD-11, DSM-5 and the National Institute of Mental Health's Research Domain Criteria (RDoC). *Psychological Science in the Public Interest*, 18(2), 72–145.

Cohen, A. (2013). Kant on doxastic voluntarism and its implications for epistemic responsibility. *Kant Yearbook*, 5(1), 33–50.

Csukly, G. et al. (2011). Are patients with schizophrenia rational maximizers? Evidence from an ultimatum game study. *Psychiatry Research*, 187, 11–17.

Davis, L. J. (1995). *Enforcing normalcy*. London: Verso.

Dennett, D. (1995). *Darwin's dangerous idea: Evolution and the meanings of life*. New York: Simon & Schuster.

Dennett, D. C. (1979). Intentional systems. In D. C. Dennett (Ed.), *Brainstorms: Philosophical essays on mind and psychology*. Montgomery, VT: Bradford Books.

Dennett, D. C. (1987). True believers. In D. Dennett (Ed.), *The intentional stance*. Cambridge, MA: MIT Press.

Dennett, D. C. (1998). *Brainchildren: Essays on designing minds*. Cambridge, MA: MIT Press.

Dworkin, R. (2011). *Justice for hedgehogs*. Cambridge, MA: The Belknap Press of Harvard University Press.

Edmond, G. (2012). Is reliability sufficient? The Law Commission and expert evidence in international and interdisciplinary perspective (Part 1). *International Journal of Evidence and Proof*, 16(1), 30–65.

Edwards, C. (2009). Ethical decisions in the classification of mental conditions as mental illness. *Philosophy, Psychiatry, and Psychology*, 16(1), 73–90.

Foucault, M. (1961). *Folie et déraison. Historie de la folie à l'âge classique*. Paris: Plon.

Frierson, P. (2009a). Kant on mental disorder. Part 1: An overview. *History of Psychiatry*, 20(3), 267–289.

Frierson, P. (2009b). Kant on mental disorder. Part 2: Philosophical implications of Kant's account. *History of Psychiatry*, 20(3).

Gage v HM Advocate [2011] HCAJC 40, para 28.

Glenn, A. L., Ravi, I., Graham, J., Koleva, S., and Haidt, J. (2009). Are all types of morality compromised in psychopathy? *Journal of Personality Disorders*, 23(4), 384–398.

Golob, S. (2017). Kant and thought insertion. *Palgrave Communications*, 3(16108), 1–8.

Graham, J. (2002). Recent work in philosophical psychopathology. *American Philosophical Quarterly*, 39(2), 109–134.

Hacking, I. (1990). *The taming of chance*. Cambridge, MA: Cambridge University Press.

Haidt, J., and Graham, J. (2007). When morality opposes justice: Conservatives have moral intuitions that liberals may not recognize. *Social Justice Research*, 20(1), 98–116.

Halligan, P. W. Marshall, J. C., and Wade, D. T. (1995). Unilateral somatoparaphrenia after right hemisphere stroke: A case description. *Cortex*, 31, 173–182.

Hempel, C. G. (1965). Fundamentals of taxonomy. In C. G. Hempel (Ed.), *Aspects of scientific explanation and other essays in the philosophy of science*. New York: Free Press.

Horowitz, A. V. (2015). The normal pain of the social brain: Confusing depressive disorder with normal sadness. In R. K. Schutt, L. J. Seidman, and M. S. Keshavan (Eds.), *Social neuroscience: Brain, mind, and society*. Cambridge, MA: Harvard University Press.

Horowitz, A. V., and Wakefield, J. C. (2007). *The loss of sadness: How psychiatry transformed normal sorrow into depressive disorder*. New York: Oxford University Press.

Jaspers, K. (1963). *General psychopathology* (1913[1]) (J. Hoenig and M. W. Hamilton, trans.). Manchester: Manchester University Press.

Johnson, D. L. (1960). The moral judgment of schizophrenics. *The Journal of Nervous and Mental Disease*, 130(4), 278–285.

Johnson, S. C., and Elbogen, E. B. (2013). Personality disorders at the interface of psychiatry and the law: Legal use and clinical classification. *Dialogues in Clinical Neuroscience*, 15(2), 203–211.

Julian, M. V. (1970). The determinist's perspective of criminal responsibility. *Alberta Law Review*, 8(3), 376–388.

Kant, I. (1764/2007). Essay on the maladies of the head. In G. Zöller and R. B. Louden (Eds.), *The Cambridge edition of the works of Immanuel Kant in translation*. Cambridge, MA: Cambridge University Press.

Kant, I. (1798/2007). Anthropology from a pragmatic point of view. In G. Zöller and R. B. Louden (Eds.), *The Cambridge edition of the works of Immanuel Kant in translation*. Cambridge, MA: Cambridge University Press.

Kendell, R. E, et al. (1986). What are mental disorders? In A. M. Freedman, R. Brotman, I. Silverman et al. (Eds.), *Issues in psychiatric classification: Science, practice and social policy*. New York: Human Sciences Press.

Kennedy, H. G. (2005). Limits of psychiatric evidence in criminal cases: Morals and madness. *Medico-Legal Journal of Ireland*, 11(1), 1–17.

Kirgis, P. F. (2002). The problem of the expert juror. *Temple Law Review*, 75(3), 493–538.

Kirmayer, L. J., and Young, A. (1999). Culture and context in the evolutionary concept of mental disorder. *Journal of Abnormal Psychology*, 108(3), 446–452.

Kitcher, P. (2001). Real realism: The Galilean strategy. *The Philosophical Review*, 110(2), 151–159.

Kooijmans, T., and Meynen, G. (2017). Who establishes the presence of a mental disorder in defendants? Medicolegal considerations on a European Court of Human Rights Case. *Frontiers in Psychiatry*, 8(199), 1–6.

Lyre, H. (2018). Socially extended cognition and shared intentionality. *Frontiers in Psychology*, 9, Article 831.

Manwell, L. A. et al. (2015). What is mental health? Evidence towards a new definition from a mixed methods multidisciplinary international survey. *British Medical Journal Open*, 5, (6), 1–11.

Math, S. B., and Kumar, C. N., and Moirangthem, S. (2015). Insanity defense: Past, present, and future. *Indian Journal of Psychology and Medicine*, 37(1), 381–387.

McCormick, M. (2011). Taking control of belief. *Philosophical Explorations. An International Journal for the Philosophy of Mind and Action*, 14(2), 169–183.

McGuire, J., Langdon, R., and Brüne, M. (2014). Moral cognition in schizophrenia. *Cognitive Neuropsychiatry*, 19(6), 495–508.

Mitchell, C. N. (1986). Culpable mental disorder and criminal liability. *International Journal of Law and Psychiatry*, 6, 273–299.

Mitchell, E. W. (1999). Madness and meta-responsibility: The culpable causation of mental disorder and the insanity defence. *Journal of Forensic Psychiatry*, 10(3), 597–622.

Moore, M. S. (2009). *Causation and responsibility: An essay in law, morals, and metaphysics*. Oxford: Oxford University Press.
Morse, S. J. (2000). The moral metaphysics of causation and results. *California Law Review*, 88(3), 879–894.
Morse, S. J. (2007). The non-problem of free will in forensic psychiatry and psychology. *Behavioral Sciences and the Law*, 25(2), 203–220.
Morse, S. J. (2008). Determinism and the death of folk psychology: Two challenges to responsibility from neuroscience. *Minnesota Journal of Law Science & Technology*, (9)1, 19–34.
Morse, S. J. (2009). Against control tests for criminal responsibility. In P. H. Robinson, A. P. Garvey, and K. K. Ferzen (Eds.), *Criminal law conversation*. New York: Oxford University Press.
Morse, S. J. (2011). Mental disorder and criminal law. *The Journal of Criminal Law & Criminology*, 101(3), 884–968.
Morse, S. J. (2018). Mental disorder and criminal justice. *Faculty Scholarship at Penn Law*, 1751, 251–329.
Nicolson, D., and Auchie, D. P. (2017). Assessing witness credibility and reliability: Engaging experts and disengaging Gage? In P. R. Duff and P. R. Ferguson (Eds.), *Scottish criminal evidence law: Current developments and future trends*. Edinburg: Edinburgh University Press.
Nuevo, R. et al. (2012). The continuum of psychotic symptoms in the general population: A cross-national study. *Schizophrenia Bulletin*, 38(39), 475–485.
O'Reilly, K., O'Connell, P., O'Sullivan, D., Corvin, A., Sheerin, J., O' Flynn, P., . . . Kennedy, H. G. (2019). Moral cognition, the missing link between psychotic symptoms and acts of violence: A cross-sectional national forensic cohort study. *BMC Psychiatry*, 19(1), 1–24.
Putnam, H. (1992). *Renewing philosophy*. Cambridge, MA: Harvard University Press.
Putnam, H. (2002). *The collapse of the fact/value dichotomy and other essays*. Cambridge, MA: Harvard University Press.
Quine, W. V. (1969). Naturalized epistemology. In W. V. Quine (Ed.), *Ontological relativity and other essays*. New York: Columbia University Press.
Quine, W. V. (1987). *Quiddities: An intermittently philosophical dictionary*. Cambridge, MA: Harvard University Press.
Rai, T. S. Valdesolo, P., and Graham, J. (2017). Dehumanization increases instrumental violence, but not moral violence. *Proceedings of the National Academies of Sciences*, 114(32), 8511–8516.
Regier, D. A., Kuhl, E. A., and Kupfer, D. J. (2013). The DSM-5: Classification and criteria changes. *World Psychiatry*, 12, 92–98.
Reimer, M. (2010). Only a philosopher or a madman: Impractical delusions in philosophy and psychiatry. *Philosophy, Psychiatry, & Psychology*, 17(4), 315–328.
Roberts, A. (2012). Expert evidence on the reliability of eyewitness identification: Some observations on the justifications for exclusion: *Gage v HM Advocate*. *The International Journal of Evidence & Proof*, 16, 93–105.
Rose, D., Buckwalter, W., and Turri, J. (2014). When words speak louder than actions: Delusion, belief, and the power of assertion. *Australasian Journal of Philosophy*, 1–18.
Rössler, W. (2013). What is normal? The impact of psychiatric classification on mental health practice and research. *Frontiers in Public Health*, 1(68), 1–4.
Roux, E. (2018). Function, dysfunction, and normality in biological sciences. *Biological Theory*, 13(1), 17–28.
Santana, C. (2017). Why not all evidence is scientific evidence. *Episteme*. Cambridge University Press. www.cambridge.org/core.

Sass, L. (1994). *The paradoxes of delusion: Wittgenstein, Schreber and the schizophrenic mind.* Ithaca, NY: Cornell University Press.
Scheiner, S. M. (2004). Experiments, observations, and other kinds of evidence. In M. L. Taper and R. L. Subhash (Eds.), *The nature of scientific evidence: Statistical, philosophical, and empirical considerations.* Chicago: University of Chicago Press.
Schultze-Kraft, M., Birman, D., Rusconi, M., Allefeld, C., Görgen, K., Dähne, S., et al. (2016). The point of no return in vetoing self-initiated movements. *Proceedings of the National Academy of Science USA*, 113, 1080–1085.
Schurger, A., Mylopoulos, M., and Rosenthal, D. (2016). Neural antecedents of spontaneous voluntary movement: A new perspective. *Trends Cognitive Science*, 20, 77–79.
Scolten, M. (2016). Schizophrenia and moral responsibility: A Kantian essay. *Philosophia*, 44, 205–225.
Sifferd, K. L. (2006). In defense of the use of commonsense psychology in the criminal law. *Law and Philosophy*, 25, 571–612.
Singh, D., and Sinnott-Armstrong, W. (2015). The DSM-5 definition of mental disorder. *Public Affairs Quarterly*, 29(1), 5–31.
Sisti, D. A. (2012). Was Kant a normativist or naturalist for mental illness? *Journal of Ethics in Mental Helth*, 7, 1–7.
Spitzer, M. (1990). Kant on schizophrenia. In M. Spitzer and B. A. Maher (Eds.), *Philosophy and psychopathology.* New York: Springer Verlag.
Stein, D. J., Phillips, K. A., Bolton, D., Fulford, W. M., Sadler, J. Z., and Kendler, K. S. (2010). What is a mental/psychiatric disorder? From DSM-IV to DSM-V. *Psychological Medicine*, 40(11), 1759–1765.
Stone, A. A. (2008). The ethical boundaries of forensic psychiatry: A view from the ivory tower. *Journal of the American Academy of Psychiatry and the Law*, 36(2), 167–174.
Szasz, T. S. (1960). The myth of mental illness. *American Psychologist*, 15, 113–118.
Vecina, M. L., Marzana, D., and Paruzel-Czachura, M. (2015). Connections between moral psychology and intimate partner violence: Can IPV be read through moral psychology? *Aggression and Violent Behavior*, 22, 120–127.
Vincent, N. A. (2015). A compatibilist theory of legal responsibility. *Criminal Law, Philosophy*, 9, 477–498.
Wachbroit, R. (1994). Normality as a biological concept. *Philosophy of Science*, 61(4), 579–591.
Wakefield, J. C. (1992). The concept of mental disorder. On the boundary between biological facts and social values. *American Psychologist*, 47(3), 373–388.
Wakefield, J. C. (1999). Evolutionary versus prototype analyses of the concept of disorder. *Journal of Abnormal Psychology*, 108(3), 374–399.
Wakefield, J. C. (2000). Aristotle as sociobiologist: The 'function of a human being' argument, black box essentialism, and the concept of mental disorder. *Philosophy, Psychiatry, and Psychology*, 7, 17–44.
Wakefield, J. C. (2007). The concept of mental disorder: Diagnostic implications of the harmful dysfunction analysis. *World Psychiatry*, 6, 149–156.
Wakefield, J. C., and First, M. B. (2013). Clarifying the boundary between normality and disorder: A fundamental conceptual challenge for psychiatry. *The Canadian Journal of Psychiatry*, 58(11), 603–605.
Watson, D. (2005). Rethinking the mood and anxiety disorders: A quantitative hierarchical model for DSM-V. *Journal of Abnormal Psychology*, 114(4), 522–536.
White, M. D. (2012). Kantian moral psychology and criminal behaviour. *Journal of Criminal Psychology*, 2(1), 67–76.

Wilkinson, S. (2000). Is 'normal grief' a mental disorder? *The Philosophical Quarterly*, 50(200), 289–305.

Wischniewski, J., and Brüne, M. (2011). Moral reasoning in schizophrenia: An explorative study into economic decision making. *Cognitive Neuropsychiatry*, 16(4), 348–363.

Young, A. W. (1999). Cognitive theories of mental illness. *The Monist*, 82(4), 571–589.

10

THE DARK SIDE OF LANGUAGE

Valentina Cardella and Alessandra Falzone

1 Introduction

Language is one of the most remarkable features of human species. Nothing can compare its infinite possibilities of meaning, its combinatory potential, its capacity to invest and shape all other human activities. It allowed *Homo sapiens* to spread worldwide, to create tools, to use symbols and rituals, it made cumulative transmission possible, transformed our specific sociality, made us one of the most adaptive species in the history of evolution. Philosophers, linguists, psychologists, experts in artificial intelligence, ethologists, all have explored different aspects of human language, showing how the most complex system of communication dramatically contributes to the distinctiveness of the human species. But language is not a simple tool for communication. It has some distinctive and amazing power. Since the dawn of Western philosophy, language has been viewed as a sort of magic device: "speech is a powerful lord that with the smallest and most invisible body accomplishes most godlike works. It can banish fear and remove grief and instil pleasure and enhance pity", stated Gorgias more than 2000 years ago (1982: H8). Language is invisible, has no material body, but it can do miracles. And we experience its magic in our everyday life. Words make us laugh, cry, fall in love, move, scare, shake, they unite people and split them apart, build barriers and cancel them, create worlds and stories and make us believe them; in sum, language is one of the most powerful capacities mastered by the human brain.

But what would happen if language was affected by some sort of virus? A virus that doesn't damage the language's biological bases, like linguistic articulation (as in those syndromes resulting from brain damages), but a much higher level, more difficult to detect, which lies at the intersection of semantic and pragmatics capacities? In this case, language would not only be the host of the virus, but also be some sort of trigger for the spreading of the virus itself. The question could be regarded as bizarre, or specious. But here's an example of this strange kind of virus:

- How are you?
- To relate to people about new-found talk about statistical ideology. Er, I find that it's like starting in respect of ideology, ideals change, and ideals present ideology and new entertainments new, new attainments. And the more one talks about like, ideal totalitananism, or hotelatarianism, it's like you want new ideas to be formulated, so that everyone can benefit in mankind, so we can all live in our ideal heaven. Presumably that's what we still want, and with these ideas it can be brought about. I find the it's like a rose garden.

(McKenna and Oh, 2005: 43)

What happened to language in this example? We are not facing any alteration which affects the articulatory capacity, or the rules of grammar, or lexical and syntactical abilities. What is profoundly disturbed here, is the flow of speech, its coherence, its cohesion, and its meaning. And we can identify the virus that makes people talk this way: its name is schizophrenia.

In our chapter, we'll examine the impact that language has on this mental disorder. We claim that schizophrenia is, in a strong sense, a *linguistic experience*. Language plays a crucial role in this psychosis. It is directly involved, in that disorganized language is one of the most important features of schizophrenia, but it is also indirectly involved in the other distinctive schizophrenic symptoms: delusions and hallucinations. What we will try to show is that, in schizophrenia, language can short-circuit, and, in doing so, contribute to maintaining the mental disorder itself. In some sense, thus, schizophrenia can be viewed as a language's virus that shows the dark side of this remarkable feature of mankind.

2 Schizophrenic language

Schizophrenia is one of the most severe forms of mental disorder that involves a large series of symptoms affecting attention, language, perception, volition, affect, and behaviour. According to the DSM-V (APA, 2013), the common signs of schizophrenia are delusions, hallucinations, disorganized language, negative symptoms, and disorganized behaviour. Delusions are false beliefs, usually bizarre, which are not amenable of change in the light of conflicting evidence. Persecutory delusions are the most common. In some cases, delusions involve extraordinarily bizarre beliefs, e.g., having a completely see-through mind, with telepathically accessible thoughts, or having a microchip in the brain by which alien entities control what the subject says or does. From a linguistic point of view, delusions are particularly important; therefore, we will come back to this topic later in this chapter (see Section 4). The hallucinations are more common in the auditory form, and they are one of the most distressing symptoms of schizophrenia (patients can hear voices almost constantly). For their linguistic nature, hallucinations can reveal the importance of language in schizophrenia: this will be the topic of the last paragraphs.

The term 'disorganization' refers to a group of various symptoms that comprise disorganized speech and bizarre behaviour. In most cases, schizophrenic patients look clearly 'strange', because they behave in a bizarre, unusual, affected, unnatural way. They can display inappropriate affect (for example, laughing in sad circumstances), show unfitting social conduct (such as indecent exposure), put too many clothes on, not follow basic hygienic rules, be extremely agitated in unpredictable ways, or exhibit negative symptoms. Those symptoms involve a withdrawal of some functions or traits, as in anhedonia – the inability to experience pleasure; catatonia – motor immobility, and abulia – impaired ability to perform voluntary actions.

In disorganized speech, language changes in one of the most bizarre and peculiar way. Schizophrenia exhibits a specific cluster of linguistic features, including derailment, tangentiality, and incoherence, which represent the different ways schizophrenic people can lose track of conversations. Here's an example of disorganization:

> They're destroying too many cattle and oil just to make soap. If we need soap when you can jump into a pool of water, and then when you go to buy your gasoline, my folks always thought they should get pop, but the best thing to get is motor oil, and money. May totalitarianism as well go there and trade in some pop caps and, uh, tires, and tractors to car garages, so they can pull cars away from wrecks, is what I believed in.
>
> *(Andreasen, 1979: 1319–1320)*

The first observations on the peculiar way schizophrenic patients speak date back to Krapelin and Bleuler; the former, who is in every respect the father of the modern concept of schizophrenia, noted that in this disorder 'the train of thought does not progress at all in any one direction, but only wanders with numerous and bewildering digressions in the same general paths' (Kraepelin, 1913: 40), while the latter talked of a 'loosening of associations', which, by the way, he considered the basic disturbance of schizophrenia (Bleuler, 1950). Derailment, tangentiality, and loss of goal are the core expressions of disorganized speech: the links among the parts of discourse get weaker and weaker, the replies of the patient touch the topic for only a second, and then go on following unpredicted directions, the conversation drifts slowly away from the initial thread, and the subject seems completely unaware that she's going off the track (Cardella, 2017). Here's another example of this peculiar language:

P.: My mummy is very upset, yes. [laughs]
T.: Nothing to laugh about.
P.: No, yes, it's sad [laughs], it's sad the owl said, and it looked at his young and it was an owl itself.

T.: I didn't get that.

P.: It's sad the owl said, and it looked at his young and it was an owl itself. Don't you understand? I don't either anymore and I won't say it again, you know, I'm going to eat my apple to store vitamins for telling stories, otherwise I'll crumble to pieces.

(De Decker and Van de Craen, 1987: 252)

The most severe form of this disorganization is incoherence, where speech becomes almost incomprehensible, like in the following examples:

Lukewarm is real free, hot or cold-warm is false.

Lukewarm is false?

Lukewarm is real in a manhood. Hot isn't in a man, a woman uses cold. One, the Bible says, Revelation says, 'you're neither hot or cold, lukewarm'. That's the rewritten-wrote down all that suffer stuff an'all the plagues. I know who it was – Michael.

Michael?

Well, this friend of mine. He calls himself the arcmain. I call him the arcmain. He didn't know who he was. Didn't keep reminding himself. He fell. Jim James took over. He's more, ah, we call adequaa. He knows Jesse James.

(Carpenter, 1982: 562)

Moreover, there are other typical features which contribute to make the schizophrenic speech so bizarre and difficult to understand, that is, neologisms and paralogisms. Schizophrenics use the terms of their language with wide freedom: they can create new words (neologisms), and they can use existing words in an inappropriate way (paralogisms). Neologisms are usually created to express concepts linked to delusional or hallucinatory experiences: these are subjective events that patients need to convey through the invention of designated words. The neologism's use is therefore quite stable in schizophrenia, with the new word acquiring a permanent place in the patient's vocabulary. For example, Bleuler (1950) wrote of a patient who claimed that voices were brought to her by an 'aero-telephone'; Cummings and Mega (2003) reported a schizophrenic who used the word 'seisometer' to indicate a device behind his right eye that received and transmitted information; one patient analysed by Carpenter (1982) termed the voices emanating from his body *heart-voices*; another one called trafusion (*trafusione* in the original) the torture she suffered by hands of her relatives (Cardella, 2013). Paralogisms, on their hand, are due to unusual use of words; for instance, a patient used the term 'hill' to indicate a letter, another one called 'cuttlefish', a means of transport and 'fishing' his personal assets, and one more used 'suggestive' to mean caused by suggestion (Cardella, 2017). Words are employed privately, and there is no doubt that this kind of language, with this strange employ of words and the often bizarre neologisms, clearly affects the possibility to understand schizophrenic people, and contributes to creating a sense of extraneity between us, 'normal people', and 'them'.

We are beginning to see that language is an important part of schizophrenic disorder. But, of course, there are other disorders which involve language (brain disorders, degenerative illnesses, and so on), and this doesn't mean that language plays a peculiar role in them: it is only a secondary effect of the disease, that would remain more or less the same, independently from the linguistic side. But is this the case of schizophrenia? Is schizophrenia a disorder that has in language one of its striking aspects, nothing more?

To answer this question, we'll start considering the peculiar attitude schizophrenic patients have towards language. Their words seem to unveil that there is in language a powerful, almost magic dimension, which can yet turn into a dark side.

3 A hyper-reflexive attitude towards language

> What about a cougar? What would you associate a 'gar' with? What is a 'gar?' See this is what I'm telling you about these letters coming together. I separate them out. They indicate people's desires.
>
> *(Oltmanns, 1984: case n.3)*

Many authors noted that schizophrenic patients seem to show a hyper-reflexive attitude towards language, as if they were considering it an object of study, rather than a tool for communication (Goss, 2011). Tanzi (1905) was one of the first researchers who highlighted the cult that schizophrenics have for words and their special power; basing on this kind of 'from the outside' language's observation, individuals with schizophrenia begin to show idolatry for words, that are regarded as something sacred and enigmatic. Schizophrenic patients manipulate language, divide it into its different elements ('I separate them', like in the foregoing quotation), and can also adapt their behaviour to what the 'words' tells them. A famous example of this sort of 'linguistic oracle' is that of Lola Voss (Binswanger, 1957), a girl who was 'controlled' by language, since she used the unbundling of words (performed between two languages, Spanish and English) and the interpretation of the consequent message as a guide for action. For instance, when she was worried, watching someone putting his hand on his face had a relaxing effect on her, because face in Spanish is *cara*, that sounds like *care*, the second syllable of the Spanish word *mano* (hand in Spanish) is *no*, so the final result was *no care*, don't worry. Thus, the words guided her behaviour, building up a different reality.

By virtue of this peculiar attitude towards language, schizophrenic patients deconstruct it, manipulate it, find new ways to interpret it. As noted by Phillips, "the schizophrenic . . . becomes acutely aware of his or her own words or gestures as words or gestures, they suddenly reveal their nature as signs – or semiotic things" (2000: 19). This deep linguistic awareness leads to a paradoxical result: trapped in the language's world, fascinated by language games, schizophrenics lose the possibility to communicate something, in that the linguistic level detaches from reality and lives a life of its own, as in the following examples:

> What is contentment? Well, uh, contentment, well the word contentment, having a book perhaps, perhaps your having a subject, perhaps you have a chapter of reading, but when you come to the word "men" you wonder if you should be content with men in your life and then you get to the letter T and you wonder if you should be content having tea by yourself or be content with having it with a group and so forth.
>
> *(Lorenz, 1961: 604)*

> I don't like television, I would like the tele but not the vision, more the sion than the vi, because the vi reminds me of the letter V that is in the TV that means television and I don't like it.
>
> *(Piro, 1992: 44)*

The so-called *clanging* is one of the aspects involved; schizophrenic patients can rhyme, rather than talk, paying more attention to sound associations than to the meaning they want to convey:

> My mother's name was Bill. [pause] . . . and coo? St. Valentine's Day is the official startin' of the breedin' season of the birds. All buzzards can coo. I like to see it pronounced buzzards rightly. They work hard.
>
> *(Chaika, 1974: 260)*

> I'm not trying to make noise. I'm trying to make sense. If you can make sense out of nonsense, well, have fun. I'm trying to make sense out of sense. I'm not making sense (cents) anymore. I have to make dollars.
>
> *(Andreasen, 1979: 478)*

> Does water saunter? As to protein, might one tote-it-in? Is it a hydro-car-boat or a carbohydrate? As to any vitamin, might one invi- te-them-in? Is the dinner-all there with mineral? Is the bulk cellulose or the hulk swell-you-host? Might the medicine have met-us-some? Is it a platypus or adipose? Is the seasoning pleasing? Is food reserved to be preserved? Is one glad-to-give an additive?
>
> *(McKenna and Oh, 2005: 49)*

> Today is the day that I say March, April, and May without delay, if I may say. High-powered transmitters permitters me to know no way. Yesterday was a rain delay – a damp, lamp.
>
> *(Sacks, 2005: www.unc.edu/~sacksm/Schizhan.html)*

The parallel with poetic language must not be misleading: schizophrenics don't *choose* to talk this way. As noted by Chaika:

> Preoccupation with definition, abnormal rhyming, and inappropriate word associating have long been recognized as features of schizophrenic speech. In fact, typically they are the concern of poets. Of course, poets make these their concern by especially focusing on them. In their usual conversations, poets, like most people, ignore such features, or at least they do not allow them to interfere with the topic at hand in their surface utterances. The schizophrenic, however, does not seem to be able to suppress his notice of the features of words.
>
> *(Chaika, 1974: 269)*

In other words, in schizophrenia, differently from poetry, there is an *inability* to get beyond the signifier.

> only the symbol remains, but, because of the absence of its relation to the signified, it loses its true value as a signifier, a symbol. It is no longer anymore than an image taken for reality. The imaginary has become the real.
>
> *(Lemaire, 1970: 233)*

These observations accord to Freud's intuition that the strangeness of the symptom in schizophrenia is due to "the predominance of the word-relation over that of the thing" (Freud, 1915: 147)

The connection between schizophrenia and language is thus much narrower than one could think. Language in schizophrenia goes around in circles, devours itself, gets stuck preventing any possibility to mean something: a virus, then, that lies in language (and that it's impossible to imagine without language), and that doesn't infect language only, but the whole schizophrenic existence.

4 Nothing is exactly what it seems: the world of delusion

As already remarked, one of the main features of schizophrenia is delusion, that is, a false belief not amenable to change even in the light of conflicting evidence. For their bizarreness, and the peculiar obstinacy they are defended with, delusions have drawn the attention of all researchers since the origin of modern psychiatry. A wide range of literature focused on the most spectacular aspect of delusion, that is, the possibility to believe in impossible things, and the apparent lack of rationality that make delusional subjects hold their beliefs despite any contrary evidence. But there is another side of the delusion which often passes unnoticed: its linguistic side. In delusions too, language plays a crucial role, since words always tell something more, something different.

To clarify this point, we have to step backwards for a moment, to the early stages of delusions. Schizophrenic patients, before 'officially' entering the domain of delusion, often begin to perceive the world differently. External reality suddenly seems to have lost its familiarity, and objects, places, even people start looking unreal, creepy, frightening, enigmatic. More precisely, patients don't claim that things and people have changed from the perceptual point of view, rather than, whilst staying the same, all have changed in meaning. The pre-delusional atmosphere (the so-called Whanstimmung, cf. Jaspers, 1913) is primarily an overwhelming loss of meaning. Patients testify these early stages of delusion's linguistic side: they declare that the terms of language can't be read with their usual meaning, and that behind the words lie a hidden sense. They feel that the words' meaning has changed, but they don't know how to replace it. Someone even begins to think that people around him are speaking in code, rather than speaking the *normal* language (Timlett, 2011; Cardella, 2017), while other patients don't seem to recognize the usual references of the words, like this schizophrenic girl who complained that, when she saw a chair, or a pot, she didn't recognize their function, she didn't saw a chair to sit on, or a pot to hold water, "they had lost their name, their meaning, their function, they had become things" (Sechehaye, 1950: 55). This sense of unreality seems to be due to the pragmatics, semantic and affective components connected to the objects recognition. The meaning is suspended, and things, lacking a recognizable function, become mysterious and strange; patients attend to this event with unspeakable angst.

This loss of meaning regards people, too, who look like mannequins, automatons, or robots. The schizophrenic girl we just quoted reported to be frightened by her roommate because she looked inhuman (ivi: 165), like some sort of android, another one noted that, when she saw the face of someone, the face started to look weird, and she failed to find meaning in it (Kaysen, 1996: 43). This loss of meaning, which involves both things and people, and is often interpreted as if something terrible is going to happen, is thus perceived as extremely scary and threatening.

But when the world becomes unfamiliar and seems to gradually lose its meaning, where is it possible to recover what we are losing? The answer is easy: in the inner world. It comes as no surprise, then, that schizophrenic patients manage to get out from this insufferable state of suspension only when the delusional idea rises. The delusion comes when the loss of meaning is at its peak, and it reverses the condition, producing an *overload* of meaning. The delusional idea fixes the situation, and fills in everything with meaning: before, it was impossible to interpret anything, and now, everything becomes interpretable; before, every possibility to understand was suspended, and now, one understands everything. This world *suffused* with meaning is clearly described by this patient:

> Schizophrenia is a disease of information. And undergoing a psychotic break was like turning on a faucet to a torrent of details, which overwhelmed my life. In psychosis, nothing is what it seems. Everything exists to be understood beneath the surface. A bench remained a bench but who sat there became critical. Like irony, the casual exchange of words between a stranger or a friend meant something more than was being said. The movies, TV,

> and newspapers were alive with information for those who knew how to read. Without warning my world became suffused with meaning like light. In response, I felt as if I had been only half conscious before, as ignorant of reality as a small child. Although my sense of perception remained unaffected, everything I saw and heard took on a halo of meaning that had to be interpreted before I knew how to act. An advertising banner revealed a secret message only I could read. The layout of a store display conveyed a clue. A leaf fell and in its falling spoke: nothing was too small to act as a courier of meaning.
>
> *(Weiner, 2003: 877)*

As one could see, the condition is turned upside down, and the schizophrenic subject is suddenly overwhelmed by the meaning's dimension. Speeches mean more than what they literally say. Each conversation, even among strangers, is a clue to something, or refers to the subject.

> Additionally, I had begun to see hidden meanings in everything, from graffiti to architecture and to everyday speech. People in Ann Arbor were so intellectual that they used symbolic speech! This was a great discovery for me, and I henceforth began an attempt to discern what people actually were talking about behind their banal conversations. Initially, thinking this way was beneficial to me in my architecture classes, where one analyzed every little detail, but it soon led to great distortions when I began applying it to everyday life.
>
> *(Reina, 2010: 4)*

Eventually, each word seems to get a special meaning:

> When I half-heard a conversation in the distance or the honking of a car, I would think it held special significance for me. I would randomly open a dictionary and find a word ('die', 'liar', 'evil') and interpret how the word had special meaning for me.
>
> *(Chapman, 2002: 547)*

We can look to this phenomenon differently: the delusion prevents things to happen by chance, in that everything is connected. Delusional subjects spend the vast majority of their time decoding and interpreting every single gesture, every single word. The delusional belief is so powerful that it will enter all of the schizophrenics' conversations, it will dominate their thoughts and speeches with overwhelming strength. Thus, when asked to explain the idiomatic expression 'a drowning man will clutch at a straw', one patient, dominated from mystic delusions, answered: "Duh. Help! Is anyone going to save him. I could say I'm a drowning man right now. Anyone who asks for help. Ask and you shall receive. Seek and you shall find it. It all has to do with Christ" (McKenna and Oh, 2005: 14). A schizophrenic girl, who believed in magic, and was convinced that some of her college's teachers were witches, one day, sitting on the lobby of her college, saw a poster displaying students and saying "At the University of Michigan I learned of worlds that I had never known to exist", and immediately thought that "this was clear proof that magic, ie, the other worlds, existed" (Reina, 2010: 4). In the realm of delusion, the subject is overwhelmed from a flood of information, all concerning the subject's delusional idea, and all having the same importance. All speak, to whom who knows how to listen. Once again, it's hard to overrate the relevance of language; every single word, in delusions, is full of meaning, and each conversation, even the most trivial, has to be systematically over-interpreted. One way or another, the words pronounced by the others confirm to the patient the delusion's truth, confirm his belief to be persecuted, to be cheated, to be special, and there's no way out from this confirmatory cycle.

The delusion fills up with meaning the same reality which had become obscure and unfamiliar in the stages preceding the delusion. It is a private belief, impossible to share, but its massive capacity to signify fascinates the people who hold it. As reported by this patient:

> A note about becoming 'sane': medicine did not cause sanity; it only made it possible. Sanity came through a minute-by-minute choice of outer reality, which was often without meaning, over inside reality, which was full of meaning. Sanity meant choosing reality that was not real and having faith that someday the choice would be worth the fear involved and that it would someday hold meaning.
>
> *(Anon., 1992: 335)*

Thus, schizophrenia has strongly to do with language. The latter is specifically affected and transformed, and schizophrenic subjects show a peculiar attitude towards it: they manipulate it, play with it, and can also get trapped in a world of rhymes, associations, and linguistic games. In delusion, schizophrenic people usually overinterpret language, and each conversation, each word become full of meaning. It's time to show how language occurs in another important symptom of schizophrenia, that is, auditory hallucinations. We will focus on this feature in the next sections.

5 The language within: the phenomenon of inner speech

In the previous sections, we have discussed the role of language in the characterization of schizophrenia: schizophrenic language is disorganized, derailed, and, above all, is the cognitive trigger that the linguistic experience of the schizophrenic is built on. The reports and linguistic testimonies of schizophrenic experiences clearly express the power and fascination that language exerts on cognition and representation of the world. This relationship is evident in a very common aspect of the linguistic experience – inner speech, or internal dialogue. First, we will discuss this phenomenon, its characteristics, and its pervasiveness in everyday experience. Then we will illustrate the close connection between inner speech and one of the most obvious symptoms of schizophrenia: auditory verbal hallucinations (Rosen et al., 2018). Our aim is not to go fully into the debate on the mechanisms and functioning of inner speech, but to argue that inner speech is a genuine linguistic experience, which demonstrates the power of language over other cognitive processes. In this perspective, schizophrenia is the testing ground for the power of language.

Inner speech can be considered one of the most intimate and natural linguistic experiences. Each one of us has experiences of internal dialogue, although not always explicitly. At different times of the day, we find ourselves talking to ourselves in our minds. Some people experience inner speech while they are doing sports, or a cognitive task, meeting a friend, planning their day, or remembering an episode. Inner dialogue can also occur while resting (mind-wandering: Perrone-Bertolotti et al., 2014; see Irving and Glasser, 2020 for a philosophical approach) as a form of flow of thoughts not necessarily associated with external stimuli or other cognitive processes.

Basically, "human beings talk to themselves every moment of the waking day" (Baars, 2003: 7).

In both scientific and philosophical literature, it is often referred to as internal dialogue, inner language, inner speaking, self-talk, internal monologue (Morin et al., 2011). In general, inner speech can be defined as the ability of the subject to speak to himself in a silent manner (Geva and Warburton, 2018), in his/her own mind, in the absence of linguistic articulation (Alderson-Day and Fernyhough, 2015).

According to many authors, it is a central cognitive phenomenon, ubiquitous but poorly examined by classical cognitive psychology and cognitive neuroscience for two main reasons. First, it has complex relationships with other cognitive functions such as planning, reasoning, and problem-solving (Baldo et al., 2015); self-regulation and memory (Morin et al., 2011); self-motivation (Geva and Fernyhough, 2019); self-awareness (Morin, 2009, 2012); creativity (Smallwood and Schooler, 2014); consciousness and self-reflection (Alderson-Day and Fernyhough, 2015), to name but a few. Secondly, there are some methodological issues (Morin and Uttl, 2013; Fernyhough, 2008), mainly concerning the ecological validity of the quanti-qualitative tools for its evaluation (Hurlburt, 2011).

An interesting approach is proposed by Hurlburt and colleagues stating that inner speech "naturally occurs in natural situations" and it is a "pristine" phenomenon, i.e., "it naturally occurs before a specific attempt to alter it" (Hurlburt et al., 2013: 1480). For this reason, they proposed a qualitative method to describe pristine inner speech based on randomly sampled inner experience (Descriptive Experience Sampling) which does not include the manipulation by experimental procedures (Heavey and Hurlburt, 2008). According to Hurlburt et al. (2013), some aspects of the methodological issue on inner speech arise because of its ubiquity and importance and its several manifestations. In their study, sampling health college students, they reported five types of inner experience (inner speech, feelings, mental imagery, sensory awareness, and unsymbolized thinking). Some objections have been raised about this method, because it is not so clear if the methodology grasps the real nature of inner speech (Alderson-Day and Fernyhough, 2014), i.e., if this method assesses events that involve non-inner speech occurrences (Morin et al., 2011).

Nevertheless, researchers have identified the fundamental characteristics of inner speech, drawing on the phenomenology of this pervasive phenomenon. Inner speech is covert speech, i.e., it doesn't involve the voice but it can vary in pitch, frequency, type of voice, vividness (Wilkinson and Alderson-Day, 2016; Vilhaurer, 2017) just like the overt, but the way phonological/lexical characteristics emerge during inner speech varies from that of overt speech (see Oppenheim and Dell, 2008, but in contrast Corley et al., 2011). The quality of the inner voice can vary depending on the external context, the task in which the subject is involved, emotions, and direct or indirect reporting (Yao et al., 2015). Typically self-reported inner speech focuses on the speaker or people close to them (Morin et al., 2011) and the inner voice is attributed to the speaker her/himself (Rosen et al., 2018) as the agent of the internal speech attributed to the subjects that "produce" the voice (Gallagher, 2007).

Neuroscientists have investigated inner speech to describe its function with respect to overt speech and other cognitive processes. Inner speech neural processing involves overlapping areas in respect to those activated during overt speech (classical linguistic regions, i.e., Broca's and Wernicke's areas, inferior parietal lobule in the specialized left hemisphere), but inner speech and overt speech are not the same neural process. While overt speech elicits a greater activation of motor and premotor cerebral regions as compared to inner speech, covert speech involves other specific areas (left precentral gyrus, left middle frontal gyrus, left or right middle temporal gyrus, left superior frontal gyrus, right cingulate gyrus, left or right inferior parietal lobe, left dorsal frontal cortex, left parahippocampal gyrus, right cerebellum – see Perrone-Bertolotti et al., 2014 for a review).

Perrone-Bertolotti et al. (2014) reviewed neuroscientific studies comparing brain activations during overt speech and covert/inner speech conditions, observing that "inner speech seems to recruit some cerebral regions that are not recruited in overt speech. Some of these activations can be attributed to inhibition of overt responses or response conflict" (2014: 230). In fact, despite the first studies that seemed to incline towards a description of inner speech as overt speech without a motor component, the main research about the relationship between overt/covert speech rejects this impoverished view.

The most plausible proposal is that these areas involved exclusively in inner speech are part of an inhibition system (Wilkinson and Fernyhough, 2018) that allows control of internal functions by eliciting agency (see Corollary Discharge model, Frith, 2019; Subramanian et al., 2019). In a recent article, using electroencephalography (EEG) and functional near-infrared spectroscopy (fNIRS), Stephan and colleagues (2020) have demonstrated that the brain prepares overt and inner speech differently: their results are consistent with the hypothesis that a cerebral inhibitory mechanism works during inner speech.

The variability in the phenomenology of inner speech leads many authors to propose multi-component models to describe this process. Following Vygotskij's theory of functional language stages that consist of progressive processes of interiorization of language from open dialogue (infants), through private speech (verbalized dialogue with themselves as toddlers) to asymbolized and inaudible inner speech (adolescents) (Vygotskij, 1934–1987), Fernyhough (1996, 2008, 2009) has proposed a four-level model in which inner speech is the result of a progressive internalization process of dialogue. There is the first level (external dialogue) starting from the first sounds and consisting of overt dialogues with caregivers, a second level (private dialogue) during which children conduct an overt inner dialogue with themselves, gradually subvocalizing it, a third level (expanded inner speech) in which inner speech is completely internalized keeping its dialogical structure, and a fourth level (condensed inner speech), in which inner speech is characterized by the syntactic and semantic abbreviation in respect to overt or covert dialogic structure.

Inner speech is not simply a stage of our language development but a modality through which we construct our inner life and consequently our experience (Lœvenbruck, 2018).

How is inner speech linked to experience? Several scholars, philosophers as well as psychologists have questioned the nature of inner speech. As we have seen previously, inner speech has several characteristics, the main one being that in the vast majority of cases, it has a content, that is, it refers to a part of the experience. Although there is much debate on the intentional or unintended nature of our inner speech (see Irving and Glasser, 2020), several authors agree with the idea that inner speech is about an experience of the world. Whether in its condensed or extended form, the 'interior monologue' refers to some form of experience in the world (abstract or concrete, lived or future). In essence, inner speech "is something that we do, and which we have an experience of" (Wilkinson and Fernyhough, 2018: 2).

In this way, inner speech is a cognitive tool through which we experience our (internal and external) 'world knowledge' (Hagoort et al., 2014; Falzone, 2016). Inner speech, therefore, is considered a form of eminently linguistic experience, not in the sense of verbal content (we are not referring to how "mental sentences" are constructed or the accuracy with which the utterances of inner speech are expressed), but in the sense of linguistic-representational content. Although inner and overt speech are not super-imposable processes, many studies show that inner speech is an eminently linguistic process. But the sense of this characterization is not so immediate.

The experience level which we refer to is not simply that of motor practice or motor simulation, but the representational level. For instance, Netsell and Bakker (2017) showed that the inner speech in people who stutter is reported as fluent even though their vocalized speech presents many word-order and word-onset errors. Researchers have investigated inner speech in non-hearing subjects to comprehend if they have inner speech and the possible form it has. Wilson and Emmorey (1998) have shown that Sign Language is processed on the basis of its articulatory properties rather than its visual-gestural modality, supporting a multimodal characterization of inner speech in the deaf. Other studies conducted with neuroscientific methods have argued for similarity in circuits underpinning inner speech in hearing and non-hearing subjects (McGuire et al., 1997). According to Wilkinson and Fernyhough (2018), an experience of inner speech represents an interior linguistic act and it concerns the mental state expressed by that linguistic act and, consequently, it concerns the individual possessor of that mental state, that is, the speaker: thus when one asserts something in inner speech, the conscious experience of that represents their belief in what they have asserted, and, somewhat trivially, represents it as belonging to them. This much can also be said about hearing someone (oneself or someone else) sincerely assert something in outer speech (Wilkinson and Fernyhough, 2018).

Another example of the linguistic nature in the sense of linguistic cognition is represented by the experience of voices in the reports of profoundly deaf people: the profoundly deaf, even the congenitally deaf, report hearing voices in their heads. Such voices can comment positively, they can be reassuring, or they can constitute a negative experience. Hallucinations are also present in the deaf population, as demonstrated by numerous studies. What researchers have questioned is whether the voice reported by the profoundly deaf with hallucinations is a type of experience similar to that experienced by people who are not deaf. Some scholars argue that these are non-auditory experiences and that the representation of these hallucinations is actually not auditory, but multimodal: when the deaf hallucinate voices, they actually hallucinate multimodal experiences.

Yet, in numerous detailed reports, deaf signing people with hallucinations describe having clearly audible hallucinatory experiences, although they declared themselves to be (and were) completely deaf (du Feu and McKenna, 1999). According to Atkinson (2006), in reality these are not voices but messages without a defined agent. It is still unclear whether hallucinatory voices experienced by deaf people are the result of motor mechanisms' activation (given the iconic-visual nature of sign language gestures). What appears evident from the reports is that hallucinations are experienced as linguistic information that conditions the subject's experience and describes it.

This data enables us to formulate two observations: the first, inner speech is a cognitive phenomenon that must be investigated by adopting a method that takes into account the first-person perspective (Fernyhough, 2016). The reports of people who hear voices have provided essential information both for the structuring of experimental protocols and for the formulation of theoretical models relating to the functioning of inner speech and the cognitive abilities with which it is connected. The second, the essential phenomenological aspect that characterizes inner speech is the voices. This phenomenon, as we have described previously, can be both positive and negative. The voices in one's head can play a fundamental role in daily experience, just as they can prove to be a danger when such voices are not recognized as being owned by the person who experienced them. And this is the case with some psychopathologies, schizophrenia in particular.

6 The power of language: schizophrenia and inner speech

The voice we hear in our head is our voice. It can have different verbal characteristics and vary in tone, it can be expressed in the form of a syntactically correct utterance and be explained in its entirety or it can be condensed, elliptical. It may rehearse the voice of someone we know, but in any case this voice is perceived as originating from ourselves. Numerous studies have tried to understand why the vast majority of healthy people hear voices in their heads. A proposed distinction concerns the difference between the experience of speaking to oneself (as self-speaker) and the experience of listening to a voice in one's head (as self-listener). There is no agreement on how the two processes are connected (which may also involve partially different neural systems), or if in reality it is a single process (inner speech) modulated through different perceptual pathways. What the studies converge on is the perception of the voice's agency: whether it is a sort of one's own 'dematerialized' and condensed voice, or whether it is a form of memory, not necessarily faithful, to a heard voice, but the voice is considered to belong to the subject who perceives it. In some cases, this attribution is not so obvious, as in auditory verbal hallucinations (AVHs). An increasing number of studies demonstrate that this phenomenon can be interpreted as a form of modification of the normal process of attributing inner speech to oneself. As we have described in the previous sections, AVHs are a telltale symptom of psychosis, particularly schizophrenia. As Fernyhough (2014: 1090) stated "if schizophrenia is, as in Thomas Szasz's coinage, the 'sacred symbol of psychiatry', then this [AVH] is the sacred symbol of the sacred symbol". AVHs are the main clinical feature of schizophrenia, manifesting in hearing a voice (or voices) that judges the patient's behaviour, encourages him to carry out actions, or offends him. AVHs are sometimes so upsetting and pervasive for the patient's existence that the patient feels 'lived by another' (Fernyhough, 2016).

AVHs have characterized schizophrenic disorder since its first definitions (Bleuler, 1950) and reveal a very high diagnostic value (Cardella, 2017). There are various hypotheses about the cause of this symptom. One of the most accredited assigns these AVHs in schizophrenics to a deficit in monitoring their own actions. According to Frith (2019), the AVHs are a consequence of the modification of the functioning of the cognitive system that controls self-produced actions. This system monitors whether the actions are produced by the subject or if they come from outside, preventing the subject from perceiving his actions as performed by others (see Blakemore et al., 2000). Self-talk, that is the language produced and directed to oneself, also falls within this system. When we produce inner speech, the areas of language involved in the process of producing language aloud are activated and send an efference copy to the part of the auditory cortex responsible for decoding language. This message alerts the areas that decode the linguistic message that respond with a lower intensity of activation than that required for the understanding of external verbal productions.

It is as if this efference copy 'attenuated' the decoding activity of linguistic areas (Ford and Mathalon, 2004; Whitford et al., 2011). In this way, the monitoring of one's inner speech activity would be achieved: the inhibitory message sent from the Broca area (responsible for linguistic coding) through the arched file would immediately reach the Wernicke area (responsible for linguistic decoding) therefore inhibiting its activation. Thus, our brain processes the voice produced by the Broca area as an internal voice.

According to this hypothesis, AHVs in schizophrenic subjects are produced by a change in the inner speech control system. It seems that schizophrenic patients have unusual patterns of connectivity between the frontal regions (in which the Broca area is located) and the temporal regions (in which the Wernicke area is located). Such patterns modify the communication from the frontal to the temporal lobe, so the schizophrenic subject perceives the internal voices as produced by someone else, or in any case as not belonging to himself (for a discussion, see Parlikar et al., 2019). Several objections have been raised to this model, most of which derive from the nature of the control system (mainly motor or in any case connected to the action). Other scholars, for example, argue that inner speech is the product of functional connectivity activated during the resting state (default mode network). In patients with schizophrenia, the normal DMN is hyperactivated in respect to controls both in speech perception and in verbal thought generation (Rapin et al., 2012; Perrone-Bertolotti et al., 2014).

Also, in this case, various objections have been raised regarding the methodologies used to investigate the mind-wandering state. To date, not enough evidence has been collected to support one of these hypotheses exclusively, but in the last 30 years, research in psychiatry has considered inner speech as a raw material for auditory verbal hallucinations. Let us consider two elements: AVHs can also occur in non-psychotic subjects (Larøi, 2012). In this case, the experience is equally upsetting, but typically the subject considers that experience to be an alteration, an experience that is not part of everyday life and is linked to contingent situations (such as substance abuse). Furthermore, in the phenomenological field, there is a copious amount of literature in which healthy persons report hearing voices, often comforting or encouraging, as in the case of those who practice sports that require constant concentration but motor activity only at certain times or in writers (in literature these subjects are identified with the term voice-hearer, see Fernyhough, 2016).

If we look at the experiential level, several elements suggest that the experience of voices is not only associated with moments of psychotic alteration, prompting researchers to describe the experiences of voices as a continuum: schizophrenia is placed at an extreme where interior linguistic experiences are experienced as belonging to another rather than oneself.

In this perspective, internal voices constitute the testing ground of the cognitive power of language. The studies we have discussed previously assign the role of raw material for AVHs to internal language. In the perspective we have offered, inner speech is an essential phenomenon for the construction of the self, connected with many other cognitive processes. Carruthers (2002, 2018) argues that language, and in particular inner speech, is a process that holds together domains of cognition that would otherwise be separate.

Reflecting on the role of language in human cognition and in relation to other cognitive processes, Carruthers formulates an idea of inner language "as a mental lingua franca: a medium for representing items of information drawn from distinct domain-specific modules in the brain" (Nelson, 2002: 694). Without this process, the outputs of cognitive activities will remain autonomous, separated, "disconnected", and "fragmentary". Accordingly, Wilkinson and Fernyhough (2018) stated that inner speech is a fundamental process for self-knowledge, the way everyone reflects on (and constructs) her/himself. Inner speech, therefore, is a constructor of ipseity, which, in the schizophrenic subject, is modified, different, other (Sass and Parnas, 2003).

The voices in the heads of schizophrenics communicate with each other using the same mechanisms of vocal speech, generating a sense of external agency that in healthy persons corresponds to themselves. Often schizophrenic subjects listen to the speech of their own voices and analyse them in content, pragmatic adequacy and in relation to their own self. This analysis does not concern the formal and syntactic correctness of the utterances of the internal voices, but their very presence. Schizophrenics hear internal voices as third entities that invade their mental life, although they are often aware that such voices can only be a product of their own mind. Adam, one of the voice-hearers of the "Hearing the Voice" project (Fernyhough, 2014), when interviewed about the difference between his ordinary thoughts and his voices, he answered:

> It becomes so confusing when you have it for so long. You're talking to yourself, but you're getting a response. You're talking to yourself, but you're getting asked questions. Which can be very difficult, because say if you think of something, you aren't sure if it's you who's thinking it. . . . I have another person living inside my head. . . . It isn't me, but it is me.
>
> *(Fernyhough, 2016: 270)*

The disorientation that the experience of voices causes in the existence of schizophrenics is often connected with a consequent detachment from reality that leads the subjects to question themselves about what is more natural, what a healthy subject usually takes for granted: who is thinking what it's on my mind? Is it me or is it someone else? This tendency is called hyper-reflexivity, i.e., a form of exaggerated awareness of "oneself that would normally remain in the background of awareness" (Sass, 2014: 369; Stephensen and Parnas, 2018; see also the chapter by Pennisi and Gallagher in this book). Sass (2014) outlines how the schizophrenic usually observes his own inner world from the outside, and his own language as an object of alien reflection (see also Goss, 2011). This determines the break with the world and the belief that others cannot understand what is inside their lived life.

It could then be hypothesized that the schizophrenic's internal linguistic life consists only of voices. But is the inner speech of schizophrenics made up exclusively of voices? Several studies have shown that patients can distinguish their own voice from that produced by others and their thoughts. Thus, patients know that hallucinated voices, however similar they may be to those produced by themselves (inner speech) or heard externally during a conversation, are something else (Leudar and Thomas, 2000).

Voices are perceived as real as people, but the subject is aware that they do not have a body, they are voices that live within their soul (Fernyhough, 2016). Schizophrenics may have a clear perception that voices inhabit their body, they are not external voices of someone who utters them. The awareness of this third party of hallucinated voices has prompted researchers to wonder why, once such awareness is achieved, the voices are still retained. Often, in the experience of the schizophrenic, even after therapy, the voices remain present, continue to talk to each other, and the schizophrenic chooses not to feed them. Some reports also indicate a certain ability to control the situations and topics on which the voices intervene. For example, Garrett and Silva report the case of a patient who hears the voice of a child in a 2003 study. They describe this patient during a clinical assessment who claimed that the child's voice was real only when the patient was in a condition of emotional need; "she hesitated to say the baby was real because she said she would then have to worry about its need for care. They quoted the patient as saying "she's like my imaginary baby. She's real to me in some senses. I love her" (Garrett and Silva, 2003: 450). She "calls" the baby real only when this served her emotional needs.

Patients try to experiment on their own if the voices they hear are real. They question them and test them, thus confirming their real existence and their importance within the patient's cognitive life. Experiences such as those described previously show that the schizophrenic subject's inner speech is one of the elements in maintaining the voices themselves. The different way of constructing one's inner speech for schizophrenics is as painful and tiring as it is powerful. According to the analysis of phenomenological psychiatry, schizophrenics idolize words, they consider them something sacred (Pfersdorff, 1935). If we consider inner speech as a proof that language is a cognitive tool that allows one to build their inner life and organize it thoroughly, then schizophrenic voices are the proof of this exponential power.

8 Conclusion

We started this chapter stating the importance of language for the human species. It allows us to communicate in very sophisticated ways, but its power is terrific, since language is much more than just a tool for communication. Schizophrenia turns the power of language into its dark side. The metalinguistic function, one of the most brilliant and exclusive features of human language, where the language is used to talk about language itself, in schizophrenia is pushed to extreme consequences, in that the linguistic level detaches from reality and lives a life of its own. Thanks to language, we can convey meaning. But, in schizophrenia, the process of interpreting becomes potentially infinite, with devastating effects. Each word, each piece of conversation, as trivial as it may be, gets full of meaning, and means always something more. In delusion, this over-interpreting activity is directed to only one direction: the delusional belief. Finally, language accompanies us in all our activities, with an inner dialogue that helps us to plan our activities, solve problems, and build our self-image. In schizophrenia, the inner speech becomes something external, that the subject doesn't recognize anymore, and it starts haunting the patient, harassing her with endless voices.

And maybe this is the way to describe the linguistic experience of this mental disorder: schizophrenic patients, in different ways, are haunted by language, and show us its dark, dangerous, and even frightful side.

Authors contribution

For the specific constraints of the Italian Academy, we specify that Valentina Cardella wrote Sections 1, 2, 3, 4, and 8; Alessandra Falzone wrote Sections 5, 6, 7 and 8.

References

Alderson-Day, B., and Fernyhough, C. (2014). More than one voice: Investigating the phenomenological properties of inner speech requires a variety of methods. Commentary. *Consciousness and Cognition*, 24, 113–114.

Alderson-Day, B., and Fernyhough, C. (2015). Inner speech: Development, cognitive functions, phenomenology, and neurobiology. *Psychological Bulletin*, 141, 931–965.

American Psychiatric Association (APA). (2013). *Diagnostic and statistical manual of mental disorders* (5th ed.). Washington, DC: American Psychiatric Association.

Andreasen, N. C. (1979). Thought, language, and communication disorders I. *Archives of General Psychiatry*, 36, 1315–1321.

Anon. (1992). Portrait of a schizophrenic. *Schizophrenia Bulletin*, 18(2), 333–336.

Atkinson, J. R. (2006). The perceptual characteristics of voice-hallucinations in deaf people: Insights into the nature of subvocal thought and sensory feedback loops. *Schizophrenia Bulletin*, 32, 701–708.

Baars, B. J. (2003). How brain reveals mind. Neural studies support the fundamental role of conscious experience. *Journal of Consciousness Studies*, 10(9–10), 100–114.

Baldo, J. V., Paulraj, S. R., Curran, B. C., and Dronkers, N. F. (2015). Impaired reasoning and problem-solving in individuals with language impairment due to aphasia or language delay. *Frontiers in Psychology*, 6, 1523.

Binswanger, L. (1957). *Der Fall Lola Voss. Studien zum Schizophrenie Problem*. Pfullingen: Verlag Neske.

Blakemore, S. J., Smith, J., Steel, R., Johnstone, C. E., and Frith, C. D. (2000). The perception of self-produced sensory stimuli in patients with auditoryhallucinations and passivity experiences: Evidence for a breakdown in self-monitoring. *Psychological Medicine*, 30(5), 1131–1139.

Bleuler, E. (1950). *Dementia praecox or the group of schizophrenias* (J. Zinkin and N. D. C. Lewis, trans.). New York: International University Press.

Cardella, V. (2013). *Perdersi nei giochi linguistici. Schizofrenia, filosofia del linguaggio e scienze cognitive*. Roma: Corisco.

Cardella, V. (2017). *Language and schizophrenia: Perspectives from psychology and philosophy*. London: Routledge.

Carpenter, K. (1982). Neologisms in 'word salad': How schizophrenic speakers make themselves misunderstood. In *Proceedings of the eighth annual meeting of the Berkeley Linguistics Society* (pp. 562–571). Berkley, CA: The Berkley Linguistics Society.

Carruthers, P. (2002). The cognitive functions of language. *Behavioural and Brain Sciences*, 25(6), 657–725.

Carruthers, P. (2018). The causes and the contents of inner speech. In P. Langland-Hassen and A. Vincente (Eds.), *Inner speech: New voices*. Oxford Scholarship Online. https://doi.org/10.1093/oso/9780198796640.003.0002.

Chaika, E. (1974). A linguist looks at schizophrenic language. *Brain and Language*, 1, 257–276.

Chapman, R. K. (2002). First person account: Eliminating delusions. *Schizophrenia Bulletin*, 28, 3, 545–553.

Corley, M., Brocklehurst, P. H., and Moat, H. S. (2011). Error biases in inner and overt speech: Evidence from tongue twisters. *Journal of Experimental Psychology on Learning Memory and Cognition*, 37(1), 162–175.

Cummings, J. L., and Mega, M. S. (2003). *Neuropsychiatry and behavioral neurosciences*. Oxford: Oxford University Press.

De Decker, B., and Van de Craen, P. (1987). Towards an interpersonal theory of schizophrenia. In R. Wodak and P. Van de Craen (Eds.), *Neurotic and psychotic language behavior*. Clevedon: Multilingual Matters.

du Feu, M., and McKenna, P. J. (1999). Prelingually profoundly deaf schizophrenic patients who hear voices: A phenomenological analysis, *Acta Psychiatrica Scandinavica*, 99, 453–459.

Falzone, A. (2016). Neurocerebral foundamentals. In A. Pennisi and A. Falzone (Eds.), *Darwinian biolinguistics: Theory and history of a naturalistic. Philosophy of language and pragmatics*. Cham: Springer.

Fernyhough, C. (1996). The dialogic mind: A dialogic approach to the higher mental functions. *New Ideas in Psychology*, 14, 47–62.

Fernyhough, C. (2008). Getting Vygotskian about theory of mind: Mediation, dialogue, and the development of social understanding. *Developmental Review*, 28, 225–262.

Fernyhough, C. (2009). Dialogic thinking. In A. Winsler, C. Fernyhough, and I. Montero (Eds.), *Private speech, executive functioning, and the development of verbal self-regulation*. Cambridge: Cambridge University Press.

Fernyhough, C. (2014). Hearing the voice. *Lancet*, 384, 1090–1091.

Fernyhough, C. (2016). *The voices within: The history and science of how we talk to ourselves*. London: Profile Books Ltd.

Ford, J. M., and Mathalon, D. H. (2004). Electrophysiological evidence of corollary discharge dysfunction in schizophrenia during talking and thinking. *Journal of Psychiatric Research*, 38(1),37–46.

Freud, S. (1915). The unconscious. In P. Rief (Ed.), *The collected paper of Sigmund Freud: General psychological theory*. New York: MacMillan Publishing Company.

Frith, C. D. (2019). Can a problem with corollary discharge explain the symptoms of schizophrenia? *Biological Psychiatry of Cognitive Neuroscience and Neuroimaging*, 4(9), 768–769.
Gallagher, S. (2007). Sense of agency and higher-order cognition: Levels of explanation for schizophrenia. *Cognitive Semiotics*, 32–48.
Garrett, M., and Silva, R. (2003). Auditory hallucinations, source monitoring, and the belief that "voices" are real. *Schizophrenia Bulletin*, 29(3), 445–457.
Geva, S., and Fernyhough, C. (2019). A penny for your thoughts: Children's inner speech and its neuro-development. *Frontiers in Psychology*, 10, 1708.
Geva, S., and Warburton, E. A. (2018). A test battery for inner speech functions. *Archives of Clinical Neuropsychology*, 34(1), 97–113.
Gorgias. (1982). *Encomium of Helen* (BCP Greek Texts) (D. M. Macdowell, trans.). London: Bristol Classical Press.
Goss, J. (2011). Poetics in schizophrenic language: Speech, gesture and biosemiotics. *Biosemiotics*, 4, 291–307.
Hagoort, P., Hald, L., Bastiaansen, M., and Petterson, K. M. (2014). Integration of word meaning and world knowledge in language comprehension. *Science*, 304, 5669, 438–441.
Heavey, C. L., and Hurlburt, R. T. (2008). The phenomena of inner experience. *Consciousness and Cognition*, 17(3), 798–810.
Hurlburt, R. T. (2011). *Investigating pristine inner experience: Moments of truth*. Cambridge: Cambridge University Press.
Hurlburt, R. T., Heavey, C. L., and Kelsey, J. M. (2013). Toward a phenomenology of inner speaking. *Consciousness and Cognition*, 22, 1477–1494.
Irving, Z. C., and Glasser, A. (2020). Mind-wandering: A philosophical guide. *Philosophical Compass*, 2020(15), e12644.
Jaspers, K. (1913). *Allgemeine psychopathologie*. Berlin: Springer Verlag.
Kaysen, S. (1996). *Girl, interrupted*. New York: Vintage Books.
Kraepelin, E. (1913). *Dementia praecox and paraphrenia*. Edinburgh: Livingstone.
Larøi, F. (2012). How do auditory verbal hallucinations in patients differ from those in non-patients? *Frontiers in Human Neuroscience*, 6, 25.
Lemaire, A. (1970). *Jacques Lacan*. London: Routledge.
Leudar, I., and Thomas, P. (2000). *Voices of reason, voices of insanity: Studies of verbal hallucinations*. London: Routledge.
Lœvenbruck, H. (2018). What the neurocognitive study of inner language reveals about our inner space. *Epistémocritique, épistémocritique: littérature et savoirs*. Langage intérieur – Espaces intérieurs/Inner Speech – Inner Space, 18. hal-0203966.
Lorenz, M. (1961). Problems posed by schizophrenic language. *Archives of General Psychiatry*, 4, 603–610.
McGuire, P., Robertson, D., Thacker, A., David, A. S., Kitson, N., Frackowiak, R. S., et al. (1997). Neural correlates of thinking in sign language. *Neuroreport*, 8, 695–698.
McKenna, P. J., and Oh, T. (2005). *Schizophrenic speech: Making sense of bathroots and ponds that fall in doorways*. Cambridge: Cambridge University Press.
Morin, A. (2009). Self-awareness deficits following loss of inner speech: Dr. Jill Bolte Taylor's case study. *Consciousness and Cognition*, 18, 524–529.
Morin, A. (2012). *Inner speech encyclopedia of human behavior* (pp. 436–443). Cambridge: Academic Press.
Morin, A., and Uttl, B. (2013). Inner speech: A window into consciousness. *The Neuropsychotherapist*. https://doi.org/10.12744/tnpt.14.04.2013.01
Morin, A., Uttl, B., and Hamper, B. (2011). Self-reported frequency, content, and functions of inner speech. *Procedia – Social and Behavioral Sciences*, 30, 1714–1718.

Nelson, K. (2002). Developing dual-representation processes. *Behavioral and Brain Sciences*, 25(6), 693–694. https://doi.org/10.1017/S0140525X02430129

Netsell, R., and Bakker, K. (2017). *Fluent and dysfluent inner speech of persons who stutter*. Springfield, MO: Missouri State University.

Oltmanns, T. (1984). Schizophrenic disorders: Case #3. In C. Lamar (Director), *Psychopathology: Diagnostic vignettes* [Videocassette]. Bloomington: Radio and Television Services of Indiana University.

Oppenheim, G. M., and Dell, G. S. (2008). Inner speech slips exhibit lexical bias, but not the phonemic similarity effect. *Cognition*, 106, 528–537.

Parlikar, R., Bose, A., and Venkatasubramanian, G. (2019). Schizophrenia and corollary discharge: A neuroscientific overview and translational implications. *Clinical and Psychopharmacological Neurosciences*, 17(2), 170–182.

Perrone-Bertolotti, M., Rapin, L., Lachauxc, J.-P., Baciua, M., and Lœvenbruck, H. (2014). What is that little voice inside my head? Inner speech phenomenology, its role in cognitive performance, and its relation to self-monitoring. *Behavioural and Brain Research*, 261, 220–239.

Pfersdorff, C. (1935). Les catégories du langage aphasique et la dissociation schizophrénique. *Annales of Medical Psychologie*, 93.

Phillips, J. (2000). Peirceian reflections on psychotic discourse. In J. Muller and J. Brent (Eds.), *Peirce, semiotics, and psychoanalysis*. Baltimore and London: The Johns Hopkins University Press.

Piro, S. (1992). *Parole di follia*. Milano: Franco Angeli.

Rapin, L., Dohen, M., Loevenbruck, H., Whitman, J. C., Metzak, P., Woodward, T. (2012). Hyperintensity of functional networks involving voice-selective cortical regions during silent thought in schizophrenia. *Psychiatry Research: Neuroimaging*, 202, 110–117.

Reina, A. (2010). The spectrum of sanity and insanity. *Schizophrenia Bulletin*, 36(1), 3–8.

Rosen, C., McCarthy-jones, S., Chase, K. A., Humpston, C. S., Melbourne, J. K., Kling, L., and Sharma, R. P. (2018). The tangled roots of inner speech, voices and delusions. *Psychiatry Research*, 264, 281–289. https://doi.org/10.1016/j.psychres.2018.04.022

Sacks, M. (2005). *Examples of delusions and disorganization of thinking and speech*. www.unc.edu/~sacksm/Schizhan.html.

Sass, L. A. (2014). Explanation and description in phenomenological psychopathology. *Journal of Psychopathology*, 20, 366–376.

Sass, L. A., and Parnas, J. (2003). Schizophrenia, consciousness, and the self. *Schizophrenia Bulletin*, 29(3), 427–444.

Sechehaye, M. (1950). *Journal d'une schizophrène*. Paris: Presses universitaires de France.

Smallwood, J., and Schooler, J. (2014). The science of mind wandering: Empirically navigating the stream of consciousness. *Annual Review of Psychology*, 66. https://doi.org/10.1146/annurev-psych-010814-015331

Stephan, F., Saalbach, H., and Rossi, S. (2020). The brain differentially prepares inner and overt speech production: Electrophysiological and vascular evidence. *Brain Science*, 10, 148.

Stephensen, H., and Parnas, J. (2018). What can self-disorders in schizophrenia tell us about the nature of subjectivity? A psychopathological investigation. *Phenomenological and Cognitive Sciences*, 17, 629–642.

Subramanian, D., Alers, A., and Sommer, M. A. (2019). Corollary discharge for action and cognition. *Biological Psychiatry: Cognitive Neuroscience and Neuroimaging*, 4(9), 782–790.

Tanzi, E. (1905). *Trattato delle malattie mentali*. Milano, Napoli, Roma: Società editrice libraria.

Timlett, A. (2011). Language games, paranoia and psychosis. *Schizophrenia Bulletin*, 37(6), 1099–1100.

Vilhaurer, R. P. (2017). Characteristics of inner reading voices. *Scandinavian Journal of Psychology*, 58, 269–274.

Vygotskij, L. S. (1934–1987). Thinking and speech. In R. W. Rieber and A. S. Carton (Eds.), *The collected works of L. S. Vygotskij*, Vol. 1. New York: Plenum, 1987 (original work published in 1934).

Weiner, S. K. (2003). First person account: Living with the delusions and effects of schizophrenia. *Schizophrenia Bulletin*, 29(4), 877–879.

Whitford, T., Mathalon, D., Shenton, M., Roach, B., Bammer, R., Adcock, R., . . . and Ford, J. (2011). Electrophysiological and diffusion tensor imaging evidence of delayed corollary discharges in patients with schizophrenia. *Psychological Medicine*, 41(5), 959–969.

Wilkinson, S., and Alderson-Day, B. (2016). Voices and thoughts in psychosis: An introduction. *Review of Philosophy and Psychology*, 7, 529–540.

Wilkinson, S., and Fernyhough, C. (2018). When inner speech misleads. In P. Langland-Hassan and A. Vicente (Eds.), *Inner speech: New voices*. Oxford: Oxford University Press, Chapter 9. www.ncbi.nlm.nih.gov/books/NBK538965/

Wilson, M., and Emmorey, K. A. (1998). "Word length effect" for sign language: Further evidence for the role of language in structuring working memory. *Memory and Cognition*, 26, 584–590.

Yao, B., Scheepers, C., Frazier, L., and Gibson, E. (Eds.). (2015). Inner voice experiences during processing of direct and indirect speech. In *Explicit and implicit prosody in sentence processing: Studies in honor of Janet Dean Fodor* (Studies in Theoretical Psycholinguistics, Vol. 46). New York: Springer Nature.

11

IDENTITY, NARRATIVES, AND PSYCHOPATHOLOGY: A CRITICAL PERSPECTIVE

Pietro Perconti

Prospero

We are such stuff
As dreams are made on; and our little life
Is rounded with a sleep.

William Shakespeare, The Tempest, *Act 4, Scene 1, 148–158*

1 Mental disorders and the stories

To capture the spirit of our times, the celebrated statement by Prospero could be reformulated slightly differently, saying that the human being's mind is made by *stories*, instead of dreams. Considering stories and dreams as a fingerprint of mankind, however, is not a Shakespeare's prerogative. History was also a *leitmotiv* in the classical German age. In a sense, the *Phänomenologie des Geistes* by Georg Wilhelm Friedrich Hegel can be considered as the attempt to show the structure of the human mind from a *historical* perspective. And, with his *Über die Aufgabe des Geschichtschreibers*, Wilhelm von Humboldt was trying to discover the "grammar" of what stories are and to highlight their role in human life. This very idea was equally celebrated in the Victorian era and it is also the basis of the theory of natural selection by Charles Darwin, which in the end is a general theory of biological *change*. The popularity of stories in the culture of the last decades, however, is possibly more and more increasing, by influencing almost every field of human civilization. From art to politics, every human artefact has been considered as the result of our capacity to shape stories. Everything is a story: "Narrative is the primary form by which human experience is made meaningful" (Taylor, 1996). Mental disorders are no exception.

To find what really counts as a cause for a mental disorder, many scholars claim that most of the deficits could be considered as the result of the inability to manage personal stories in the right way. Consider Multiple Personality Disorder and the typical difficulty to handle a consistent autobiography. In Borderline Personality Disorder, people are characterized by life stories which are significantly more incoherent than healthy controls (Lind et al., 2018). The same occurs with Dissociative Identity Disorder, schizophrenia, and many other mental disorders. From a therapeutic point of view, talk therapies can be basically considered as various attempts to reconstruct, or imagine *ex novo*, alternative narratives able to give sense to the patient's life in terms of a consistent story. Narrative coherence is considered as a good measure of well-being and telling stories in a very incoherent manner is related to psychopathology (Vanden Poel and Hermans, 2019; Mitchell et al., 2020). According to Roy Schafer, psychoanalysis is nothing but a "narrational project" (1980: 83) and the therapist and her patients are mutually engaged in shaping a non-dysfunctional story, within previous difficulties can be managed in a new light (Schafer, 1981, 1992). In a word, wrong and broken stories are the mark of mental illness, while consistent narratives are the sign of a healthy inner life.

If individuals' personal identity is considered as a result of a given narrative, this latter should be gone wrong, when the individual experiences some form of mental disorder. There is a widespread hypothesis in psychotherapy, often implicitly, according to which the idea that human identity has an essentially narrative nature is linked with the expectation that an adult and healthy person should be an individual able of exercising full control over his or her mind and behaviour (White, 2007; Dickerson, 2016). Narrative psychotherapy, moreover, is based on a kind of story-based pedagogy. According to Dan Hutto, children are naturally predisposed to categorize the world narratively. The basic idea of his Hypothesis of Narrative Practice is that through the stories offered to children by their parents in interactive contexts, they become familiar with the basic structure of common sense psychology and the possibilities to exercise it concretely, learning how and when to use it (Hutto, 2007; Hutto, 2008). In other words, nature predisposes human beings to stories and education develops this trend in an orderly and productive way (Goodson and Gill, 2011).

In such a view, however, there is a risk of implicitly manifesting an unjustified preference for a particular type of personality. Why, after all, should it be preferable being a kind of person which is completely in charge of her own behaviour? Why would "losing control" be a disvalue or something to be considered as dysfunctional? And why should it be desirable to be both the author and the main character of one's own autobiography? On what basis should we adopt a psychotherapeutic treatment that assumes such theses as desirable, without any further justification?

2 Narrative and episodic lifestyles

The popularity of narratives is mainstreaming, but not ubiquitous. Galen Strawson's *Against Narrativity* (2004) is a celebrated exception. According to him, the popularity of the stories depends on the combination of two theses: the psychological narrativity thesis and the ethical narrativity thesis. In his words:

> There is widespread agreement that human beings typically see or live or experience their lives as a narrative or story of some sort, or at least as a collection of stories. I'll call this the psychological Narrativity thesis, using the word 'Narrative' with a capital letter to denote a specifically psychological property or outlook. The psychological Narrativity thesis is a straightforwardly empirical, descriptive thesis about the way ordinary human beings actually experience their lives. This is how we are, it says, this is our nature. The psychological Narrativity thesis is often coupled with a normative thesis, which I'll call the ethical Narrativity thesis. This states that experiencing or conceiving one's life as a narrative is a good thing; a richly Narrative outlook is essential to a well-lived life, to true or full personhood.
>
> *(Strawson, 2004: 428)*

The two aforementioned theses provide four main combinations as shown in Figure 11.1.

The ethical and psychological version of the thesis of narrativity requires different reasons and leads to different theoretical commitments. Generally speaking, it is a matter of appreciating the idea that it is different to believe that our inner life has an essentially narrative nature and to believe that cultivating this psychological

	Psychological Narrativity thesis +	Psychological Narrativity thesis –
Ethical Narrativity thesis +	A. Human beings are narrative creatures. Narratives are crucial for a good life.	B. Human beings are not narrative creatures. But, they should have a narrative inner life to have a good life.
Ethical Narrativity thesis –	C. Human beings are narrative creatures, but narratives are an obstacle to a good life.	D. Human beings aren't narrative creatures and this isn't a bad thing. Many non-narrative individuals have a good life.

FIGURE 11.1

characteristic should be considered as a value. In this way, indeed, we end up preferring lifestyles that emphasize our narrative nature and discourage the more episodic ones. For example, children are encouraged to keep a diary, but not in the style of James Joyce's *Finnegans Wake* or *The Big Lebowski* in the crime comedy film directed by Joel and Ethan Coen.

By imagining how personal identity could be shaped without stories and storytelling, Jeffrey "The Dude" Lebowski, with his typical jumping from an isolated experience to another one, can be taken as a champion. Lebowski's days go by without following a particular pattern. He certainly has preferences and projects, but the overall sense of his existence, if any, does not seem to derive from those preferences and plans, but from temporary episodes, which seem to happen without any particular reason. According to the mainstream trend, this kind of scattered lifestyle is less worthy than one that accomplishes a storyline. Yet, in the perspective here proposed, some people don't narratively experience their lives and yet are virtuous (whatever it means – who decides?). It's a kind of personality that we could call "episodic", to distinguish it from narrative and diachronic. Individuals who have an episodic personality do not try to structure their stream of consciousness in such a way as to make sure that it is the same individual who takes part in it (Strawson, 2007, 2017).

David Hume is celebrated for proposing a concept of the self that does not match the expectations of coherence which are typical of the narrative perspective. He is often regarded as a sceptic, but perhaps he is simply suggesting a non-narrative view of what introspection is:

> For my part, when I enter most intimately into what I call myself, I always stumble on some particular perception or other, of heat or cold, light or shade, love or hatred, pain or pleasure. I never can catch myself at any time without a perception, and never can observe anything but the perception. . . . If anyone, upon serious and unprejudiced reflection, thinks he has a different notion of himself, I must confess I can reason no longer with him. All I can allow him is, that he may be in the right as well as I, and that we are essentially different in this particular. He may, perhaps, perceive something simple and continued, which he calls himself; though I am certain there is no such principle in me.
>
> *(Hume, 1739–40: 252)*

It could be argued that, after all, Lebowski's experiences also form a story, as does the kaleidoscope of events found in James Joyce's *Finnegans Wake* or *Ulysses*. That is a good point. However, it overestimates the objection to the thesis of the ubiquity of narratives. This latter, indeed, is not intended to maintain that there are experiences that are impossible to describe narratively. More modestly, the point is that those experiences are not lived in a massively narrative way and that they can be told using a particular narrative style in the attempt to give back what it means to have a non-narrative experience.

3 Not only episodes: non-conceptual (self-)knowledge

Considering the possibility of a style of personality not based on narratives, which is indeed highly episodic, and yet morally virtuous, or neutral, it's definitely a way of contrasting the thesis of the ubiquity of narratives. But, perhaps, it is not radical enough. The problem with episodes is that, after all, by definition they are only segments of a story. They are constituent elements, indeed, like beaded necklaces. Otherwise, they are episodes of what? It is doubtful whether an episode should be understood as the minimum element endowed with meaning in a story (a sort of 'narratological morpheme') or whether it's even a more elementary one, like a simple green card in a mosaic, without an inherent sense. In any case, however, an episode is such because it is a constituent element of a story. Defending the idea that even an episodic lifestyle can be ethically virtuous, or neutral, is, therefore, a way of arguing that even the constituents of stories can have the same value that we are ready to accord to the story as a whole.

The logical feature that makes the episodes the constituent parts of a narrative is the fact that their content can ever be *described*. Like the stories, precisely, only in a simpler way. The underlying rationale of the narrative perspective is that personal identity, after all, is a kind of identity and that "identity" is a conceptual and linguistic matter. The joint job of language and concepts are traditionally intended to provide a referential criterion made up by satisfying conditions, i.e., a set of conditions able to designate a given state of affairs in the world in a non-equivocal way. Definite descriptions are the linguistic champions of this use of language to refer to individuals. "The capital of the People's Republic of China" refers to Beijing because this latter is the only city which satisfies the condition of being the capital of the People's Republic of China.

This perspective, however, is more controversial than one could expect. First of all, language and concepts are not the only way to refer to something in a univocal manner. This picture, indeed, does not take into the right consideration the role of the demonstrative reference. Gareth Evans (1982) famously argued for the idea that reference can occur also in another way, by using demonstrations, like pointing and gaze following. Demonstratives, i.e., words like "this" and "that", are the linguistic counterpart of this way of referring. Their typical use of demonstrations (Kaplan, 1977) shows how linguistic resources are not able to refer successfully in every circumstance. There is another way to refer, like in the case of indexicals and demonstratives, where these non-linguistic devices are necessary and sufficient conditions for the linguistic reference.

Furthermore, the ability to detect more perceived objects than our language can describe is another evidence that concepts and definite descriptions are not the only cognitive devices to univocally refer to individuals in the world. Consider, for example, our common ability to discriminate between colours of a certain colour range. Red, therefore, can be "ruby", "Pompeian", or "bordeaux", and many other *nuances* without a name. This capacity for discrimination is amplified by education and culture. Thus, a painter will probably be able to identify more colours than ordinary people. Furthermore, however great this ability may be, it will still be greater than the corresponding descriptive ability. It's kind of a recursive process. It is always possible, indeed, to identify one more shade of red than all those for which we have a description. And it is also always possible to identify that point of red employing a new description. But it is also always possible to further expand our discriminating ability beyond the descriptions and vocabulary available at a given moment, alluding to a new chromatic tone, perhaps simply a little more saturated than the one for which we had just found a name or a description. The scope of non-conceptual experiences, therefore, is by definition much broader than that of linguistic description and conceptual articulation. It also constitutes the largest part of the human experience.

But what about *ourselves*? Is self-reference simply a case of traditional linguistic reference, or do we need to suppose something else? If concepts and definite descriptions are not the only way to gain the identity of the external individuals, we can suppose that the same happens also in the case of the self. It is possible to refer to ourselves using descriptions. But it is very different from the case of the *essential* self-reference (Perry, 1979). Here is an example by John Perry:

> I once followed a trail of sugar on a supermarket floor, pushing my cart down the aisle on one side of a tall counter and back the aisle on the other, seeking the shopper with the torn sack to tell him he was making a mess. With each trip around the counter, the trail became thicker. But I seemed unable to catch up. Finally it dawned on me. I was the shopper I was trying to catch. I believed at the outset that the shopper with a torn sack was making a mess. And I was right. But I didn't believe that I was making a mess. That seems to be something I came to believe. And when I came to believe that, I stopped following the trail around the counter, and rearranged the torn sack in my cart. My change in beliefs seems to explain my change in behavior.
>
> *(Perry, 1979: 3)*

On the whole, there two ways to have 'de se' thoughts, the first using a description which univocally refers to the speaker, and the second using an essential indexical (Perconti, 2013).

There is, therefore, alternative way in which people shape their self, compared to the narrative perspective, and this is made of psychological episodes and non-conceptual experiences. Héctor-Neri Castañeda (1989), John Perry (2001), and many others argued that self-reference works, thanks to the logical rules of pronouns and indexicals, i.e., the capacity to refer to the speaker in a manner which is (more or less) independent from the speaker's intention and the mechanism of satisfying conditions. They claim that self-reference is not a matter of concepts and stories; rather, it is a matter of logical rules and the ability to handle the context in the right way.

The relationship between moral norms, which are more or less widely accepted in a community, and what should be considered as a mental disorder, is a major problem in psychopathology. Foucault (1972) identified in this link one of the main repressive mechanisms embodied in the social structure. It is well known how controversial is the relation between the Viennese ethics of the late nineteenth century and Freud's psychoanalysis (Goodman and Severson, 2016). The popularity of the notion of 'dysfunctional' in psychopathology can be seen just as an attempt to bypass this problem through a hopefully ethically neutral notion. But, of course, it is just an illusion. This is demonstrated by the numerous nosographic changes in the various editions of the *Diagnostic and Statistical Manual of Mental Disorders* (DSM V, 2013). Consider, for example, the various sexual disorders in relation to social change and it will easily be seen how this relationship is still highly controversial. The case of narrative and episodic personality styles I discussed so far can be considered as a chapter in this long book.

The point is that, according to today's prevailing ethical stance, it is a value for individuals having the absolute and conscious control over their preferences and behaviour. This control usually takes the form of a story, made up of autobiography and public narratives which are consistent with the story of one's own life. A fully developed individual would be able to hierarchize his or her preferences, making plans to accomplish them, by cooperating or competing with other people. Stories are what hold together all the just mentioned elements. They give them a sense and allow people to monitor the progress of their projects by comparing the events in their personal lives into a comprehensive account. Films, novels, social media, and intersubjective relationships are part of an overall story, partly private and partly public, that measures the quality of one's life. What it was argued earlier is that this picture is both a widely accepted assumption in psychopathology and a claim that is lacking in justification which is offered to interlocutors explicitly.

References

American Psychiatric Association. (2013). *Diagnostic and statistical manual of mental disorders (DSM-5®)* (5th ed.). Arlington, VA: American Psychiatric Publishing.

Castañeda, H.-N. (1989). Self-consciousness, I-structures and physiology. In M. Spitzer and B. A. Maher (Eds.), *Philosophy and psychopathology*. Berlin: Springer.

Dickerson, V. (2016). *Poststructural and narrative thinking in family therapy*. New York and Berlin: Springer.

Evans, G. (1982). *The varieties of reference*. Oxford: Clarendon Press.

Foucault, M. (1972). *Histoire de la folie à l'âge classique*. Paris: Gallimard.

Goodman, D. M., and Severson, E. R. (2016). *Viennese ethics of the late 19th century and Freud's psychoanalysis*. London: Routledge.

Goodson, I. F., and Gill, S. R. (2011). *Narrative pedagogy: Life history and learning*. New York: Peter Lang.

Hume, D. (1739–40). *A treatise of human nature*. Oxford: Oxford University Press, 1978.

Hutto, D. (2007). The narrative practice hypothesis. Origins and applications of folk psychology. In D. Hutto (Ed.), *Narrative and understanding persons*. Royal Institute of Philosophy Supplement. Cambridge: Cambridge University Press.

Hutto, D. (2008). *Folk psychological narratives: The sociocultural basis of understanding reasons*. Cambridge, MA: The MIT Press.

Kaplan, D. (1977). Demonstratives: An essay on the semantics, logic, metaphysics, and epistemology of demonstratives and other indexicals. In J. Almog, J. Perry, and H. Wettstein (Eds.), *Themes from Kaplan*. Oxford: Oxford University Press.

Lind, M., Jørgensen, C., Heinskou, T., Simonsen, S., Bøye, R., and Thomsen, D. (2018). Patients with borderline personality disorder show increased agency in life stories after 12 months of psychotherapy. *Psychotherapy*, 56(2), 274–284. https://doi.org/10.1037/pst0000184.

Mitchell, C., Reese, E., Salmon, K., and Jose, P. (2020). Narrative coherence, psychopathology, and wellbeing: Concurrent and longitudinal findings in a mid-adolescent sample. *Journal of Adolescence*, 2079, 16–25.

Perconti, P. (2013). The role of motivational force and intention in first-person beliefs. In N. Feit and A. Capone (Eds.), *Attitudes De Se: Linguistics, epistemology, metaphysics*. Stanford: CSLI Publications.

Perry, J. (1979). The problem of essential indexical. *Noûs*, 13(1), 3–21.

Perry, J. (2001). *Reference and reflexivity*. Stanford: CSLI Publications.

Schafer, R. (1980). Action and narration in psychoanalysis. *New Literary History*, 12, 61–85.

Schafer, R. (1981). Narration in the psychoanalytic dialogue. In W. J. T. Mitchell (Ed.), *On narrative*. Chicago and London: University of Chicago Press.

Schafer, R. (1992). *Retelling a life: Narration and dialogue in psychoanalysis*. New York: Basic Books.

Strawson, G. (2004). Against narrativity. *Ratio (New Series)*, XVII.

Strawson, G. (2007). Episodic ethics. In D. Hutto (Ed.), *Narrative and understanding persons*. Cambridge: Cambridge University Press.

Strawson, G. (2017). *The subject of experience*. Oxford: Oxford University Press.

Taylor, D. (1996). *The healing power of stories: Creating yourself through the stories of your life*. New York: Doubleday.

Vanden Poel, L., and Hermans, D. (2019). Narrative coherence and identity: Associations with psychological well-being and internalizing symptoms. *Frontiers in Psychology*, 10, 1171.

White, M. (2007). *Maps of narrative practice*. New York: Norton & Co.

12

BODIES THAT LOVE THEMSELVES AND BODIES THAT HATE THEMSELVES: THE ROLE OF LIVED EXPERIENCE IN BODY INTEGRITY DYSPHORIA

Antonino Pennisi and Alessandro Capodici

1 Introduction

Ordinarily, each of us experiences the primary and implicit *sense of body ownership*, a belongingness that accompanies every conscious experience. Our body is, as Sartre said, "passed by in silence" (Sartre, 1943, tr. 1956: 330). Sometimes, however, this tacit harmony between body and mind can be problematic and emerge to consciousness and thematization. This discrepancy in bodily self may occur in neurological and psychopathological disorders; the scientific literature presents a variety of clinical cases in which subjects express feelings of estrangement towards their body as a whole or parts of it. In many of these disorders, there is a cognitive dissonance between the subject's body image and his body consciousness.

This work focus on the phenomenology of a condition in which subjects aspire to amputation or functional/sensory deprivation of a healthy body part. In most cases, the target of desire concerns the amputation of the lower limbs. However, this may also involve amputation of the upper limbs, paralysis, or damage to the visual and auditory organs. People with BID are not typically affected by specific mental disorders, such as depression, paranoia, schizophrenia, or neuroses. In this pathology, there is an alteration in the relationship between the imagined/narrated body and the real body. The specific desire for amputation, for example, involves that the ideal body denies the real body "until he wants to physically eliminate it, abolish it, kill it not metaphorically but *carnally*" (Freedberg and Pennisi, 2020: 16).

Most of these people claim that only amputation path will allow their body to match their body image (Kasten, 2009: 17). In this scenario, the argument of surgeries is still highly controversial (Bayne and Levy, 2005; Müller, 2009). Since professionals are not authorized to remove or inhibit healthy body parts, individuals with this disorder often go to extremely risky self-mutilation practices. To date, psychological therapies have rarely been effective (Thiel et al., 2011). In contrast, some people who have achieved the desired disability have reported an improvement in their quality of life (Smith, 2004), although in some cases the desire reappeared later focusing on other body parts (Sorene et al., 2006; Berger et al., 2005).

Currently, the desire for disability is not present in the DSM-V, but it has been listed with the Body Integrity Dysphoria label (code 6C21) in the ICD-11, which will officially come into effect in January 2022. In line with this classification, in this chapter we will adopt the last expression (BID) to highlight the first-person perspective of those who experience this disorder. In particular, we have conducted a qualitative study through a questionnaire that aims to bring out different aspects of the lived experience of these subjects.

2 The body as a target of love and hate

As already mentioned, BID variants imply a dissonance between the real body and the imagined one, i.e., the body constructed through internalized narratives.

In this regard, it is also possible to think about anorexia, vigorexia, and body hacking (Pennisi, 2020). The gaze of these subjects immersed in their body reflected in the mirror can transform the anorexic body into an obese body, the body of a superpalestrate into a slender body, the fully tattooed body in someone who realizes that it is still possible to colour his own sclera (eyeball tattoo).

One could hypothesize that under these dysphoric behaviours can be traced the will to improve one's body to make it attractive to others: a mental mirror in which lies the universal biological principle of sexual selection. Even among non-human animal species, in fact, something very similar happens: peacock, under the pressure of natural selection, has developed a wonderful colourful tail adorned with showy shapes, but this anomalous genetic evolution has made it lose the ability to fly and sing. The same can be said of the superb antlers of the alpha-male moose that ended up damaging its ability to move in forests full of low branches.

One could continue to list a dense series of other 'marvellous monstrosities' that have benefited sexual selection but, at the same time, have drastically limited other bodily possibilities of the more genetically showy subjects. Here it will suffice, however, to observe that among non-human animals, the selection process takes place through gradual modifications of the body structure between generations without any contribution of a voluntary individual choice.

BID does not follow the same criteria of the bodies 'who love themselves'. In these cases, the body image is always oriented towards the conservation and idealization of the body picture. It is the body that wants to love itself that produces conflicts. If we didn't love our body, we wouldn't take care of it, we wouldn't do anything to improve it, to adorn it, to keep it intact. It is sexual selection that naturally pushes us in this direction (Freedberg and Pennisi, 2020: 13).

On the other hand, there are also bodies that hate themselves. The *Misoplegia* (now *Somatoparaphrenia*), e.g., described by Critchley in 1955, is a condition in which patients with hemiplegia refer disdain or even hatred for paralyzed limbs.

Misoplegics verbally attack their diseased limb and often strike it with their hands or with an object. In this pathology, neurocerebral alterations cause a failure in the sense of belonging of limbs: somatoparaphrenics can attribute their arm to others or demand its removal; they can insult and hate the part or pamper it to convince it to die (Loetscher et al., 2006). However, "the misoplegic has serious reasons to hate his body: there are no 'mystifications' of this body, they are not mental images generated exclusively by ruminations or inner narratives", but a neurocerebral alteration that causes a lack of bodily consonance (Freedberg and Pennisi, 2020: 13).

Pennisi (2020) reports a second dimension of bodies that hate themselves; these cases concern apparently healthy bodies, whose dysphoric condition is attributable to a discrepancy between the body and its image, a disharmony that inevitably generates psychic and social repercussions.

In previous studies (Pennisi, 2020; Freedberg and Pennisi, 2020), it has been pointed out that body image disorders result from an altered complex system involving biological and psychosocial factors, including cultural and social customs, libidinal pressures, and sexual repression. Unlike self-loving bodies – which adapt and modify (through food, training, resistance to pain) while always remaining themselves – self-hating bodies are immersed in an inexorable path that can only end up making them different from how they were born. The suicides that occur in the population with *Gender Dysphoria* (GID) make it clear how unsustainable it can become to survive these unbridgeable bodily dissonances. According to data surveyed by the National Transgender Discrimination Survey (NTDS) and published in September 2019 (UCLA) in the United States, as many as 80% of them have seriously thought about suicide while 42% among MTF (male-to-female) and 46% among FTM (female-to-male) actually attempted it. People with gender dysphoria commit suicide ten times more than other people (4.5%).

Unlike anorexia and other 'bodies that love themselves', it is plausible to assume that in BID and GID there may be the involvement of organic processes and substrates, which favour the evolution of body identity.

3 Which approach in the field of BID studies?

The nomenclature used to refer to this condition has changed over time in line with the approaches adopted for its investigation (Sedda and Bottini, 2014). The first scientific report was proposed by Money (1977) with the label 'apotemnophilia', in which the investigation has focused primarily on the sexual and paraphilic components of desire.

Subsequently, both 'Amputee Identity Disorder' (Furth and Smith, 2000) and 'Body Integrity Identity Disorder' (First, 2005) labels attempted to highlight the hiatus that can occur between the anatomy and identity of these subjects, stressing that sexual arousal is not a primary motivation.

In the neuroscientific field, instead, McGeoch and colleagues (2011) proposed the term 'Xenomelia' to qualify a congenital dysfunction of the right upper parietal lobule and its projections with the insula (Ramachandran and McGeoch, 2007; Brang et al., 2008). This anomaly causes a decoupling between the body image in the right parietal lobe and the actual physical body. This discrepancy was detected by both magnetoencephalography (MEG) and skin conductance response (SCR).

As for the latter, Ramachandran and colleagues – starting from the observation that many subjects with BID report a specific cut height – conducted a SCR study by applying on each leg small electrical stimuli above and below the desired amputation line (on feet and thighs). Subjects who desired an amputation under the right knee exhibited a double difference in SCR between the left and right legs below the amputation line, another double difference through the desired amputation line on the right leg, but no observed difference in normal limb. In xenomelics who desired a double amputation both under the left knee and under the right thigh the differences recorded were greater: there was a triple difference below the amputation line compared to above in both the left and right legs. Of course, nothing similar occurred in the control subjects. According to the researchers, these results prove that Xenomelia derives from the congenital malfunction of the upper right parietal lobule, which receives and integrates inputs from various sensors in the areas and from the insula to form a coherent sense of body image.

Magnetoencephalography studies have also gone in this direction, reinforcing cerebral hypothesis. McGeoch and colleagues (2009) showed an absence of activity in the upper right parietal lobe following tactile stimuli on the unwanted limb in subjects with BID. This implies that although individuals with BID can feel the target body parts, these may not be integrated into the body image, eliciting the desire for amputation.

In the scientific literature, it is possible to trace constant behaviours which seem to confer plausibility to brain-based hypothesis. Many of those who experience this condition are extremely convinced that there are no alternatives to the epilogue that involves body damages. Another aspect that could be mentioned is the disproportion between the amputation requests. Many subjects, indeed, aspire to left leg amputation, while fewer subjects experience a desire focused on the right leg or both legs. Furthermore, a large number of subjects pose the onset of desire during childhood. These data seem to suggest an interference in neurodevelopment processes, which may have occurred, perhaps, during embryogenesis.

The embodied cognition approach aims to go beyond the brain considered in isolation, highlighting the role of the dynamic brain-body-environment relationship (Gallagher and Zahavi, 2008; Shapiro, 2011; Capodici and Russo, 2019, Capodici, 2019). Therefore, the purpose of this study is not to reject neuroscientific hypotheses, but to emphasize some recurrent aspects of the lived experience of these subjects that cannot be neglected. The idea is to move away from a purely reductionist view of this phenomenon, as already expressed by Brugger and colleagues (2013, 2018; Brugger and Lenggenhager, 2014), who suggested that it is necessary to consider not only neurological factors but also psychological and social ones.

In the perspective of these researchers, for example, it is not possible to neglect the sexual component of the desire for disability, as the insula is not only involved in enteroception but also plays an essential role in somatoesthetic and sexual arousal (Brugger, 2013). Furthermore, as we will see later, neurological theories cannot satisfy all the occurrences of the phenomenon: sometimes it happens that the target of desire can change from one leg to another (Kasten and Stirn, 2009), or that desire can re-emerge in other forms after a first amputation (Sorene et al., 2006). Moreover, Brugger and colleagues invite the scientific community to pay attention to the phenomenon of brain plasticity which, lasting over time during the development of each individual's life, could explain the connection between neurobiology, environment, and sociocultural influences (including those of telematic spaces).

Such an approach allows investigating aspects of BID that deserve more attention, such as – among others – exposure to amputees during childhood, pretending behaviour, and virtual places in which users meet to confront their experiences; events and practices that imply the presence of other people, objects, and a social environment. Therefore, the hypothesis is that experience can retroact and influence some of those processes involved in the onset and maintenance of BID.

4 The self-narrative questionnaire

The study aims to investigate the first-person perspective of those living with the BID through a qualitative questionnaire in order to highlight different aspects of these lived experiences. The questionnaire consists of six sections: five of them propose three open-ended questions, while the last one is formulated as a closed-ended question (the items can be consulted in § Appendix 1, while the quantitative data extracted and distributed in tables are shown in § Appendix 2). The research has been authorized by the Ethics Committee of the Department of Cognitive, Psychological, Pedagogical and Cultural Studies of the University of Messina.

Participants were recruited through different web platforms (Reddit, Facebook, Tumblr). Initially, the study involved 69 participants, but we excluded three minors from the results. The youngest of them was 13 years old while, of the 66 remaining participants, the oldest is 75 years old. We divided the participants into three age groups, as can be seen in Table 12.1.

Our data about the provenance of the participants overlap with those already found in the literature. In Table 12.2, it is possible to see a distribution of participants by continent of origin. It seems that there is a prevalence of the phenomenon in Western cultures (Lawrence, 2009); however, these data may derive from more limited economic possibilities, from the existence of specific networks linked to the country of origin or – as highlighted by Blom (2016) concerning Eastern cultures – from intrinsic cultural characteristics.

As shown in many other studies (Johnson et al., 2011; Blom et al., 2012), a substantial number of participants are male (43 subjects), 14 are female, and the last 9 declared other dimensions of gender identity, such as non-binary (Table 12.3).

In general, the most desired form of disability (Table 12.4) is amputation (71.2%), followed by paralysis (15.2%) and sensory deprivation (7.6%). It was necessary to create the 'mixed' category that includes 3 participants (4.5%) and which we will describe later. Lastly, a participant was placed in the category 'Not better specified' (N.B.S.) because he did not indicate the form of his desire.

The most common form of disability (Table 12.5) among male subjects is leg amputation (37 participants), followed by paralysis (3 participants) and sensory deprivation (1 participant desires blindness). Two subjects reported a mixed desire: the first stated that he desires to become wheelchair dependent, regardless of the type of disability needed for this purpose. The second declared that he sometimes feels the desire to be a DAK amputee and sometimes to be a paraplegic.

Among female participants, the most common desire is for paralysis (6 participants), followed by amputation (5 participants) and sensory deprivation (2 participants desire blindness). It was not possible to trace the desire of 1 participant (N.B.S). These data confirm the prevalence of desire for amputation in the male population and desire for paralysis in the female population (Brugger et al., 2016: 1176). In the latter case, however, our study shows a minimal gap between the desire for paralysis and the desire for amputation.

Finally, the most common desire in the 'Other' category concerns amputation (5 participants), sensory deprivation (2 participants), paralysis (1 participant), and a mixed desire (1 participant) that concerns a leg and genitals. This participant has already reached eunuch condition. In literature, however, the inclusion of the desire for emasculation or castration in the BID spectrum is highly controversial (Wassersug et al., 2007; Lawrence, 2010; Johnson et al., 2010).

Some participants' answers will be reported integrally in the next paragraphs, while an overview of the data can be found in §Appendix 2. However, this study has limitations, such as the fact that the sample recruited on the web has not been previously tested and differentiated. Besides, the quantitative data presented in this work emerges from the descriptive answers given by the participants to the open questions, so we have schematized the data to extract objective results. For this reason, these data are necessarily incomplete. When quantitative data could not be determined, we opted for the expression 'Not better specified' (N.B.S). Therefore, it will be necessary to integrate this research with other quantitative and experimental methods.

5 Growing with a growing desire

At age 5 I knew. I remember it well. It is my strongest memory. I saw a one-legged woman on crutches. And I was nailed to the floor, unable to move, think or anything else. I was completely awestruck. I couldn't take my eyes of off her. And when she left my eyesight I could act again (*a participant's response to our questionnaire*).

In scientific literature, childhood-related stories are quite recurrent. In our study, in fact, 72.7% of the participants placed the onset of the disorder in childhood (Table 12.7). This prevalence had already emerged from the two cases presented by Money (1977), both of which reported an early onset of the disorder. However, 20 years later, Bruno (1997) emphasized more prominently the role of exposure to the sight of amputees in childhood. He proposed the expression "Factitious disability disorder" to describe a desire for disability ascribable to the emotional sphere, in which the lack of parental love and the envy felt towards caring for disabled people would translate into the desire to acquire disabilities and attentions related to it:

> My earliest memories are probably in 4th grade – which was a time of my life marked by big changes. . . . I felt ignored and 'un-special', so I began limping to see if anyone would notice. At the time, I had a brother who had an ankle brace so I thought I could garner enough attention for my parents to coddle me and take me to a doctor, where I would be thoroughly looked after. Over time, I guess, this desire for love and attention (hopefully I don't come across as narcissistic – I was just a lonely kid living in a chaotic situation) evolved into an obsessive search for ways to earn love and affection. People are much kinder to you when you are physically disabled.
>
> *(a participant's response to our questionnaire)*

However, many individuals with BID deny that a search for compassion drives their request for disability. Indeed, as pointed out by some authors, people with BID often idolize people who are successful in life despite their disability (Kasten, 2019: 33).

I was terrified that . . . strangers would ridicule me or accuse me of being an attention seeker (even though attention to this aspect of my life was the absolute last thing I could ever want) (*a participant's response to our questionnaire*).

Furthermore, from a study focused on the childhood of subjects with BID (Obernolte et al., 2015), no significant evidence emerged relating to inadequate parental care, neither in terms of physical abuse nor as overprotective control. Therefore, the purpose of this chapter is not to describe BID as a Factitious Disorder; nonetheless, we believe that Bruno's hypotheses are interesting above all for the attention paid to the emotional dimension.

Enactive theories emphasize *how we affect each other*, that is, how the encounters we make in the course of our lives contribute to the constitution of subjectivity: "social interactions not only modulate us, they partly make us into who we are" (De Jaegher, 2015: 125).

Obernolte and colleagues (2015) reported that subjects with BID tend to remember a higher number of experiences with disabled subjects, compared to the control group. In particular, BID sufferers vividly remind contacts with amputated or paralyzed people (and not, for example, with those affected by mental retardation). However, the authors specify that it is difficult to determine whether the subjects with BID were exposed more frequently to disabled subjects than the control group or if they remember these events better due to the continuous thematization around their own corporeality. In accordance with the key-lock principle, Obernolte and colleagues (2015) show that, since childhood, subjects with BID react with a positive attitude to the first sight of disabled subjects.

As already mentioned, it seems that for many subjects, early exposure to amputees represented a kind of trigger for the apprehension of the disorder. According to some authors, this interpretation seems to follow the concept of 'maternal impression', which correlates the pregnant woman's exposure to the sight of amputees to a high risk of giving birth to a child affected by congenital limb deficiencies (Aoyama et al., 2012: 106). Aoyama and colleagues specify that, although this theory is superstitious and childhood-related stories could be considered as retrospective reconstructions, it should not be excluded that an intense emotional experience may influence the representation of the body (*ibidem*).

Therefore, empathy could play a significant role. In this regard, a study has shown that visual exposure to the actions of an amputee influences our sensorimotor responses (Liew et al., 2013). In more detail, Liew and colleagues wondered what happens when we see a body in action that does not match to our body. In particular, they conducted an fMRI study on subjects with minimal experience with amputees, showing them short videos of an amputee woman (both arms above elbow) performing a series of actions with her residual limbs and videos of actions performed with the hands by a physically ordinary woman. Surprisingly, the observation of the amputee woman decreed a greater sensorimotor resonance in the AON (*action observation network*), particularly in the right inferior and superior parietal lobule, especially in the most empathic subjects (Liew et al., 2013: 144). A second fMRI session conducted after prolonged exposure to both video categories showed an attenuation of the difference in the AON in response to the residual limbs and hands, except in the right superior parietal lobe and occipito-temporal regions, suggesting the updating of the internal model of the participants. Although this experiment focuses on action view and motor response, it can provide interesting insights. First of all, it allows us not to exclude possibilities of incorporation of other's bodies into one's own body representations. Secondly, the evidence that empathic subjects could be more susceptible to this eventuality could strengthen some hypotheses already expressed in the context of the BID.

In particular, some authors mentioned that a hyperempathic response to the sight of an amputee might predispose subjects with BID to the integration of these bodily defects in their own representations of the body (Hilti et al., 2013; Brugger et al., 2016). The authors highlighted these aspects by describing the 'mirror-touch synaesthesia' phenomenon, i.e., the experience of healthy subjects who, observing tactile stimulations on the body of others, feel the sensation of being touched. The interesting aspect is that this sensation also emerges on the phantom limb of amputees, although their physical body does not match with the observed one. Moreover, Hilti and Brugger (2010) considered the BID as a 'negative phantom', that is the counterpart of the *aplasic phantom limb*, in which subjects, observing the movement of others' limbs, perceive the presence of their absent limbs. Therefore, in BID "observing the absence of another person's limb could unmask a congenital underrepresentation of the person's own present limb" (Brugger et al., 2016: 1182).

Our questionnaire shows that the sight of amputees could be considered by subjects as a trigger factor (at least for the apprehension of the disorder) even if the event did not occur in presence. In fact, some participants remember seeing amputees on TV or on the web during childhood or adolescence:

> I think it was when I watched this one episode of CSI or Law and order or one of those kinds of shows. A perpetrator took part of a limb from people when they came to him for a different type of surgery, I think. I was very young and I don't know if I had it at that moment because of it, or if it was in line with what I already 'wanted/needed'. Like beforehand maybe it was a passive thought, and the episode made it a conscious thought.
>
> *(a participant's response to our questionnaire)*

Although the power of images over the body – with a particular mention to those that depict human bodies – represent a theoretical area that should be more investigated experimentally (Freedberg and Pennisi, 2020), it is difficult to conclude that the aetiology of BID can be reduced to the impact of the sight of disabled people. If this were the case, one could hypothesize the involvement of empathic factors that could reassemble the mirror neuron system's neural prerequisites and their effects on imitative activity.

This thesis has been strongly contested by Ramachandran in all the writings that we have reported previously, to the point of ridiculing it ("others have proposed that seeing an amputee at a young age has caused this to be somehow 'imprinted' onto the sufferer's psyche as the 'ideal body image'", Brang et al., 2008: 1305). Notwithstanding the fundamental disagreement, in another essay Ramachandran however resorts to a reconstructive hypothesis involving mirror neurons in the origin of the formation of body self-awareness. The self is not for him a holistic property of the brain but a function of specific sets of interconnected brain circuits. Its main characteristic is recursion, that is, the property of turning within the self, of turning one's own attention to one's mental image.

The specific neurocerebral components on which this property would be based have their roots precisely in the mirror neurons which are highly concentrated in the lower parietal lobule of great apes and in humans. With the evolution of the brain in hominids, the lobule divided into two turns – the supramarginal gyrus and the angular gyrus. The first specialized in reflecting on the body pattern that allows to anticipate the actions necessary to avoid damage in the spatial movement. The second in the management of the body image and, probably, in the social and linguistic aspects of the left hemisphere of our cerebral self. Hence the emergence of self-awareness.

Of course, Ramachandran immediately takes precautions against the naive interpretations of this thesis by declaring that mirror neurons are not sufficient for the emergence of the self, otherwise the self-awareness of the other primates should also be supported. The recursive predisposition of mirror neurons is indeed intertwined in human animals with language brain areas (in particular with the Wernicke's area that allows their understanding) and with part of the frontal lobes.

These hypotheses could represent an explanatory cue not only for the pathology but also for the physiology of body image and self-identification processes. The perspective that considers ontogenetic development, in fact, allows conjugating biological aspects of the brain-body and those of the non-brain-body, and so psychological, cultural, and social factors.

6 Enacting disability

In the scientific literature on BID, the simulation of disability is undoubtedly one of the most recurrent aspects. Traditionally, this practice is defined with the expression 'pretending behavior'. However, when questioning subjects with BID on this issue, it becomes clear that this terminological choice is not unanimously appreciated:

> First of all, I'd like to argue that the word 'pretending' is not fully applicable (and potentially harmful) for our condition. Two reasons: first of all the media attention this disorder gets is usually of a sensational nature, which is in a way understandable. But if we are to get other people to be more accepting of BIID I think a different term would be better. This sketches an image of people using medical aid equipment 'for fun' or to 'get free handicapped parking spaces'. Unfortunately this also makes it easy to confuse BIID with medical fetishes. I know those two aren't mutually exclusive, but for the outside world this isn't so easy to understand.
>
> *(a participant's response to our questionnaire)*

> I actually feel very strongly that we should *not* use the word 'pretending'. To me, the word 'pretending' implies that the actions are make-believe, unnecessary, and/or deceitful. I think this is extremely harmful to those who are already living with a lot of shame from BIID and who are most likely struggling with the idea of ever being open and honest about their situation. I prefer to think about using various assistive devices or binding a limb, etc. as coping behaviours or management of the BIID discomfort. When both the community of researchers and people affected by BIID use the word 'pretending', in my opinion it sends the signal that these behaviours must be kept a secret (and that is not a healthy way to move forward). I have been trying to change the discourse within my community, but I also hope that perhaps you could amplify this request both to researchers studying BIID and to those struggling with it
>
> *(a participant's response to our questionnaire)*

The study conducted by First (2005) showed that 92% of the participants practiced or had practiced the simulation of disability. Our data on disability simulation can be observed in Table 12.8: the 'Yes' category shows that 63.6% of the participants currently practice simulation. This category also includes participants who have been amputated but who simulate further disabilities. The category 'Not anymore' includes participants who stopped simulation practices (15.2%) due to the following reasons: frustration, futility, reinforcement of desire, the achievement of the desired disability. Furthermore, we chose to include the category 'Not yet' (4.5%) which concerns participants who have had explicitly stated their intention to engage in the simulation in the near future (as soon as conditions allow or when they can get the necessary devices). Finally, 9 participants (13.6%) stated that they had never practiced and for 2 participants (3%) it was not possible to determine the category (N.B.S.).

The disability simulation consists in mental images or motor actions related to the desired mode of existence, so the subjects try to inhibit the functionality and the presence of the unwanted body part, avoiding to involve it in the movement (Brugger et al., 2013; Blom et al., 2012). Often, even these practices start from childhood, as one of our participants described:

> I have had it for as long as I can remember, but the first time I remember thinking of it was when I was five and I found that I could pretend using a crutch. I remember thinking that I wasn't meant to walk and also I felt a need to hide that because I felt ashamed of what I felt, so I only 'played' when I walked on crutches or used a wheelchair when no-one was watching.

According to some authors, the (congenitally or developmentally) alterations of body representations in BID could be strengthened by mental images and simulation practices (Giummarra et al., 2011). By inhibiting the unwanted part, the remaining limbs assume the total load of motility. It has been hypothesized that this functional switch could lead to a reprogramming of the motor representation of the limbs, reducing the representation of the unwanted body part (Hänggi et al., 2016). Langer and colleagues (2012) showed that immobilizing a limb for two weeks is enough to induce a rapid reorganization of the sensorimotor system and – through a motor imagery task – Meugnot and colleagues (2014) demonstrated that 24 hours of sensorimotor deprivation through hand immobilization can decree changes in its cognitive representation.

Regarding BID, the scientific literature presents some cases in which simulation behaviours led to alterations strictly related to limb inhibition. For example, Storm and Weiss (2003) showed the case of a subject who, due to the persistent use of tourniquet, reported a sensory decrease to light touch and pinprick on the ankles, reduced vibratory sensitivity at the big toes, weakened ankle and plantar flexion, and absent ankle reflexes. In relation to the role of lived experience, Giummarra and colleagues (2012) discussed a more significant case, which shows how simulating a disability could culminate in the amplification of the desire itself. In particular, a subject with a desire for paralysis, accustomed to wearing steel orthoses, has developed (in addition to leg deterioration and atrophy) the desire to amputate both legs at the level corresponding to the top of the orthosis (Giummarra et al., 2012).

However, although the simulation of disability appears to be a relief from a discomfort experienced since childhood, some authors point out that, over time, its palliative effect fades (Aner et al., 2018). In this regard, we asked our participants to describe what the simulation represents to them. Our question about the feelings aroused by the simulation included the words 'frustration', 'palliative', and 'relief'. In most cases, the subjects followed these categories to describe their experiences. Cases departing from these categories were differentiated into 'Relief and shame', 'Relief (but strengthens BID)', 'Fun' (Table 12.9). Our questionnaire, in sum, reports ambivalent feelings:

> I used it for several reasons: 1) it did good and felt so good, it brought lust, 2) I needed to try how it is to use a wheelchair, 3) it seemed to lower the stress, the tension to some degree. But then I found that in the long run it increased the BID pressure, it made it more different to push my desires, fantasies, etc.
>
> For me it's mostly a relief. For once, even though it's just for a moment, I can feel more whole as a human being. But at the same time it might add frustration because in the back of my head I still (of course) know that my legs work and I get upset with the fact that my body isn't how I would like it to be.
>
> Pretending is like a momentary relief, but that relief is never complete, it is like being hungry and eating, but never feeling satiated. So, in a way, it ends up being a kind of suffering, an eternal search for something that never comes.
>
> It slows the episodes but when I stop pretending, they get worse. It's like a drug addict who gets a huge hit of heroin . . . for a few minutes, all is perfect until the high wears off and the need comes back twofold.

Within the sample simulating disability (42 participants, as shown in Table 12.8), 12 stated that they simulate it every day, 8 several times during the week, 12 occasionally (from a few sessions per month to more extended periods between simulations), while 4 stated that they still practice the simulation but to a lesser extent than in the past and, lastly, 6 participants did not provide any indication of the frequency of these practices (Table 12.10).

Since some individuals have stopped practicing it, while others – with the words of one of our participants – 'do it as much as humanly possible', it might be interesting to set up a study entirely dedicated to the evaluation of neural correlates in the two groups. Recently, a study conducted by Saetta and colleagues (2020) showed a strong correlation between brain alterations and disability simulation. We will return to this study later on.

From an identity point of view, disability-related devices become an integral part of the being-in-the-world of these subjects (Heidegger, 1927). Everaerd (1983) presented a particular case, in which the desire for amputation was closely linked to the use, to the *incorporation* we might say, of a wooden leg. Moreover, the latter represented for the subject the real pillar of desire; without it, as he declared, amputation would have been in vain. As already mentioned, this could be considered a very uncommon case. Indeed, it is necessary to specify that most of the subjects interviewed in our questionnaire only described the functional value of these objects – in terms of useful tools or as synonymous of the achievement of disability, something that would complete their disabled identity. In Xenomelia (the specific desire for leg amputation), the intention is not to destroy the functionality of the body. Typically, the functional component subtracted by the absence or inhibition of the target body part is compensated through the use of prostheses that allow behavioural continuity. Marie, a 20-year-old with BID and GID, has described this phenomenon as "transabled paradox". Malafouris (2013: 154) defines the blind man's stick – and technology in general – as an "enactive cognitive prosthesis". One might wonder whether the artificial objects used during the simulation – or after amputation – by subjects with BID can be defined, to a certain degree and on an affective level, as existential prostheses.

However, what emerges is that, in some cases, material and visual culture can also play a role:

> I always felt different – but I saw Robocop at about age 13 and was fascinated by losing limbs and having them replaced with prosthetics. I realized that my feet were not really part of me and as such I'd rather have plastic feet that weren't so 'disgusting'.
>
> *(a participant's response to our questionnaire)*

7 Thinking (and talking) about desire

From a phenomenological point of view, the intriguing aspect is that in BID the *judgement of ownership* remains intact. However, there is a lack of *feeling of ownership*, the implicit experience that permeates one's own body and the coincidence with it as a harmonious premise of the existence (Romano et al., 2015: 141).

In many cases of phantom limb, it is the body that perceives to possess or even seeks a disappeared part. The mind feels the weight of a 'loss' and it is possible to imagine or experimentally demonstrate all the paths it has taken to reconstruct not only a representation, but also an embodied simulation by refocusing the mental states of the past. Less well-known and studied are the cases in which it is precisely this loss that the body consciousness invokes. It is a question of anticipating an event that will happen, that must necessarily happen, and therefore imagine a future state of mind. However, this does not make this state of mind, expected for the future, less embodied than the ones induced by the cases of a loss of what has already been possessed in the past. Actually, this urge to lose a limb is stronger than the desire of those who want to regain a missing part of the body (Freedberg and Pennisi, 2020: 21).

The BID presents a singularity, which has emerged since the study conducted by First (2005). So far, academic attention has focused mainly on sensations that reflect the incompleteness of the body, as happens in the phantom limb. In BID, on the other hand, individuals are tormented by a feeling of *hypercompleteness*.

In First's questionnaire, as much as 77% of the BID subjects of the sample indicates 'feel whole, complete, set right again' (First, 2005: 923) as the main cause of their choice to amputate. Furth and Smith (2000) also suggest that the subjects interviewed by them consider the idea of amputating a way to feel more skilled and more fully functioning, more whole, more complete.

The logical argument is very clear: I feel *excessively* complete with that leg and, therefore, the amputation serves to bring my body back to completeness, becoming regular again as it should be. The function of that limb (or other organ) remains in the state of cognitive normality and, therefore, is re-implanted in the amputated part activating it through a mechanical substitute. The transition of functional ability therefore constitutes a transition from bodily technology to extracorporeal technology.

It is not the functional component that defines the conflicted relationship between mind and body. This component works both before and after the amputation and must still be satisfied. The xenomelic wants to hit the body, or rather: his *brain-body* wants to hit his *not-brain-body*, to use the terminology of Alva Noë (2009; in Hutto and Myin, 2017: *neural body and non-neural body*). The natural organs of this body are apparently fully functional. However, they are not perceived as harmonic parts of one's body: they are alien, depersonalized clippings, extraneous to both the scheme and the body image.

The problems that absorb the full-blown xenomelic are all technical: 'will I be able to convince a doctor to amputate? how much will it cost me? And if I can't convince any surgeon how can I amputate myself without dying?'

Moreover, BID forces the subject to immerse himself in a condition of social bodily solipsism. Some of the authors previously mentioned have hypothesized that not only concrete simulations can decree neuroplastic effects, but also the imaginative activity of these subjects could contribute. Modern cognitive science does not consider mental images as 'pictures in the mind', but emphasizes their embodied nature, primarily grounded in a partial reactivation of the sensorimotor system (Iachini, 2011; Meugnot et al., 2014).

The imaginative faculty animates a still-open debate. McGinn (2009) made a clear distinction between cognitive and sensory imagination. The first concerns a propositional attitude (that involves beliefs and concepts), while the second is based on the sensory dimension. In response to this dichotomy, other authors proposed a *multimodal spectrum of imagination* (Thomas, 2014).

Going into these topics goes beyond the scope of our work; however, we believe that also top-down processes can, at least, contribute to intensifying the desire for disability. As pointed out by some authors: "The more often a person thinks about being disabled, the more real the desire to fulfil this wish becomes" (Aner et al., 2018: 35).

As already mentioned, psychological therapies do not appear to be resolutive. Kröger and colleagues (2014) presented a questionnaire to 25 participants to investigate the effects of various therapeutic approaches, showing that 64% of these subjects never turned to psychotherapists or took psychopharmaceutical drugs. In our study, the percentage of those who have never turned to specialists is 56.1% (Table 12.11). Although it was not possible to determine the various therapeutic approaches followed by the participants, 50% of those who did psychotherapy (Table 12.12) stated that it did not help them, 25% stated that it did not help them with BID per se, and 10.7% stated that the psychological path helped them to accept the disorder, mitigating their feeling of being bizarre. Instead, 4 participants did not provide any indication of the effects of psychotherapy (14.3%).

In other studies, some patients with BID reported that adopting psychotherapeutic methods helped them relieve anxiety and depression (Blom et al., 2012), while others claimed that these sessions resulted in increased desire; according to Noll and Kasten (2014), this happens because talking about BID induces patients to focus their attention even more on the desire, which persists and strengthens.

Recently, Grocholewski and colleagues (2018) showed that BID – like *Body Dysmorphic Disorder* (BDD) – is characterized by a more significant number of mental images than the control group. Besides, contrary to what happens to individuals with BDD, it seems that mental images in BID are less intrusive and permeated by a positive attitude, so "parallel to real, everyday life, intentionally evoked mental images may often run as a permanent mental movie in the brain, which shows life as a person with the desired disability" (Grocholewski et al., 2018: 9).

However, a significant presence of intrusive thoughts – which seem to decrease after amputation – has also been found in BID (Oddo et al., 2009). Not surprisingly, some studies have investigated the similarities between BID and *obsessive-compulsive disorder* (OCD) (Braam et al., 2006), assuming the possibility that BID can be considered a subtype of OCD, in which the simulation of disability could be considered as a control compulsion in response to repetitive ruminations about desire (Link and Kasten, 2015).

We asked our participants to describe the intensity and impact of these thoughts in their lives. For some of them 'the feelings go up and down like an angry sea', in relation to stress levels, the attention paid, the type of activity performed and other circumstances:

> For me I guess BIID is a constant thing but at the same time it's kind of in the background? It's just feeling weird/off always to some degree but it's so amorphous it's difficult to pin it down. If I think about it too much it can be overwhelming and then all I want to do is get rid of the limb so I won't have to deal with it anymore.
>
> They come up regularly. Weekly, or more than weekly. If I am not stressed, but have a lot of work, they come up weekly. If I am stressed and a lot of work, they come up daily or hourly. The thoughts transfer me into an alternate reality.
>
> I have noticed that the extent of disconnection to my legs depends quite strongly on factors that would be expected to alter my brain's functioning. For example, a lack of sleep and even extremely small amounts of alcohol are two of my biggest triggers. Additional triggers include intense fright, and

> possibly excessive caffeine intake and stress (though these are more minor factors compared to the first three). Although I believe this is likely to be at root a neurological problem, I have lived the vast majority of my life with the belief that my legs should not function as they physically are able to. It is very possible that this has conditioned my brain to change the way it perceives my legs to the point where it is now impossible to distinguish cause from correlation.

Other participants responded that they are always 'hyperaware' of their bodily dissonance:

> The intensity fluctuates, but it's always there. Everywhere I walk, I imagine I'd be in a wheelchair; when I'm in bed I feel miserable about the fact that I'll have to get up again and when I sit down I imagine I'm in my wheelchair. This affects my mood, it feels like it is always a fight to push those thoughts away. It distracts immensely from everything else, work, friends, creativity etc. I think this makes that I'm not always performing to the best of my capabilities, because I spend so much time and energy on this internal fight.
>
> I am surprised when I catch myself not thinking about it. I think about it every hour of every day. Not constantly every day, but the thoughts are always there in the background at least. The only time I have had relief is when pretending to be a high level quadriplegic with assistance. . . . Allowing myself to have the BIID thoughts has flipped a switch and made the suicidal ideation disappear. Of course allowing myself to have these thoughts also takes up a great amount of my time. I think it has contributed to the loss of one job and made it extremely difficult to start another job. I specifically chose my current job because it allows me time every hour or so to think of anything that I want. It is also structured enough that if I find myself completely distracted from my work I can figure out where I was and get right back into it. I spend my free time mainly online with others who understand me, chatting and role playing, or consuming related media. My relations in person have been neglected because of this.

The Internet has represented a powerful turning point for minorities and, more specifically, for those suffering from this disorder (Bruno, 1997; Davis, 2012). As Berger and colleagues (2005) pointed out, without the advent of the web, it would have been difficult for people with BID to establish such a network of information and contacts.

In this regard, we asked our participants what online communities represent to them and we have summarized the answers in three categories (Table 12.13). We have included in the 'Positive' category answers such as '*It is a lifesaver! I have met other people like me and it is comforting that I can finally communicate with people like me*', or answers from those who have spent a lot of time on these platforms. In the 'Neutral' category, we inserted answers like '*Just communities*'. Lastly, in the

'Negative' category, we inserted answers like '*I now keep a minimal online presence in the BIID community as my past experience with it has been more about wallowing in depression than attempting to help each other*'. As we shared the questionnaire within social networks, we believe that 'not users' were invited to fill in the questionnaire by other participants.

The desire for disability has been defined by Charland (2004: 340) as "the first psychiatric disease manufactured in cyberspace". We disagree with this assumption. Some of our participants are over 70 years of age and report experiencing this discomfort since childhood. However, the reflections proposed by Davis (2011) might be interesting in relation to what we mentioned in the previous paragraph, about the engagement with material and digital things. Far from considering users (*prosumers*) and their content as separate elements, Davis argues that it is necessary to recognize that shared content itself can shape individuals' identity. In this view, participation in these communities would contribute to the prosuming of 'transabled identity' and, at the same time, to the construction of the category 'transableism' as a cultural variable of identity (Davis, 2011: 8–9).

Navigating these communities, we learned that the term 'transabled' is not welcomed by all users, especially after it has rebounded in the mass media attracting feelings of blame from public opinion.

Finally, we assume that intersubjectivity, the sharing of one's experiences and self-recognition within a horizon of personal and collective meaning, can contribute to the apprehension and the maintenance of desire:

> I've had these feeling for several years, but they became more intense once I learned about the term BIID. It's nice to finally have an explanation/definition for what I'm feeling, but it also makes me more aware of it.
>
> *(a participant's response to our questionnaire)*

Beyond the digital spaces, we asked the participants if they talked about their desire in the context of concrete relationships (Table 12.14). From our dates, it emerges that 60.6% spoke about their condition (in Table 12.15 it is possible to observe specifically with whom they did so).

8 Conclusion

Recently, Saetta and colleagues (2020) published the most comprehensive experimental study focused on BID. The principal evidence found by the researchers were as follows: a lack of intrinsic functional connectivity in the right paracentral lobule (rPCL) and the right superior parietal lobule (rSPL), interpreted as an inadequate anchoring of limb representations; atrophy of the left premotor cortex (lPMv) and the right superior parietal lobule (rSPL) which would suggest a deficit in multimodal integration; both functional and structural alterations in the rSPL, which would reflect an impaired body image at the highest level of integration (Saetta,

2020: 3). Furthermore, the authors correlated increased atrophy in the rSPL with a greater inclination to disability simulation, which would be the attempt of these subjects to mitigate the perceived discrepancy between their actual body and the desired one.

This study is precious, especially because it is conducted by a team of neuroscientists who have always underlined the importance of the psychological and sociological aspects inherent in this condition. For this reason, we wonder if the correlation between rSPL atrophy and disability simulation could also be read from the perspective of neuroplasticity.

Recently, Kasten (2019) pointed out the limitations of some brain theories, as these would not explain all cases of BID. According to the author, if the discrepancy between the physical body and the mental body resulted from a congenital dysfunction or damage in early development, there should be a congruent number of desires for legs and arms; moreover, the latter should be more recurrent, since the cerebral representation of the arm is more exposed in the cortex than that of the leg, and therefore would be more vulnerable (Kasten, 2019). In this respect, our study shows a decisive disproportion between requests for amputation (Table 12.6). While the desire to amputate the legs was indicated by 35 participants (one leg or bilateral legs), only 4 participants indicated the desire to amputate the arms (one arm or bilateral arms). Also, 5 participants reported a mixed desire for amputation of legs and arms (one leg and one arm, bilateral legs + one arm, quadruple amputation).

Also, as Kasten pointed out, sometimes the focus of desire can change over time or be directed to other parts after amputation (Sorene et al., 2006; Berger et al., 2005). In this regard, 60.6% of our participants stated that desire has never changed. Instead, 21.2% reported that desire has changed and 9.1% that it can change (Table 12.16).

The category 'Changed' includes the following changes: 1) from the right leg the desire also extended to the left and right arm, 2) from paralysis to bilateral amputation (with an intermittent desire directed to the arms and sensory deprivation); 3) an initial doubt between right and left leg; 4) from one arm the desire also extended to one leg; 5) from bilateral amputation to one leg; 6) from the left leg to the right leg; 7–8) from the right leg has also extended to the left; 9) from the right leg to the left leg; 10) from paraplegia to tetraplegia; 11) a desire that over time has translated into the desire to be visually more impaired than before; 12) from the left arm to the right leg; 13) the height of the cut; 14) not specified.

The category 'It can change' includes: 1) a participant who declared that the desire sometimes concerns amputation and sometimes paraplegia; 2) a desire for bilateral amputation which sometimes becomes a desire to be as deficient as possible; 3) a desire for paralysis which could be replaced by a bilateral amputation in order to live in a wheelchair; 4) bilateral amputation which sometimes becomes a wish for quadruple amputation; 5) indecision about being blind in one eye or both; 6) in addition to the left leg, sometimes the participant desires amputation of the right leg and right arm.

Furthermore, Kasten (2019) mentioned some cognitive-based changes, in which the preference of the limb to be amputated is related to functional limitations resulting from its absence. A small number of our participants responded as follows:

> I have always found several types of amputations interesting, however, bilateral amputation below the knee has solidified over time. But when I was younger, I was interested in arm amputations, paraplegia, and blindness as well. However, I imagine that the functional restrictions imposed by these deficiencies would be too great and I would not be happy to be so. But in a way, there is a desire in me to be as deficient as possible, in the sense that if there was a functionally perfect prosthesis of the arm, I think I would like this amputation too. And like the amputation of the legs, in intimate moments I would not like to use either the prostheses of the legs or those of the arms.
>
> *(a participant's response to our questionnaire)*

It changed from the right leg to the left leg after I started having problems with the left foot.

The last participant, however, reported that he had achieved amputation in his left leg and never regretted it. In this regard, we asked our participants if they have ever damaged any of their own body parts (Table 12.17). Participants in the category 'Yes' have achieved the desired disability or have come very close to it (12.1% of participants). None of them said they regretted their choice. The category 'Minor damage' refers to those cases involving mutilation or minor damage to the toes, fingers, eyes, calves (7.6%). 15.2% said they tried without success and 6% did not answer the question. Finally, 59.1% did not damage any body parts.

There is also another aspect that needs to be emphasized. We explicitly asked the participants whether the acquisition of a disability other than the aspired one could mitigate the desire to amputate or inhibit the unwanted parts. Out of 66 participants, it was found that only 13.6% of them said that this eventuality could 'satisfy' them (Table 12.18).

Finally, in the last part of our study – the only closed-answer question – we presented the following scenario:

> *Imagine a method which could fully restore your body integrity (with no collateral effects). Would you use it or would you still prefer to proceed with your desire?*
>
> - Yes, I would opt for a therapeutic method.
> - No, I would prefer to pursue my desire.

Our survey shows that 74.2% of respondents would prefer to achieve the desired disability (Table 12.19). This data could be a preliminary approximation of the degree of participation relative to a hypothetical rehabilitation horizon. In a

BID-centred book that also contains the patients' point of view, an academic physician with this condition wrote:

> It is reasonable to ask an individual with BIID whether (s)he would like to be cured of the desire for an amputation. Some may choose this. Many, including myself, do not want to be cured. When something has been part of one's psyche for as many years as BIID has been of mine – since my childhood – asking me to be cured of it is tantamount to asking me to change who I am.
>
> *(in Gheen, 2009: 97–98)*

However, as can be seen, a minority of participants are open to alternatives to surgery. About online communities, one of our participants said:

> People talk about how sexy they think they are, or obsess over what assistive devices they want/like, or justify their demands for surgery by falsely comparing what we go through to what trans people go through. Very rarely does anyone want to talk about how to just . . . live and learn to heal from it? It's alienating, especially when some BIID people are so aggressive about the surgery thing that they actually refuse to talk about anything ⋆but⋆ amputation.

In this study, we have tried to outline how body image can be, to a certain degree, a plastic process. In addition to a possible neurological origin, we have tried to highlight the role of a first phase of vulnerability in childhood, the neuroplastic retroaction related to simulation, the potential influence of culture and sharing of experiences. The primary purpose of this research was to reunite the brain with the living body, narratives, and environment:

> The brain is formed by mental life; from early childhood on, mental structures come to be imprinted in the brain's structure, and the individual increasingly shapes his own brain through his actions and interactions. . . . It constitutes a *system of open loops* that have been formed in the course of earlier interactions, and that are functionally closed each time the organism is interacting with a certain object or situation that it has dealt with before.
>
> *(Fuchs, 2011: 197–198)*

References

Aner, L. L., Schmitt, F., and Kasten, E. (2018). The beauty and the BIID. *International Journal of Research in Humanities and Social Studies*, 5(5), 33–53.

Aoyama, A., Krummenacher, P., Palla, A., Hilti, L. M., and Brugger, P. (2012). Impaired spatial-temporal integration of touch in xenomelia (body integrity identity disorder). *Spatial Cognition and Computation*, 12(2–3), 96–110.

Bayne, T., and Levy, N. (2005). Amputees by choice: Body integrity identity disorder and the ethics of amputation. *Journal of Applied Philosophy*, 22(1), 75–86.

Berger, B. D., Lehrmann, J. A., Larson, G., Alverno, L., and Tsao, C. I. (2005). Nonpsychotic, nonparaphilic self-amputation and the internet. *Comprehensive Psychiatry*, 46(5), 380–383.

Blom, R. M., Hennekam, R. C., and Denys, D. (2012). Body integrity identity disorder. *PLoS One*, 7(4), e34702.

Blom, R. M. (2016). Body integrity identity disorder crosses culture: Case reports in the Japanese and Chinese literature. *Neuropsychiatric Disease and Treatment*, 12, 1419–1423.

Braam, A. W., Visser, S., Cath, D. C., and Hoogendijk, W. J. (2006). Investigation of the syndrome of apotemnophilia and course of a cognitive-behavioural therapy. *Psychopathology*, 39(1), 32–37.

Brang, D., McGeoch, P., and Ramachandran, V. (2008). Apotemnophilia: A neurological disorder, *Cognitive Neuroscience and Neuropsychology*, 19(13), 1305–1306.

Brugger, P., Christen, M., Jellestad, L., and Hänggi, J. (2016). Limb amputation and other disability desires as a medical condition. *The Lancet Psychiatry*, 3(12), 1176–1186.

Brugger, P., Kurthen, I., Rashidi-Ranjbar, N., and Lenggenhager, B. (2018). Grey matter or social matters? Causal attributions in the era of biological psychiatry. *European Psychiatry*, 52, 45–46.

Brugger, P., Lenggenhager, B., and Giummarra, M. J. (2013). Xenomelia: A social neuroscience view of altered bodily self-consciousness. *Frontiers in Psychology*, 4, 204.

Brugger, P., and Lenggenhager, B. (2014). The bodily self and its disorders: Neurological, psychological and social aspects. *Current Opinion in Neurology*, 27(6), 644–652.

Bruno, R. L. (1997). Devotees, pretenders and wannabes: Two cases of factitious disability disorder. *Sexuality and Disability*, 15(4), 243–260.

Capodici, A. (2019). 'Sense-making': Dal 'tool' di significatività ai mondi extra-ordinari. *Reti, saperi, linguaggi*, 6(1), 131–150.

Capodici, A., and Russo, G. (2019). Map making as bodily engagement. *Reti, saperi, linguaggi*, 6(2), 223–237.

Charland, L. C. (2004). A madness for identity: Psychiatric labels, consumer autonomy, and the perils of the Internet. *Philosophy, Psychiatry, and Psychology*, 11(4), 335–349.

Critchley, M. (1955). Personification of paralysed limbs in hemiplegics. *BMJ*, 2, 284–286.

Davis, J. L. (2011). Prosuming identity: The production and consumption of transableism on transabled.org. *American Behavioral Scientist*, 56(4), 596–617.

Davis, J. L. (2012). Narrative construction of a ruptured self: Stories of transability on transabled.org. *Sociological Perspectives*, 55(2), 319–340.

De Jaegher, H. (2015). How we affect each other: Michel Henry's 'pathos-with' and the enactive approach to intersubjectivity. *Journal of Consciousness Studies*, 22(1–2), 112–132.

Everaerd, W. (1983). A case of apotemnophilia: A handicap as sexual preference. *American Journal of Psychotherapy*, 37(2), 285–293.

First, M. B. (2005). Desire for amputation of a limb: Paraphilia, psychosis, or a new type of identity disorder. *Psychological Medicine*, 35(6), 919–928.

Freedberg, D., and Pennisi, A. (2020). The body in the picture: The lesson of phantom limbs and the origins of the BIID. *Reti Saperi Linguaggi. Italian Journal of Cognitive Sciences*, I/2020, 5–50.

Fuchs, T. (2011). The brain: A mediating organ, *Journal of Consciousness Studies*, 18(7–8), 196–221.

Furth, G. M., and Smith, R. (2000). *Apotemnophilia: Information, questions, answers, and recommendations about self-demand amputation*. Bloomington, IN: 1st Books Library.

Gallagher, S., and Zahavi, D. (2008). *The phenomenological mind: An introduction to philosophy of mind and cognitive science*. New York: Routledge.

Gheen, M. (2009). Clear definitions and scientific understanding: Thoughts of an academic physician with BIID. In A. Stirn, A. Thiel, and S. Oddo (Eds.), *Body integrity identity disorder: Psychological, neurobiological, ethical and legal aspects* (pp. 94–102). Lengerich: Pabst Science Publishers.

Giummarra, M. J., Bradshaw, J. L., Nicholls, M., E., Hilti, L. M., and Brugger, P. (2011). Body integrity identity disorder: Deranged body processing, right fronto-parietal dysfunction, and phenomenological experience of body incongruity. *Neuropsychology Review*, 21(4), 320–333.

Giummarra, M. J., Bradshaw, J. L., Hilti, L. M., and Nicholls, M. E. (2012). Paralyzed by desire: A new type of body integrity identity disorder. *Cognitive and Behavioral Neurology*, 25(1), 34–41.

Grocholewski, A., Bücker, C., Kasten, E., Osen, B., and Heinrichs, N. (2018). Mental images in Body Integrity Identity Disorder (BIID) and in Body Dysmorphic Disorder (BDD): An exploratory study. *Behaviour Change*, 35(3), 174–184.

Hänggi, J., Bellwald, D., and Brugger, P. (2016). Shape alterations of basal ganglia and thalamus in xenomelia. *NeuroImage: Clinical*, 11, 760–769.

Heidegger, M. (1927). *Sein und Zeit*. Tübingen: Niemeyer, trad. it. di Chiodi, P. (1976). *Essere e Tempo*. Milano: Longanesi.

Hilti, L. M., and Brugger, P. (2010). Incarnation and animation: Physical versus representational deficits of body integrity. *Experimental Brain Research*, 204(3), 315–326.

Hilti, L. M., Hänggi, J., Vitacco, D. A., Kraemer, B., and Palla, A. (2013). The desire for healthy limb amputation: Structural brain correlates and clinical features of xenomelia. *Brain*, 136(1), 318–329.

Hutto, D., and Myin, E. (2017). *Evolving enactivism: Basic minds meet content*. Cambridge, MA: MIT Press.

Iachini, T. (2011). Mental imagery and embodied cognition: A multimodal approach. *Journal of Mental Imagery*, 35(3–4), 1–66.

Johnson, T. W., Wassersug, R. J., Roberts, L. F., and Sutherland, M. B. (2010). Desire for castration is not a body integrity identity disorder (BIID): A response. *The Journal of Sexual Medicine,* 7(2pt1), 853–855.

Johnson, A. J., Liew, S. L., and Aziz-Zadeh, L. (2011). Demographics, learning and imitation, and body schema in body integrity identity disorder. *Indiana University Undergraduate Journal of Cognitive Science*, 6, 8–15.

Kasten, E. (2009). Body Integrity Identity Disorder (BIID): Befragung von Betroffenen und Erklärungsansätze. *Fortschritte Neurologie Psychiatrie*, 77, 16–24.

Kasten, E. (2019). Which leg shall i cut off? Body Integrity Dysphoria (BID) is not only a neurologic disease: Results of five case-studies. *Case Studies Journal*, 8(12), 31–34.

Kasten, E., and Stirn, A. (2009). Body integrity identity disorder (BIID). *Zeitschrift für Psychiatrie, Psychotherapie und Psychologie*, 57, 55–61.

Kröger, K., Schnell, T., and Kasten, E. (2014). Effects of psychotherapy on patients suffering from body integrity identity disorder (BIID). *American Journal of Psychology*, 3, 110 115.

Langer, N., Hänggi, J., Müller, N. A., Simmen, H. P., and Jäncke, L. (2012). Effects of limb immobilization on brain plasticity. *Neurology*, 78(3), 182–188.

Lawrence, A. A. (2009). Parallels between gender identity disorder and body integrity identity disorder: A review and update. In *Body integrity identity disorder: Psychological, neurobiological, ethical and legal aspects* (pp. 154–172). Lengerich: Pabst.

Lawrence, A. A. (2010). Desire for castration is not a body integrity identity disorder: Comment on Johnson et al. (2007), Brett et al. (2007), and Roberts et al. (2008). *The Journal of Sexual Medicine*, 7(2pt1), 852–853.

Liew, S. L., Sheng, T., and Aziz-Zadeh, L. (2013). Experience with an amputee modulates one's own sensorimotor response during action observation. *Neuroimage*, 69, 138–145.

Link, S., and Kasten, E. (2015). Xenomelia and obsessive-compulsive disorder: Similarities and differences. *American Journal of Psychiatry and Neuroscience*, 3(4), 63–69.

Loetscher, T., Regard, M., and Brugger, P. (2006). Misoplegia: A review of the literature and a case without hemiplegia. *BMJ*, 77(9), 1099–1100.

Malafouris, L. (2013). *How things shape the mind*. Cambridge, MA: MIT Press.

McGeoch, P., Brang, D., Song, T., Roland, R., Huang, M., and Ramachandran, V. (2009). Apotemnophilia – The neurological basis of a 'psychological' disorder. *Nature Proceedings*. https://doi.org/10101/npre.2009.2954.1

McGeoch, P. D., Brang, D., Song, T., Lee, R. R., Huang, M., and Ramachandran, V. S. (2011). Xenomelia: A new right parietal lobe syndrome. *Journal of Neurology, Neurosurgery and Psychiatry*, 1314–1319.

McGinn, C. (2009). Imagination. In B. McLaughlin, A. Beckermann, and S. Walter (Eds.), *The Oxford handbook of philosophy of mind* (pp. 595–606). New York: Oxford University Press.

Meugnot, A., Almecija, Y., and Toussaint, L. (2014). The embodied nature of motor imagery processes highlighted by short-term limb immobilization. *Experimental Psychology*, 61(3), 180–186.

Money, J., Jobaris, R., and Furth, G. (1977). Apotemnophilia: Two cases of self-demand amputation as a paraphilia. *Journal of Sex Research*, 13(2), 115–125.

Müller, S. (2009). Body integrity identity disorder (BIID): Is the amputation of healthy limbs ethically justified? *The American Journal of Bioethics*, 9(1), 36–43.

Noë, A. (2009). *Out of our heads: Why you are not your brain, and other lessons from the biology of consciousnes*. New York: Hill and Wang.

Noll, S., and Kasten, E. (2014). Body integrity identity disorder (BIID): How satisfied are successful wannabes. *Psychology and Behavioral Science*, 3, 222–232.

Obernolte, C., Schnell, T., and Kasten, E. (2015). The role of specific experiences in childhood and youth in the development of body integrity identity disorder (BIID). *American Journal of Applied Psychology*, 4(1), 1–8.

Oddo, S., Thiel, A., Skoruppa, S., Klinger, D., and Steis, N. M. (2009). Neurobiological and psychological aspects of BIID: An integrative approach. In A. Stirn, A. Thiel, and S. Oddo (Eds.), *Body integrity identity disorder: Psychological, neurobiological, ethical and legal aspects* (pp. 238–245). Lengerich: Pabst Science Publishers.

Pennisi, A. (2020). *Che ne sarà dei corpi. Spinoza i BIID e l'Embodied Cognition*. Bologna: Il Mulino (in stampa).

Saetta, G., Hänggi, J., Gandola, M., Zapparoli, L., Salvato, G., Berlingeri, M., . . . and Brugger, P. (2020). Neural correlates of body integrity dysphoria. *Current Biology*, 30(11), 2191–2195.

Sartre, J. P. (1943). *L'être et le néant: Essai d'ontologie phénoménologique* (*Being and nothingness: An essay on phenomenological ontology*) (H. E. Barnes, trans.). New York: Philosophical Library, 1956.

Sedda, A., and Bottini, G. (2014). Apotemnophilia, body integrity identity disorder or xenomelia? Psychiatric and neurologic etiologies face each other. *Neuropsychiatric Disease and Treatment*, 10, 1255–1265.

Shapiro, L. A. (2011). *Embodied cognition*. London and New York: Routledge.

Smith, R. C. (2004). Amputee identity disorder and related paraphilias. *Psychiatry*, 3(8), 27–30.

Sorene, E. D., Heras-Palou, C., and Burke, F. D. (2006). Self-amputation of a healthy hand: A case of body integrity identity disorder. *Journal of Hand Surgery*, 31(6), 593–595.
Storm, S., and Weiss, M. D. (2003). Self-inflicted tourniquet paralysis mimicking acute demyelinating polyneuropathy. *Muscle and Nerve: Official Journal of the American Association of Electrodiagnostic Medicine*, 27(5), 631–635.
Ramachandran, V. S., and McGeoch, P. D. (2007). Can vestibular caloric stimulation be used to treat apotemnophilia? *Medical Hypotheses*, 69(2), 250–252.
Romano, D., Sedda, A., Brugger, P., and Bottini, G. (2015). Body ownership: When feeling and knowing diverge. *Consciousness and Cognition*, 34, 140–148.
Thiel, A., Ehni, F. J., Oddo, S., and Stirn, A. (2011). Body integrity identity disorder: First success in long-term psychotherapy. *Psychiatrische Praxis*, 38(5), 256–258.
Thomas, N. J. (2014). The multidimensional spectrum of imagination: Images, dreams, hallucinations, and active, imaginative perception. *Humanities*, 3(2), 132–184.
Wassersug, R. J., Johnson, T. W., Brett, M. A., and Roberts, L. F. (2007). Eunuchs in contemporary society: Characterizing men who are voluntarily castrated (part I). *The Journal of Sexual Medicine*, 4(4), 930–945.

APPENDIX 1

- *Section one:* Living with BID
  1 Scientific literature has described BID as a paraphilia, an identity disorder or a neurological disorder. Beyond the scientific label, what does it feel like to live this condition?
  2 When did the lack of bodily integrity emerge?
  3 How intensely do BID thoughts occupy your mind? How do these thoughts affect your life?
- *Section two:* Self and Body image
  4 It appears that people who live with BIID know that the target body part belongs to their own body. Despite this, they feel it shouldn't be. Please, describe your body image.
  5 How do you feel the target body part? How does this experience differ from the experience of feeling the rest of your body? (for example, in terms of tactile, visual, motor, and emotional feelings).
  6 In your opinion, what is the cause of such a lack of consonance with the target body part to? Would you say it is caused by its functionality or its presence?
- *Section three:* Pretending behaviour
  7 What does pretending behaviour mean for you? (for example, a relief, a palliative, an additional frustration).
  8 If you usually practice it, since when and how much do you practice it?
  9 What do prostheses, wheelchairs, leg braces, crutches or similar tools mean for you? What is your relationship with these objects?
- *Section four:* Target of desire
  10 Has the target of your desire always remained the same? If not, how has it changed over time?

11 If you accidentally lost a body part other than the target one, would this event satisfy you or would you still try to pursue your desire?
12 Have you ever amputated or damaged a part of your body? If so, have you ever regretted it?

- *Section five:* Talking about desire

13 What do online communities mean for you?
14 Have you talked to friends and family about your desire? Describe your experience (for example, the reasons why you did it – or why you didn't – the reactions of people close to you, how you feel about it).
15 Have you ever followed a psychological therapy? If so, has it helped you in any way?

- *Section six:* A Hypothetical Crossroad

16 Imagine a method which could fully restore your body integrity (with no collateral effects). Would you use it or would you still prefer to proceed with your desire?

- Yes, I would opt for a therapeutic method.
- No, I would prefer to pursue my desire.

APPENDIX 2

TABLE 12.1

Age		*66 Participants*
18–30	45.45%	30
31–50	31.82%	21
51–75	22.73%	15

TABLE 12.2

Continent		*66 Participants*
Europe	45.45%	30
North America	40.91%	27
South America	7.58%	5
Oceania	3.03%	2
Asia	1.52%	1
Africa	1.52%	1

TABLE 12.3

Gender		*66 Participants*
Male	65.2%	43
Female	21.2%	14
Other	13.6%	9

TABLE 12.4

Disability desire		*66 Participants*
Amputation	71.2%	47
Paralysis	15.2%	10
Sensory deprivation	7.6%	5
Mixed	4.5%	3
N.B.S.	1.5%	1

The "mixed" category includes: 1) a participant who has stated that he wishes to become wheelchair dependent, regardless of the type of disability required for this purpose, 2) a participant who has stated that he sometimes feels the desire to be a DAK amputee and sometimes to be paraplegic, 3) a participant who has expressed the desire to remove a leg and genitals. The last participant has already reached eunuch condition.

TABLE 12.5

Gender and desire correlation						*66 Participants*
	Amputation	*Paralysis*	*Sensory deprivation*	*Mixed*	*N.B.S.*	
Male	56.1%	4.5%	1.5%	3%	–	43 participants
Female	7.6%	9.1%	3%	–	1.5%	14 participants
Other	7.6%	1.5%	3%	1.5%	–	9 participants

TABLE 12.6

Disability form		*66 Participants*
One-legged	33.33%	22
One leg, one arm	4.55%	3
One leg + genitals	1.52%	1
Bilateral legs amputation	19.70%	13
Bilateral legs + one arm	1.52%	1
Quadruple amputation	1.52%	1
One-armed	3.03%	2
Bilateral arms amputation	3.03%	2
Paraplegic	10.61%	7
Tetraplegic	4.55%	3
Blindness	7.58%	5
Dak amp./paraplegic	1.52%	1
Wheelchair goal	1.52%	1
N.B.S.	6.06%	4

TABLE 12.7

Onset of desire		*66 Participants*
Childhood (<11)	72.73%	48
Youth (12–19)	21.21%	14
Adulthood (>20)	4.55%	3
N.B.S.	1.52%	1

TABLE 12.8

Disability simulation		*66 Participants*
Yes	63.64%	42
No	13.64%	9
Not anymore	15.15%	10
Not yet	4.55%	3
N.B.S.	3.03%	2

TABLE 12.9

What it represents		*42 Participants*
Relief	50.00%	21
Frustration	2.38%	1
Relief and frustration	30.95%	13
Relief and shame	4.76%	2
Relief (but strengthens BID)	2.38%	1
Fun	2.38%	1
N.B.S.	7.14%	3

TABLE 12.10

Simulation times		*42 Participants*
Daily	28.6%	12
Weekly	19%	8
Occasionally	28.6%	12
Most in the past	9.5%	4
N.B.S.	14.3%	6

These categories have been described in the section "Enacting disability".

TABLE 12.11

Psychological therapy		*66 Participants*
Yes	42.4%	28
No	56.1%	37
N.B.S.	1.5%	1

TABLE 12.12

It has helped?		*28 Participants*
Yes (self-acceptance)	10.7%	3
No	50%	14
Not with BID per se	25%	7
N.B.S.	14.3%	4

TABLE 12.13

Attitude towards online communities		*66 Participants*
Positive	78.8%	52
Negative	4.5%	3
Neutral	12.1%	8
Not user	3%	2
N.B.S.	1.5%	1

TABLE 12.14

Talking to someone		*66 Participants*
Yes	60.6%	40
No	36.4%	24
N.B.S.	3%	2

TABLE 12.15

Talking with . . . who?		*40 Participants*
Family only	5%	2
Partner only	12.5%	5
Friends only	22.5%	9
Family and partner	2.5%	1
Family and friends	12.5%	5
Partner and friends	17.5%	7
Everyone	15%	6
N.B.S.	12.5%	5

TABLE 12.16

Change of the desire		*66 Participants*
Changed	21.2%	14
It can change	9.1%	6
Not changed	60.6%	40
N.B.S.	9.1%	6

The description of the categories "Changed" and "It can change" can be observed in their entirety in the Conclusions of this work.

TABLE 12.17

Self-damage		*66 Participants*
Yes	12.1%	8
Attempt	15.2%	10
Minor damage	7.6%	5
No	59.1%	39
N.B.S.	6%	4

TABLE 12.18

Losing another body part		*66 Participants*
Not satisfied	51.5%	34
Yes, satisfied	13.6%	9
Not sure	22.7%	15
N.B.S.	12.1%	8

TABLE 12.19

Rehabilitation or disability?		*66 Participants*
Rehabilitative method	25.8%	17
Achieving disability	74.2%	49

13

LOST IN LOVE

Why is it so painful when romance goes wrong?

Domenica Bruni

1 Mate choice from the perspective of biology

Mate choice is a very complicated matter. It is influenced by many factors: biology, environment, culture, and genetics. Mate choice is also the issue of a long and complex debate. In his seminal book, *The Descent of Man, and Selection in Relation to Sex* (1871), Charles Darwin investigated the mechanism of sexual selection and argued for the idea that females, into the wild, are the most selective gender and that sexual choice is a female matter, because in the end females are the source of the parental care.

Darwin's ideas are still surprisingly relevant for the contemporary study of sexual selection. Darwin's mechanism of sexual selection includes two aspects: the competition between male individuals and the female – or sometimes male – choice of the best partner for mating. The term 'competition' suggests a lack of cooperation in what is called *reproductive endeavour.* It could be believed that everything that has to do with mating is cooperative and supportive. In reality, there are a lot of conflicts between males and females which are difficult to eliminate also after the cultural encoding happens. In the deep time, races and competitions for mating had profound effects on both animal physiology and behaviour. Evolutionary biologists have identified how sexual selection influences how occurs human individual preferences in choosing the partner (Bruni, 2010; Buss, 1994; Pilastro, 2007). It seems that males choose all those characters which can highlight female fecundity; on the other side, the choice of females seems more complex, because it is not simply oriented towards highly masculine phenotypes.

The choice of the best mate for reproduction is the basis of the evolution of secondary sexual characteristics in both sexes. The principles governing sexual selection, indeed, are the same in males and females. However, the action of sexual selection does not have the same consequences in the two sexes of the species. To understand sexual behaviour, it is necessary to start with the basic rules of genetics. The role within both sexes is played by different investing in gametes. There are two types of gametes which are produced in most animal species: sperm and egg cells. While the former is made of very small and mobile gametes, the latter are not so mobile, and they are large and rich in nutrients. From a metabolic point of view, in the production of gametes the female investment is greater than the male. For this reason, females have to accurately protect their investment and they will be more selective in the choice of partners. This happens mainly in mammals and birds, but not in fishes. In fish, it is the males who provide parental care. In monogamous species too, males are as selective as the females because they take care of the offspring.

Males, therefore, typically compete with each other for access to females, whereas females tend to be choosy and mate only with preferred males (Bateman, 1948). As already mentioned, Charles Darwin correctly realized that female choice was an important mechanism in sexual selection.

He also understood that sexual selection can sometimes act on both sexes or more strongly on women than on men. Darwin did not, however, clearly and unambiguously identify the evolutionary reasons for female choice. Rather, he tended to refer to the presence of an aesthetic sense in animals similar to the human one.

Many questions remained unanswered, but Darwin's merit is that he offered a theoretical framework for later investigation. Overall, the study of sexual selection is a mechanism that is at the heart of contemporary studies in the field of evolutionary biology.

2 What is called 'love'

Love plays a central role in the experience and life of each of us. The romantic idea of sexuality and love includes a set of fundamental components, such as the sense of responsibility, commitment to the other, sacrifice, tenderness, and passion. It is a universal experience and as such it crosses time and cultures. Romantic love pervades many forms of our existence: poetry, music, literature, personal fantasies, and everyday life. But often the relationships, that characterize the human species, are characterized by many contradictions. Everybody can dedicate her life to finding a partner who will change, or destroy, her life because of a wrong choice.

The search for a partner with whom to build your life is a strong driving force that changes the minds and makes human behaviour unique. When a love affair ends, euphoria is replaced by depression and people may chase or persecute the lover so much that they make extreme gestures such as murder or suicide. We all talk about love all day and we all talk about it in terms of passion, pain, desire, affection, passion, and attraction. Love is declined in many ways and this makes it difficult to find a univocal and exhaustive definition. In *The Instinctoid Nature of Basic Needs* (1954), Abraham H. Maslow inserts love into the motivational system at the basis of human action in the category of the needs of social belonging.

Loving – and to be loved – is, therefore, part of the subjects' need to have a rich relational and emotional life able to produce the feeling of being part of a social context.

In 1986, Robert J. Sternberg elaborated a model that includes different types of couple love that are the result of the presence, or absence, of three variables: *intimacy* ('feelings of closeness, connectedness, and bondedness in loving relationships'); *passion* ('the drives that lead to romance, physical attraction, sexual consummation, and related phenomena in loving relationship'); and *decision/commitment*. In the short term, it refers to 'the decision that one loves a certain other', and in the long term, it refers to 'one's commitment to maintaining that love'. This model is known as the *Triangular Theory of Love* and provides seven ways in which love goes on.

According to Harry G. Frankfurt, human nature has two characteristics: rationality and the ability to love (Frankfurt, 2006). Reason and love are normative authorities that guide in the choices to be made, motivate our action, and bind it. Reason gives us the tools to realize our desires but often too many alternatives lead to paralysis. Love is taking care of oneself. Love for oneself is nothing but the spring that pushes us to search for the meaning of our life.

Helen Fisher suggests a cognitive and evolutionary explanation of love. Her main question is the simplest: 'What is love?'. According to Fisher, to answer that question we have to follow the course of our biological history. And, this latter is characterized by the development of three brain systems that make possible behaviours aimed at reproduction. The three brain systems are *lust*, *romantic attraction*, and *attachment* (Fisher, 1989, 1992, 1998, 1999, 2004). In particular, lust drives the subject to seek sexual intercourse with any partner. The romantic attraction directs and focuses this undifferentiated attention towards a particular individual. Subsequently, the man–woman attachment that has evolved to ensure protection, safety, and appropriate care for offspring comes into play. One of these three elements, i.e., romantic passion, influences *libido* (the desire for sexual fulfilment) and all the sensations that are connected to the long-term attachment (serenity, security, union). The stage of sexual attraction is associated with the production of large amounts of testosterone that drives the individual to mate. The increase in dopamine and norepinephrine would, on the other hand, be the main causes of love ecstasy together with an evident decrease in serotonin release in the brain. Affective attachment enables the formation of stable and lasting bonds between men and women. In men, the feelings of attachment are linked to the increased production of vasopressin; in women, on the other hand, it increases in oxytocin. Vasopressin and oxytocin are hormones produced by the hypothalamus, an area located in the lower part of the diencephalon.

The function exerted by the hypothalamus is twofold and is linked to survival and reproduction. The hypothalamus controls, in fact, the production of hormones and the expression of some elementary and innate behavioural patterns such as sleep-wake rhythms, nutrition, body temperature, aggression–defence mechanism, and sexual behaviour. Fisher's studies on romantic love can be compared with other research based on the identification of brain areas involved in instinctual manifestations and sexual arousal (Tiihonen et al., 1994; Beauregard et al., 2001; Karama et al., 2002). The two drives are processed in different brain areas.

Evolutionary biologists have identified in animals a large number of traits that have evolved to attract conspecifics. The brain mechanisms underlying the preferences for these traits are largely unknown. The data, however, suggest that the attraction system is associated with the dopaminergic reward system. Fisher claim that romantic love is a developed form of this attraction system. To determine the neural mechanisms associated with romantic love, Helen Fisher used functional magnetic resonance imaging (*f*MRI) on 17 subjects who had declared that they were intensely "in love" (Aron et al., 2005). The results show activation of the right ventral tegmental area and right caudate nucleus, dopamine-rich areas associated with the reward and motivation system. The reward system is a group of neural structures responsible for motivation, associative learning, and positive emotions, especially those involving pleasure (euphoria, joy, ecstasy). Therefore, romantic love is not a single emotion, but a system of motivations. It's an instinct that changes over time and it is different from the mere sexual impulse. This instinct likely evolved so that individuals would concentrate all their energy on the conspecifics to make it easier to choose the best mate for reproduction. In summary, at a functional level, we love romantically because romantic love is necessary both for reproduction and for the care of offspring, thus improving our evolutionary success. At a mechanistic level, love is obsessive, intense, and tends to impair free will. The romantic love, as described by Helen Fisher's cognitive theory, is nothing but a biological need. We feel the impulse to love and to be loved, because this makes us happy and makes us feel better, fuller, and more motivated.

3 Lost in love: a possible connection between romantic love and love addiction

Thanks to the data from the *f*MRI techniques, it is now well known that we can experience romantic love because of the activity of the brain's reward system. Lovers show all the typical symptoms underlying addictions (Acevedo et al., 2011; Aron et al., 2005; Bartels and Zeki, 2000, 2004; Fisher et al., 2003, 2005, 2010; Ortigue et al., 2007; Xu et al., 2011): persistent desire, ecstasy, salience, mood swings, emotional and physical addiction, distortion of reality, tolerance, anxiety, motivation, concentration, abstinence, craving, and fall.

By analysing the above aspects, it could be expected that romantic love is a good candidate to be considered as a typical addiction. The scientific community, however, does not agree on the unique definition of addiction, but on the fact that different behavioural traits and the complex universe of behaviours associated with the concept of addiction actually have a core of common elements and manifestations that can be legitimately brought back into this single theoretical class. Researchers are not yet ready to officially classify romantic love as an addiction insofar as they are not able to recognize its pathological and harmful aspect. Abusing substances, such as cannabis, alcohol, and tobacco, are protractedly active in the dopaminergic neurons of the 'reward system' (hyperactivation of the ventral tegmental area – VTA, ventral striatum, anterior cingulate cortex – ACC, orbitofrontal cortex – OFC, prefrontal cortex, and insula). The same happens to people in love and people rejected in love. It is this circumstance that led to the conclusion that romantic love can be treated as a kind of addiction. Addiction can be positive in the case of reciprocated love, healthy, satisfying, or negative in the case of unrequited or toxic love. Subjects who are in love or rejected in love show the same characteristics usually associated with addictions such as compulsive or craving desire and focused attention to the object they love.

Love becomes pathological when intense desire turns into necessity and pleasure into pain and suffering. Although the subjects are aware of the many negative consequences, they could persevere in the reconquest of the partner. Control systems are compromised in the same way as substance addictions. It is possible, therefore, to assume that love addiction is caused by a stiffening of the typical and natural characteristics of romantic love. Obviously, as is the case with all phenomena, romantic love needs to be placed within a much broader framework that includes other factors such as biological factors, the individual vulnerability that has been maintained throughout evolution, contextual factors (e.g., ontogenetic, historical, individual contexts), and subjective experiences. The phenomenon we are examining cannot be explained only by using the definition of 'addiction' or 'maladaptive evolution'. However, this way of investigating the phenomenon of love could offer good behavioural strategies useful to those on the borderline between attachment and dependence (see Section 5).

4 But I love you more than ever

Romantic rejection is a very common experience in everyone's life. After rejection and after the breaking of a love affair, we feel desperate, empty, stressed, angry, and scared. What is the reason for this suffering? Why can't we manage the pain and get through it in a short time? Love seems to have a dark side that can be explained by evolutionary reasons. Scientific investigations have not offered a conclusive answer to this question, but the mainstreaming hypothesis is that lovers continue to love their partners also after being rejected or after the end of a romantic relationship. A piece of evidence for this is the intense activity of the ventral tegmental area (VTA), an area involved in the brain's reward system, both physiologically and under drug stimuli (Clark, 2012; Fisher, 2004).

Love rejection could be an evolutionary response endowed with a specific function. Many psychiatrists have identified two phases of rejection: protest and despair/rejection. Each phase has specific characteristics. During the 'protest' phase, subjects are obsessed with a single idea, that is, regaining the lost object. In this phase, the greater the obstacles, the greater the love passion. Helen Fisher uses the expression "frustration-attraction" to describe this state of the mind (Fisher, 2014: 16). Let's try to analyse the two phases in greater detail. Thomas Lewis et al. (2000) believe that protest is a response present in all mammals after the breaking of social ties.

The levels of dopamine and norepinephrine in the blood increase and the animal tends to obsessively search for those who have abandoned it (usually the mother). High levels of dopamine in the blood are present also in the initial phase of romantic attraction, and this would explain why those who are left are overwhelmed by love passion despite the rejection. In addition to activating the mechanism known as "frustration-attraction", the stress system that activates dopamine production and inhibits the release of serotonin is also activated.

While individuals we love are going away from us, our brain and chemicals networks continue to create increasing intense feelings of love. There is something ironic about this feeling or, better, an incredibly powerful natural mechanism. The mechanism known as "frustration–attraction" is also triggered by other brain activities. I refer to the central components of the brain's reward system which are associated with focused attention and motivation: when an expected reward (in our case, love) is delayed, the group of neurons known as the dopaminergic–mesolimbic pathway, connecting the tegmental ventral zone (VTA) to the nucleus accumbens (NAcc), together with the GABAergic D1 neurons, extend their activity. The protest phase can also be characterized by the intense activity of the brain panic system (Panksepp, 1998), which generates concern, alarm, and separation anxiety as a behavioural response (in a similar way to what happens with newborns when the mother moves away). In addition to these continuous and intense activities, there is also the anger, which typically produces heartbeat (abandonment anger [Meloy, 1998]; hate–love [Fisher, 2004]).

Love and anger are intimately connected in our brain:

> Romantic passion and abandonment rage have much in common. Both are associated with bodily and mental arousal; both produce obsessive thinking, focused attention, motivation and goal-directed behaviors; and both cause intense yearning – either for union with or fury at the beloved (Fisher, 2004; Meloy and Fisher, 2005). Moreover, love and rage can act in tandem. In a study of 124 dating couples, Ellis and Malamuth (2000) reported that romantic love and 'anger/upset' react to different kinds of information. The lover's level of anger/upset oscillates in response to events that undermine the lover's goals, such as a mate's infidelity, lack of emotional commitment, and/or rejection. The lover's feelings of romantic love fluctuate, instead, in response to events that advance the lover's goals, such as a partner's visible social support during outings with relatives and friends or direct declaration of love and fidelity. Thus, romantic love and anger/upset can operate concurrently, adding complexity and intensity to the expression of rejection addiction.
>
> *(Fisher, 2014: 258)*

When the protest phase ends, individuals who have been abandoned move on to the second phase: the despair/reassignment. I would mention just an experiment among many. Jack Mearns (1991) evaluated 114 abandoned people in love. The results are as follows: 40% of the subjects who were tested were clinically depressed;

12% suffered from moderate to severe depression. Some of them committed suicide and others died by heartbreak or stroke. The phase of resignation/despair is present also in other mammal species among which the presence of what psychologists call the 'response to despair' has been identified. If the reward is late in coming or never comes, it decreases the level of dopamine in the blood causing lethargy, depression, and discouragement (Najib et al., 2004; Panksepp, 1998).

Depression has high metabolic and social costs. However, it also has some positive aspects, being a physical reaction that has evolved over millions of years. Many hypotheses describe the benefits of depression. Paul Watson, Paul Andrews, and Edward Hagen include depression in the list of honest signals (Hagen, 2011; Watson and Andrews, 2002). What, then, would be credible in the eyes of others? The answer, perhaps, includes the supposition that you are dealing with something deeply wrong and, therefore, you need to ask for help and be consoled. Subsequently, the subject will be able to go in search of a new partner and start again. Moreover, the kind of depression known as 'failure of denial' allows us to honestly evaluate ourselves and others, allows us to face painful truths and to implement decision-making strategies which are useful for reproductive success and survival. According to the evolutionary point of view, if we investigate the brain of people which are rejected in love, one typical feature emerges: romantic love is a powerful motivational mechanism that allows us to focus attention on a specific partner saving energy and time for mating and reproduction.

When we fail in love, we can suffer deeply and terribly for good evolutionary reasons. We feel loss (anger, fury, jealousy, panic, and stress) and we do everything we can to win back the individual we love. But, in the end, we give up completely who we love to start again the search and risk everything again to win the biggest prize in life: the partner.

5 Strategies for helping lovers: S.L.A.A., drugs, and talk therapy

Finding useful strategies to survive love suffering is not easy. However, the aforementioned studies coming from neuroscience, biology, and cognitive anthropology give us not only the vision of the brain organization of love addiction, but also some hypotheses on the strategies to be adopted to free oneself from suffering. Data from brain research suggest that rejected lovers should immediately eliminate anything that reminds them of the lost partner (photos, letters, cards, gifts, etc.). Staying tied to the past, indeed, increases the activity of dopaminergic systems linked to intense passion, thus delaying the release from pain.

Rejected lovers could also follow the twelfth steps program, a set of guiding principles that outlines a course of action for recovery from addiction, compulsion, or other behavioural problems. Specifically, they could become members of a supporting organization like 'Sex and Love Addicts Anonymous' (S.L.A.A.). S.L.A.A. is a not-for-profit organization, a voluntary support group therapy association that uses the 'twelfth steps program' to recover from sex and love addiction. S.L.A.A.

was founded in 1976 in Boston and is promoted by some members of Alcoholics Anonymous who believed that sex, emotional affairs, and love addiction were conditioning their lives just like substance addiction. According to the promoters of the association, the compulsion to sexual promiscuity or persistence in destructive relationships cannot be controlled by the force of will alone. Among the strategies to be adopted, there is also the use of some drugs: norepinephrine, prolactin, and oxytocin agonists. These drugs tend to decrease both obsessive thoughts and physical pain. Moreover, they recover the damage caused to the body by protracted stress. However, it should be taken into account that these medications cause side effects that could affect the possibility of building a new, stable, and fulfilling relationship.

Many drugs, indeed, produce addiction, apathy, weight gain, sleep disorders, or have negative effects on the emotional system and sexuality. Usually, these effects disappear after you stop taking the medicine. Therefore, it would be better for antidepressant drugs to be used for short-term therapy. Another strategy to help lovers is, of course, psychotherapy. Talk therapies can cause many changes in brain function just like the use of antidepressant drugs (Brody et al., 2001; Rosenthal, 2002). Some studies show that in those who have undergone psychotherapy, there has been new and intense activity in the insula regions that can inhibit feelings of depression. In the end, the most effective method to overcome love addiction seems to be talk therapies combined with short-term drug therapy.

It is clear that 'recovery' from love suffering takes time. As the number of days after rejection increases, the brain activity that causes the feeling of strong attachment to the loved individual decreases proportionally. It is necessary not to have more contact with those who rejected us, to build new habits in our daily life; often it is necessary to adopt a short-term pharmacological therapy and to receive a talk therapy too, if love addiction is toxic and it risks destroying our existence. According to Helen Fisher, "the brain is built to heal itself, most likely a trait that initially evolved so that our forebears could resume their search for an appropriate breeding and parenting partner" (Fisher, 2014: 274).

References

Acevedo, B., Aron, A., Fisher, H., and Brown, L. (2011). Neural correlates of long-term intense romantic love. *Social Cognitive and Affective Neuroscience*. https://doi.org/10.1093/scan/nsq092

Aron, A., Fisher, H. E., Mashek, D. J., Strong, G., Li, H. F., and Brown, L. L. (2005). Reward, motivation, and emotion systems associated with early-stage intense romantic love: An fMRI study. *Journal of Neurophysiology*, 94, 327–337.

Bartels, A., and Zeki, S. (2000). The neural basis of romantic love. *NeuroReport*, 11, 3829–3834.

Bartels, A., and Zeki, S. (2004). The neural correlates of maternal and romantic love. *NeuroImage*, 21, 1155–1166.

Bateman, A. J. (1948). Intra-sexual selection in 'drosophila'. *Heredity*, 2, 349–368.

Beauregard, K., Levesque, J., and Bourgouin, P. (2001). Neural correlates of conscious self-regulation of emotion. *Journal of Neuroscience*, 21(18), 1–6.

Brody, A. L., et al. (2001). Regional brain metabolic changes in patients with major depression treated with either paroxetine or interpersonal therapy: Preliminary findings. *Archives of General Psychiatry*, 58(7), 631–640.

Bruni, D. (2010). *Storia naturale dell'amore*. Roma: Carocci.

Buss, D. (1994). *The evolution of desire: Strategies of human mating*. New York: Basic Books.

Clark, A. M. (2012). Reward processing: A global brain phenomenon? *Journal of Neurophysiology*, 109(1), 1–4.

Darwin, C. (1871). *The descent of man, and selection in relation to sex*. London: John Murray (Princeton: Princeton University Press, 1981).

Ellis, B. J., and Malamuth, N. M. (2000). Love and anger in romantic relationships: A discrete systems model. *Journal of Personality*, 68, 525–556.

Fisher, E. (1989). Evolution of serial pairbonding. *American Journal of Physical Anthropology*, 78, 331–541.

Fisher, E. (1992). *Anatomy of love: A natural history of mating, marriage and why we stray*. New York: W. W. Norton.

Fisher, E. (1998). Lust, attraction, and attachment in mammalian reproduction. *Human Nature*, 9(I), 23–52.

Fisher, E. (1999). *The first sex: The natural talents of women and how they are changing the word*. New York: Random House.

Fisher, E. (2004). *Why we love: The nature and chemistry of romantic love*. New York: Henry Holt.

Fisher, E. (2014). The tyranny of love: Love addiction – An anthropologist's view. In L. C. Feder and K. Rosenberg (Eds.), *Behavioral addictions: Criteria, evidence and treatment*. London: Elsevier Press.

Fisher, H. E., Aron, A., and Brown, L. L. (2005). Romantic love: An MRI study of a neural mechanism for mate choice. *Journal of Comparative Neurology*, 493, 58–62.

Fisher, H. E., Aron, A., Mashek, D., Strong, G., Li, H., and Brown, L. L. (2003). *Early stage intense romantic love activates cortical-basal-ganglia reward/motivation, emotion and attention systems: An fMRI study of a dynamic network that varies with relationship length, passion intensity and gen- der*. Poster presented at the Annual Meeting of the Society for Neuroscience, New Orleans, LA, November 11.

Fisher, H. E., Brown, L. L., Aron, A., Strong, G., and Mashek, D. (2010). Reward, addiction, and emotion regulation systems associated with rejection in love. *Journal of Neurophysiology*, 104, 51–60.

Frankfurt, H. G. (2006). *The reason of love*. Princeton: Princeton University Press.

Hagen, E. H. (2011). Evolutionary theories of depression: A critical review. *Canadian Journal of Psychiatry*, 56, 716–726.

Karama, S. et al. (2002). Areas of brain activation in males and females during viewing of erotic film excepts. *Human Brain Mapping*, 161(I), 1–13.

Lewis, T., Amini, F., and Lannon, R. (2000). *A general theory of love*. New York: Random House.

Maslow, A. H. (1954). The instinctoid nature of basic needs. *Journal of Personality*, 22(3), 326–347.

Mearns, J. (1991). Coping with a breakup: Negative mood regulation expectancies and depression following the end of a romantic relationship. *Journal of Personality and Social Psychology*, 60, 327–334.

Meloy, J. R. (Ed.). (1998). *The psychology of stalking: Clinical and forensic perspectives*. San Diego, CA: Academic Press.

Meloy, J. R., and Fisher, H. E. (2005). Some thoughts on the neurobiology of stalking. *Journal of Forensic Sciences*, 50(6), 1472–1480.

Najib, A., Lorberbaum, J. P., Kose, S., Bohning, D. E., and George, M. S. (2004). Regional brain activity in women grieving a romantic relationship breakup. *American Journal of Psychiatry*, 161(12), 2245–2256.

Ortigue, S., et al. (2007). The neural basis of love as a subliminal prime: An event-related functional magnetic resonance imaging study. *Journal of Cognitive Neuroscience*, 19, 1218–1230.

Panksepp, J. (1998). *Affective neuroscience: The foundations of human and animal emotions.* New York: Oxford University Press.

Pilastro, A. (2007). *Sesso ed evoluzione. La straordinaria storia evolutiva della riproduzione sessuale.* Milano: Bompiani.

Rosenthal, N. E. (2002). *The emotional revolution: How the new science of feelings can transform your life.* New York: Citadel Press Books.

Sternberg, R. J. (1986). A triangular theory of love. *Psychological Review*, 93(2), 119–135.

Tiihonen, J. et al. (1994). Increase in cerebral blood flow of right prefrontal cortex in men during orgasm. *Neuroscience Letters*, 170, 241–243.

Watson, P. J., and Andrews, P. W. (2002). Toward a revised evolutionary adaptationist analysis of depression: The social navigation hypothesis. *Journal of Affective Disorders*, 72, 1–14.

Xu, X., Aron, A., Brown, L. L., Cao, G., Feng, T., and Weng, X. (2011). Reward and motivation systems: A brain mapping study of early-stage intense romantic love in Chinese participants. *Human Brain Mapping*, 32(2), 249–257.

14

EMBODIED AND DISEMBODIED RATIONALITY: WHAT MORBID RATIONALISM AND HYPER-REFLEXIVITY TELL US ABOUT HUMAN INTELLIGENCE AND INTENTIONALITY

Giovanni Pennisi and Shaun Gallagher

1 Introduction

Traditional conceptions of the human mind rely on the assumption that what sets us apart from the other animal species is rationality. Since Aristotle, the ability to solve problems and to understand causal relationships between different events by means of deduction, syllogistic reasoning, and inference have been considered differential marks of our ontology. Thanks to our peculiar cerebral and anatomical configuration, we are the only living creatures that develop language-based skills such as judgement making, propositional knowledge, and mind-reading. These considerations have resulted in an "intellectualist view" (Noë, 2005, 2009, 2015), namely the misconception that "rational deliberation is the most basic kind of cognitive operation" (Noë, 2009: 99). There appear to be at least two fallacies intrinsic to this position. On the one hand, it seems to imply that logical thought is the first (if not the only) "mental tool" we resort to in order to face everyday challenges such as taking a decision or carrying out intentional, goal-directed actions. On the other hand, it both rests on and reinforces the common idea that the quality of being rational can be attributed only to those acts that depend upon the use and the mastery of language.

In this chapter, we will critically challenge the principles of this intellectualist picture not only by redefining the role that some of the correlates of our linguistic rationality have with respect to more basic, embodied mechanisms, but also by arguing that such mechanisms are foundational to a peculiar kind of intelligence. We will call this intelligence "embodied rationality" (Gallagher, 2018a) and argue that this concept does not aim at downgrading the importance of our highest cognitive functions, but rather at explaining how the latter integrate with a complex system of implicit forms of non-conceptual know-how. We will develop the concept of embodied rationality by exploring a phenomenological approach to perception and skilful performance; then, we will consider the case of schizophrenia, a pathology marked by a breakdown in the process of interaction between tacit and explicit knowledge and in which the embodied aspects of rational behaviour are suffocated by "a hypertrophy of intellectual and static tendencies" (Sass, 2001: 251), that is, what Minkowski (1927) has called "morbid rationalism". We will consider the notion of morbid rationalism and compare it to that of "hyper-reflexivity" (Sass, 1992, 2000) in order to show that the analysis of these phenomena is extremely useful for both revealing the detrimental effects of a lack of embodied rationality and assessing the relationship between the latter and our highest, logical, and reflective functions.

Finally, we will introduce the concept of *disembodied rationality* to account for the inability of the schizophrenic patients to optimize their bodily and cognitive responses to environmental inputs due to the interference of their hyper-reflexive attitude. This condition is reflected in two typical symptoms, namely the breakdown in body-schematic processes (Chapman, 1966; Fuchs and Schlimme, 2009) and the disruption of the protentional function of time consciousness (Fuchs, 2007; Stanghellini et al., 2016). The correlation between these phenomena will be addressed in the final part of the chapter.

2 Rationality and normativity

Following Stanovich (2011), we distinguish between a weak and a strong sense of rationality. The weak sense, which is the one underlying the dictionary definition, refers to the quality of being in accord with reason; it has its roots in the Aristotelian conception of man as the rational animal. Because we are the only species that can be in accord with reason (and violate, consciously or not, its principles), other animal species must be considered ontologically *arational* (de Sousa, 2007). In contrast, the strong sense, which is the one used in cognitive science (Stanovich, 2011), has a prescriptive value and is opposed to *irrationality*: "rationality (and irrationality) come in degrees defined by the distance of the thought or behavior from the optimum defined by a normative model" (3). This is the working definition of rationality we use throughout this chapter.

Whereas, according to Stanovich, the idea that rationality can be delineated as the extent to which our thoughts and actions adhere to a set of established rules sparks no controversy in cognitive science, there is no consensus as to whether these rules should be considered a linguistically organized form of knowledge or not. Such a disagreement, for example, can be found in the opposition between McDowell's (1994) view on the ubiquitous presence of concepts in our normative openness to the world, and the Husserlian tradition, which holds that perception is intrinsically normative, although not structured in propositional terms (Husserl, 2001; Crowell, 2013; Doyon, 2015a). What is at stake here is the notion of normativity itself, together with the possibility of determining to what degree language is implicated in it.

Following McDowell, the relation between mind and world is normative in the sense that we, as rational animals, are in the position to assess the truthfulness of our beliefs and to make judgements about things being so and so (McDowell, 1994: xii); in doing this, we provide a regularity (a norm) to the structure of perceptual content on the basis of the conceptual one. The way the world appears to us is thus determined by our intellectual understanding of it and by the pervasive power of our propositional knowledge. Importantly, the tendency to apply the principles of our linguistic competence is a constitutive element of perception, something we cannot even try to avoid doing:

> when we enjoy experience conceptual capacities are drawn on *in* receptivity, not exercised *on* some supposedly prior deliverances of receptivity. . . . In experience . . . one's conceptual capacities have already been brought into play, in the content's being available to one, before one has any choice in the matter.
>
> *(10)*

Therefore, McDowell establishes an intimate and indissoluble connection between language and perception, which is proven not only by the fact that we are always (at least in principle) capable of providing a justification for, say, thinking that we are looking at one particular object rather than another; most notably, this link emerges as a form of "conceptual shaping" (Siewert, 2013), a relationship in which the way things like chairs, apples, and nails appear to us depends on our knowing-that, namely our understanding that apples, chairs, and nails must have certain features in order to be defined as such. However, as Siewert noted:

> [I]t is left unclear why . . . the manner in which the nails appear, from which I judge them to be a certain way, could not have been experienced by those whose lack of inferential abilities would deprive them of any *concepts* of nail or length.
>
> *(201)*

Why, then, should we consider the set of rules in virtue of which a nail is a nail (i.e., its being short, sharp, and made of steel) a language-bound kind of normativity, if the same regularities could be assessed even by those who have no clue about what a nail is? Furthermore, one might wonder: is our conceptual knowing-that about objects a necessary condition for us to grasp how to use them, that is, our know-how? And what about the relationship between our explicit knowledge of the rules we have to follow in order to carry out skilful actions and the possibility to perform them? Do we need the former to secure the latter, as the intellectualists claim? These are the questions we are going to answer in the remainder of this chapter, relying on the phenomenological approach to the issue of normativity in perception and skilful performance.

2.1 The normative character of perception

The attempt to provide an account of our experiential openness to the world that could be "both non-conceptual and yet responsive to norms" (Crowell, 2013: 127) was one of Husserl's main aims. His descriptions of perceptual intentionality, in fact, "all draw upon normative vocabulary" (ibid.: 130). Traces of such a lexicon can be found, for example, in his lectures on transcendental logic, in which Husserl (2001) claims that

> there are originally prefigured ways [norms] of possible verification . . . intrinsic to the sense of every objectivity being experienced.
>
> *(266)*

> [There is] a universal regularity encompassing the course of lived-experiences, a regularity that prefigures a firm determination for future consciousness from past consciousness.
>
> *(267)*

> [T]he spatio-temporal world and the correlative regulation of the stream of consciousness not only exists, but exists precisely for the ego, . . . as a pre-givenness, an availability, as a readiness for possibilities of cognitive activity that are to follow.
>
> *(268)*

What emerges from these passages is Husserl's fundamental idea that understanding the norms that govern our interaction with the environment (the "norms of possible verification"), allowing us to anticipate or envisage what is to come in our perceptual experience, does not rely on our capacity to internalize these rules in propositional form and then put them to the test of reality, but rather depends on the intrinsic temporal structure of our consciousness. This issue was also addressed in Husserl's lectures on the phenomenology of the consciousness of internal time (1991), in which he explained that the content of an act of perception, for example, looking at a tree or hearing a melody, is never determined by the single sensorial datum we have access to in any given moment, such as the side of the tree we are in front of or the note that is being played now (see 355; also Gallagher and Zahavi, 2021: 83). On the contrary, every act of being directed at intentional objects, whether they are physical entities like trees or event phenomena like melodies, is characterized by the impression that these objects have a temporal extension and by a related anticipatory sense of what is to follow if, say, one circles around the tree to look at a part of it that is now hidden from sight, or continues to listen to the melody.

This way of experiencing the perceptual contents as a cohesive unity that transcends the present moment, unfolding in a temporal continuum that encompasses also our future dispositions towards what is there, depends on the peculiar nature of our consciousness, which, for Husserl, has the fundamental function of structuring the flow of time in three seamlessly integrating aspects: the *primal impression*, which is a mode of appearance of the intentional object that cannot provide us any temporal information about it, as it is constituted by every single 'now' in which a portion of the object is given to the senses; a *retention*, namely a particular kind of non-representational, "primary memory that continuously attaches itself to the [primal] impression" (Husserl, 1991: 32) and that, adding to the actual 'now' of every perception, allows us to experience the intentional object as a phenomenon that extends across a time span; and a *protention*, which is the intuition that something is about to happen in the very next phase of the perceptual process, an anticipation based upon the combination of the retentional sense of the just-past moments and manifests itself as the expectation we have towards the future modes of appearance of the object. Importantly, the protentional aspect is a feature of consciousness that is constitutive of our engagement with both familiar and unfamiliar entities. In this respect, it is sufficient to think about the first time we listen to a song: "it is not that we perceive only the present (and past) of the melody and then spontaneously *postulate* a future; we *perceive* the future of the melody – though the character of that perceived future may be more or less indeterminate" (Blaiklock, 2017: 473). Although it is true that in cases like this our protentions might be guided by some normative coordinates, such as the system of rules that takes the name of musical 'style' or 'genre', it is just as true that even those who have no conceptual awareness of these rules – for instance, those who ignore what a scale is or are unable to distinguish the sound of the notes – or have a very naïve and superficial acquaintance of that genre, may have "the vaguest of protentions of the future shape of the music" (475).[1]

The crucial point of Husserl's argumentation is that our normative openness to the world, that is to say, our sense of the rules that govern our perceptual relationship with the world and that enable us to grasp what to do with and what to expect from it, is not to be understood as the direct expression of some level of knowledge of these rules in the form of a knowing-that, but rather as the natural tendency to project ourselves into the future of our perceptions, anticipating more or less predictable outcomes that will "set the standards against which the agent's performances will be measured" (Doyon, 2015a: 45). Needless to say, the accuracy of the expectations on the basis of which we adapt our bodily and cognitive responses to the intentional object may depend on many factors, such as the number of previous interactions we've had with it or the context in which the action takes place, but this is not the point. What we want to highlight here is that the normative character of perception lies in its being structured in such a way so that it predisposes us to continually attribute what Husserl calls the "norms of possible verification" to our experience, not in its alleged function of confirming (or disconfirming) our propositional knowledge about the objects and the events we have access to. Therefore, perception is to be considered as having a basic, pre-predicative and intrinsic coherence, which is interdependent with what Husserl and Merleau-Ponty call 'operative', 'bodily', or 'motor' intentionality.

2.2 Operative intentionality and coherence in skilled action

Some of the disputes over the non-conceptual yet normative character of the perception of intentional objects also concern the field of skilful performance. There is no doubt that the ability to carry out bodily activities that require a high level of expertise – for example, following a choreography, driving a car, or playing tennis – is intrinsically normative, as it presupposes a deep knowledge of how one has to move one's body in order to reach a certain goal or to successfully combine the actions that make up the whole performance. Even in this case, however, there is no consensus as to what degree language or propositional knowledge is involved in accomplishing coherent or skilled movement. Whereas, as we will see subsequently, some proponents of intellectualism support the Aristotelian claim that "what makes an action an exercise of skill, rather than mere reflex, is the fact that it is guided by the intellectual apprehension of truths" (Stanley, 2011: 174), some representatives of the phenomenological approach to skilful performance hold that skilled performance rests on at least two, closely intertwined processes, each of which is independent of the intellectual apprehension of truth: body-schematic (intrinsic) control and a performative self-awareness (Gallagher, 2005a, 2017, 2018b, 2020a; Legrand, 2007).

The body schema enables the agent to immediately and pre-reflectively adapt bodily responses to perceptual inputs and to constantly readjust the position of the body – of the head, of the limbs, etc. – in order to have the best possible "grip" on or attunement to the environment, from both a perceptual and a practical point of view (Gallagher, 1986, 2005a). Examples of how the embodied agent follows "a schema of all types of perceptual unfolding to conform to the logic of the world" (see Merleau-Ponty, 2002: 380–381) can be found in an extremely wide range of circumstances. Consider the example of eyestrain when the body makes close to automatic postural and motor adjustments even before the subject becomes aware of the oncoming headache. In such cases body-schematic processes operate "prenoetically" (Gallagher, 2005a), and pre-reflectively, as they do in everyday walking or when we make voluntary and goal-targeted movements.

Here we note that the dynamic organization of the body schema is also structured by the same Husserlian conception of intrinsic temporality – the retentional, impressional, protentional structure. Thus, Merleau-Ponty, referencing this same structure, and following the neurologist Henry Head (1920), reconfirms that each present moment of the body-schematic process is 'charged with a relation' to what has happened before so that movement incorporates past moments into the present:

> At each successive instant of a movement, the preceding instant is not lost sight of. It is, as it were, dovetailed into the present, and present perception generally speaking consists in drawing together, on the basis of one's present position, the succession of previous positions, which envelop each other.
>
> *(Merleau-Ponty, 2002: 161)*

These retentional aspects of movement are further integrated into anticipatory or prospective aspects already noted:

> Each instant of the movement embraces its whole span, and particularly the first which, being the active initiative, institutes the link between a here and a yonder, a now and a future which the remainder of the instants will merely develop.
>
> *(ibid.: 161)*

These kinds of anticipatory processes pervade motoric actions; they can be found in hand–mouth coordination in infants, where the mouth opens to anticipate the hand (Butterworth and Hopkins, 1988; Lew and Butterworth, 1995); in visual tracking (Berthoz, 2000); in postural adjustments (Babinski, 1899); in fast correction of reaching and grasping movements (Georgieff and Jeannerod, 1998; Jeannerod, 2001; MacKay, 1966). Likewise, these dynamical aspects of the body schema involve a kind of intrinsic control attuned to worldly affordances and to the intentions of the agent. That is, they are not completely automatic; rather than being blindly repetitive of the same movement in each situation, the fine-tuned and non-conscious details of the body schema adjust to changes in the environment, and to changes in agentive intention (see Section 2.3). The fact that these prospective processes "are immanent in virtually everything we think or do seems inescapable" (Haith, 1993: 237).

Although the body schema is a system that involves close-to-automatic motor responses that, ontogenetically, start to form during fetal development (Gallagher, 2005b) and are responsible for phenomena such as early mouth–hand coordination and neonate responses to caregivers (Gallagher and Meltzoff, 1996), it is also characterized by a good level of flexibility. This is shown by empirical studies that have demonstrated the incorporation of tools and instruments, like rakes, sticks, and tennis rackets into the agent's body schema (Maravita and Iriki, 2004; Fourkas et al., 2008), or by the fact that one can train one's body schema, as when a dancer works on his coordination to improve his movements or when a tennis player learns new techniques.

The functioning of body-schematic processes by themselves, however, is not sufficient to account for the complexity of skilful practices. Contrary to what some anti-intellectualists maintain,[2] in fact, the "maximal grip" (Merleau-Ponty, 2002) that the expert performer has on the situation due to his fine-tuned motor control processes is not everything he needs. Skill within a context of, say, a cricket or a basketball game requires more, because the player "has to strategically take into account the precise situation (the layout of the field, the position of other players, the speed of the ball, and so forth) that involves a mindful sense of where she is going to put the ball" (Gallagher, 2020a: 46). This 'mindful sense' is what we may call performative (Gallagher, 2005a) or 'situated' (cf. Christensen et al., 2016) awareness.

Performative awareness involves both a heedful consciousness of one's surroundings and a tacit and pre-linguistic sense of "proximity" to the purpose of one's intentional actions. It is one's awareness of bodily and environmental aspects relevant to one's ongoing action, and is functionally meshed with body-schematic processes. It has its origins in the early stages of life, allowing the infant to correct and improve coordinated movement, for example. To have a performative awareness of, say, my hand using a joystick while I play a videogame, is not to have a reflective or intellectual attitude towards my hand, or even an explicit monitoring of my hand. It is rather an awareness that accompanies a know-how, a sense of what I can do in order to achieve my goals. In this respect, children and adults are similar, insofar as they are both guided by a sense of the ongoing course of the immediate action that provides them with a good grip on whether their goal-directed gestures are on target or not. Of course, this peculiar kind of sensitivity can be enhanced over time and with training. In the course of early development, infants learn what is reachable and graspable, how best to grasp a particular object, and so on. It is no coincidence, moreover, that experienced athletes are particularly good at detecting the correctness of their movements: one thinks, for example, of the basketball player who knows he missed a shot before the ball even touches the hoop and moves accordingly to get the rebound right away, or of the tennis player, who feels he has just hit the ball too short and immediately knows what he needs to do (at least approximately) to prepare for the return (see Doyon, 2015b).

Coping with the environment sometimes involves letting the flexible nature of our body-schematic processes guide some of our actions. The importance of letting oneself be guided in a pragmatic attunement enabled by the body schema is evident in both ordinary actions – such as walking – and skilful performances.[3] A number of theorists, however, point out that this body-schematic process is not sufficient to account for the complexity of what goes on in something like dance or athletic performance, because being engaged in a skilful practice always involves the performative awareness that one is moving or doing something in terms closer to an optimum defined by the agent's intentions and by the context itself (e.g., Christensen et al., 2016; Legrand, 2007; Montero, 2015; Shusterman, 2008). As we will see, these observations about body-schematic processes and performative awareness are enough for us to refuse the intellectualist position and pave the way to the development of an embodied approach to rationality (Gallagher, 2018a).

We will deepen and extend our understanding of how the concepts of body schema and performative awareness function in the next section. In Section 3, we will then show that these phenomena are extremely problematic in schizophrenia and how this is reflected in the emergence of a *disembodied* kind of rationality. Before that, however, we need to discuss what we mean by *embodied rationality* and how this notion may fit the working definition of rationality we have adopted.

2.3 Embodied rationality

When we describe rationality in terms of the 'proximity' of our thoughts and actions to an optimum defined by a normative model, we might assume that our conceptual understanding of what is contained in this system of rules – a form of knowing-that – plays a fundamental role. As a consequence, we might be prone to think that our ability to carry out skilful performances – our know-how – *depends* on our knowing-that. There are at least two possible interpretations of such a claim: the first is that, in order to become skilled in a certain practice – say, driving – one must first be able to assess the truthfulness of some propositions, such as the ones that prescribe the exact order in which we have to press the pedals or those that tell us how to coordinate the movement of the gear stick with that of the clutch. The second is that, assuming the importance of an intellectual apprehension of the norms in order to make their application possible, we may think that the former always precedes the latter, and that our performances can be defined as skilful only when our propositional knowledge about what it is correct to do or not to do guides our actions. In this view, "knowing how to perform a skill is simply a matter of knowing the appropriate propositions governing its instantiation" (Fridland, 2014: 2737).

The distinction between these two interpretations corresponds to the difference between what Noë (2015) calls the intellectualist insight (which he endorses) and the intellectualist thesis (which he rejects). Whereas the insight is somehow implicit to the position of the intellectualists (Williamson and Stanley, 2001; Stanley, 2011; Stanley and Krakauer, 2013), the thesis represents its epistemological core and, in Noë's opinion, an unnecessary stretch. Take, for instance, the following statement, which is meant to illustrate that motor skills depend on the knowledge of facts (Stanley and Krakauer, 2013):

> Part of having skill at throwing a curve ball is having the knowledge that throwing a curveball requires picking a baseball up (as well as knowing what to do with it when it is in your hand).
>
> *(5)*

If we were to read this example in light of the intellectualist insight, we should assume that throwing a curve ball is an ability that "requires training past baseline" (4), the result of a learning process that allowed the trainer's verbal instructions on how to position the single parts of the body and to shape the hand to turn into a complex motor skill. In this sense, it is true that know-how depends on the knowledge of facts, as it can be developed only after a phase during which the novice's understanding of what he is taught plays a key role and in which his need to "consult" the propositional knowledge he has acquired takes over physical action (see Stanley, 2011: 185). If, on the other hand, we were to read the example in light of the intellectualist thesis, we should suppose that being able to throw a curve ball is the same thing as having a certain number of beliefs about what one has to do with one's hand and body. Most notably, the thesis argues that it is precisely the kind of knowledge that gets expressed in judgement that guides the action (Stanley, 2011). The difference between the thesis and the insight is slight but fundamental and can be explained with another example, which takes into account the unpredictability of a dynamical context such as a tennis game.

According to Stanley and Krakauer (2013), when an expert tennis player switches from one technique to another – say, from a groundstroke to a drop shot – based on the position of the opponent, he is "injecting" in the ongoing course of the activity a peculiar kind of knowledge about that activity (ibid.: 4). This kind of knowledge is "the knowledge of what to do to initiate actions of that sort, [which is] a feature of skill that explains the fact that the manifestations of skill are intentional actions" (ibid.: 5). Therefore, for Stanley and Krakauer, skills are intentional – and, hence, a paradigmatic example of Aristotelian rationality – insofar as they are expressions of the agent's ability to voluntarily choose among a wide range of rule-based options that he has stored in terms of knowledge of facts about that activity, a form of propositional knowledge-that. This explanation, however, does not do justice to the nuanced complexity intrinsic to the concept of skill, for at least two, closely interrelated reasons: first, for any case one might think of, "knowing how to do something implies that you have the ability to do it (and vice versa), whereas the corresponding propositional knowledge has no such practical entailments" (Noë, 2015: 6); that is, of course, unless one wants to support the unlikely hypothesis that everyone who is able to read a manual or to follow the trainer's instructions is a virtually great performer.[4]

The second reason is that even knowing what to do to initiate an action, as well as deciding whether to resort to one action rather than another, can hardly be considered as a display of the knowledge required for expert performance, at least in the sense implied by the intellectualist thesis. As Fridland (2014) notices, in fact, it is difficult to fathom how single propositions with a generic value – i.e., "I know what to do to perform a groundstroke", or "I know that when the opponent does *x*, I have to do *y*" – could ever account for the elegant, precise, and fine-grained control exhibited in various manifestations of the skilled action (see 2743–2744). Being a skilful performer is most of all a matter of being able to turn one's well-trained and rule-based motor routines into adaptive, dynamic, and context-sensitive responses when needed, "of building and accessing flexible links between knowing and doing" (Sutton et al., 2011: 95). This ability, in turn, depends on the expert's capacity to keep track of the ongoing course of the performance, exercising a mindful control over the action that is made possible by the constant emergence of performative or situated awareness (discussed later). Therefore, although the intellectualists are right when they claim that some kind of conscious control is a necessary condition for a performance to be defined as skilful, "the mistake is to think that a performance is only rational if control is exerted in the mode of judgement, as if from outside" (Noë, 2015: 7).

Many authors (Fridland, 2014; Christensen et al., 2016; Montero, 2010, 2015; Hagendoorn, 2003) have focused on the different types of conscious control involved in athletic performances, providing several accounts of skilful practice that refuse rational intellectualism – as well as the idea that being an expert is just a matter of going on automatic pilot. For instance, Fridland counters the intellectualist thesis by saying that

> when a baseball pitcher decides to throw a curveball instead of a fastball, this decision is an instance of strategic control. Also . . . knowing what one has

> to do to in order to initiate an action is part of strategic control. . . . Strategic control [is what] guides motor skill by integrating fine-grained automatic routines with the personal-level goals and intentions of the agent.
>
> *(Fridland, 2014: 2744–2745)*

What Fridland calls strategic control over skilful actions is closely connected to performative awareness. Whereas performative awareness is the tacit sense of what one can or cannot do in order to reach specific goals, given the overall contextual circumstances, strategic control is what allows the agent to modulate and implement in the course of the performance the actions called forth by performative awareness. Fridland gives several examples of how strategic control governs the activity (see 2744–2746). In similar fashion, the concept of a *meshed architecture* put forward by Christensen et al. (2016) "proposes that controlled and automatic processes are closely integrated in skilled action, and that cognitive control directly influences motor execution in many cases" (43). One of the ways in which cognitive control exerts its influence is by a "parameterization of the action, or action 'gist'" (43–44), which is

> a particular way of performing the action appropriate to the circumstances. For instance, the soccer player may form a gist in kicking a pass that aims to put the ball into a particular area with a particular weighting that will wrong-foot a defender and allow a teammate to run onto the ball.
>
> *(43)*

Action gist clearly shows that knowing-how is much more than knowing what to do (i.e., to pass a ball) and when to do it, as it is a manifestation of skill that depends upon context sensitivity, individual differences, personal sub-goals, and other elements whose combination can be explained only by an approach that takes into account the role of performative awareness and the dynamical complexity of body-schematic processes (Gallagher and Aguda, 2020).

Another important feature of skilfulness that is enabled by performative awareness and body-schematic processes is selective attention (Fridland, 2014; Wu, 2014; Sutton et al., 2011), which can be described as the expert's proficiency in focusing only on those aspects of the perceptual scene that are relevant to the achievement of his goals. Selective attention is a fully-fledged part of skilfulness insofar as it improves over time and with training, as demonstrated by the neuroscientific data on the regional brain activity of novice sportsmen, who show a high activation in the areas implicated in "the maintenance of global, rather than selective attention . . . and a lack of attentional focus . . ., which contrasts with the highly selective motor system activation in the experts" (Milton et al., 2007: 810; see also Gray et al., 2004). Selective attention is neither the result of some sort of automatic reflex or mindless process nor the outcome of the agent's top-down voluntary decision to focus on some details rather than others; it is rather the result of a bottom-up intrinsic control (Gallagher and Varga, 2020). Body-schematic processes in expert performance are already context-sensitive, open, and adaptive, rather than automatic or general, and as such they elicit selective attention, a heedful, goal-oriented form of perceptual consciousness. In this regard, the mindfulness that includes performative awareness and selective attention is not imposed as a type of top-down cognition; it's rather something closer to an attuned habit. Habit, in this case, is, as Merleau-Ponty (2002) describes it, when the body acquires the power of responding with a certain type of solution to a certain form of situation. Instead of blind automatic repetition, habit is intrinsically intelligent and reflective of an operative or motor intentionality. That is, it involves an intelligence, a rationality built into the agent's bodily movement.

To sum up, we can state that skilfulness is the result of the interaction among various elements. First of all, it depends upon the normative character of our perception and bodily action. In Section 2.1, we presented the phenomenological argument that perception is normative as it is intrinsically linked to the temporal structure of consciousness, which provides us with an anticipatory sense of the (immediate) future modes of appearance of the intentional object. Extending this observation to the example of the expert tennis player, we can say that part of his expertise consists in perceiving the various salient details of the scene – the distance from the net, the other player's body language and position on court, etc. – as bearers of a protentional sense of action possibilities to efficiently counter the opponent's shots. As Crowell (2013) puts it

> the perceptual optimum of a tennis ball in flight is relative to the best place for my body to be in order to return it; . . . perception is feelingly guided by an optimum because it takes place in the context of practices in which the body seeks to improve its stance in, and by means of, its dealings with things in the world.
>
> *(145)*

Secondly, we can say that skilfulness depends upon the integration of body-schematic processes and performative awareness. One of the ways in which the expert improves his dealing with things in the world, in fact, is by attuning and enhancing both body-schematic processes – i.e., learning new basic techniques, getting better in the overall coordination, etc. – and the sense of goal-directedness of his actions – i.e., becoming more precise in discriminating whether his movements will be on target or not, or discovering new possibilities intrinsic to his own body (see Doyon, 2015a).

Lastly, we want to stress that every account of skilfulness should address the relationship between body-schematic processes, performative awareness, and phenomena such as strategic control, action gist, and selective attention – elements of the meshed architecture that makes bodily performance intelligent. This is because, in our view, only an agent who entertains a context-related awareness that he is moving or doing something in terms closer to his aims can develop a good sensitivity towards the way in which he has to modulate the actions or orient his attention.

Moreover, action gist and selective attention provide a valid explanation for the emergence of know-how, for they both represent a kind of "cognitive control on execution [that] is *not* through 'step-by-step' [viz. reflective, or procedural] control of the movement" (Christensen et al., 2016: 44), but rather manifests itself as a pre-reflective attunement to the situation that is refined with experience, practice, and the formation of intelligent habits.

The foregoing considerations about the nature of skilfulness bring us to a final, crucial point, namely that the processes involved in the carrying out of skilful activities are the same that govern intentional and goal-directed daily actions. In saying this, we are neither qualitatively nor quantitatively equating the abilities that are displayed during a challenging performance with the physical and cognitive requirements necessary to accomplish easy, targeted, motor tasks. Rather, we want to highlight that both skilful performances and everyday intentional, goal-directed actions rely on some shared, ontogenetically determined basic mechanisms. Take, for instance, the act of grasping an object to use it: on the one hand, grasping is one of those motor programs that are enabled by innate structures that generate body-schematic processes corresponding to elemental aspects of the movement (i.e., the extension of the arm or the rotation of the wrist, see Gallagher, 2005a: 48) and processes such as a primary form of proprioceptive, pre-reflective self-awareness (p. 76); on the other hand, grasping depends on more complex capacities that are refined with practice and differ according to the purpose the agent wants to achieve, for example, adjusting the hand to the shape of a glass in order to drink from it vs. adjusting the hand to the shape of a glass in order to throw it (see Ansuini et al., 2006, 2008). Of course, we are so accustomed to grasping objects in order to use them that, once this skill is mastered, it produces an almost irrelevant cognitive effort. However, this does not imply that, at some point, action gist and selective attention do not take place, but rather that they are 'absorbed' into the intelligent habits of bodily movement and our systematic engagement with things in the world.

Examples of how conscious processes like action gist and selective attention are integrated into the habitual functioning of the body schema through practice can be found in a range of motor acts extending from the simplest (e.g., reaching, grasping) to the complex (e.g., dressing, driving). The case of grasping, however, is sufficient to illustrate why the relationship between performative awareness and phenomena such as action gist and selective attention enables us to identify "a rationality that is intrinsic in the hand" (Gallagher, 2018a: 88). As an agent reaches to grasp an object to use it, his hand shapes itself into the right posture in a way that is close to automatic but yet perfectly appropriate to his purpose, showing that "central forms of flexible and adaptive actions which are clearly not the product of deliberation or explicit reflection can nonetheless be best understood as involving certain sorts of (dynamic, embodied) intelligence" (Sutton et al., 2011: 79). This peculiar kind of intelligence is explained by the fact that the hand is part of a brain-body system that is guided by an ongoing sense of goal-directedness of one's actions and by conscious processes that both draw on and update the body schema, allowing us to have a pre-reflective attunement to most of the relevant environmental contingencies. Therefore, when we talk of embodied rationality, we mean that our efficiency in reaching an optimum in everyday situations that are clearly rule or norm-based – like all goal-targeted actions – is not conditional upon the conceptual understanding or the explicit application of these rules, but rather depends on the embodiment of conscious mechanisms that are refined by simply being in the world.

3 Schizophrenia and disembodied rationality

In the previous section, we said that when we perform intentional, goal-directed actions:

a) The intrinsic temporal structure of our perception includes a primordial and vague anticipation of the future modes of appearance of events and objects in the world.
b) There is a pre-reflective attunement to objects and things in the world, thanks to the embodied processes involving action gist and selective attention. Such processes work along with and enhances the function of our body schema – that is to say, with time and practice, we become able to effortlessly carry out an increasing amount of intentional and goal-targeted actions.

These core features belong to a basic kind of intentionality usually characterized as motor intentionality, operative intentionality, and intentionality-in-action (see Gallagher, 2012; Pacherie, 2006), and help to explain why we can talk of an "embodied" kind of rationality, namely a "sensitivity towards the worldly norms" (Doyon, 2015a: 48) that manifests itself in our ability to reach an optimum in most of our everyday activities without recurring to an explicit (reflective or conceptual) recalling of the procedural rules we have to follow in order to perform goal-targeted actions.

Embodied rationality can fail in various circumstances and often in specific psychopathologies. Here we examine schizophrenia as one such failure. If the normative character of perception and the performative aspects of motor intentional behaviour can be defined as the foundations of our 'embodied rationality', then certain symptoms of schizophrenia can be considered as involving a 'disembodied' kind of rationality. Many authors, in fact, have proposed that the early stages of the illness are characterized by (1) a breakdown in the protentional function of time-consciousness (Fuchs, 2007; Stanghellini et al., 2016) and by (2) a disruption of body-schematic processes (Chapman, 1966; Fuchs, 2005; Fuchs and Schlimme, 2009), that is, a deficit in both selective attention and action gist.

(1) The disturbances in time perception of the schizophrenic subjects have been known for a long time. In his pivotal *Lived Time* (1970), Minkowski described the peculiar temporality experienced by schizophrenics as characterized by a perpetual

feeling of immobility that has been vividly captured by the words of one of his patients:

> There is an absolute fixity around me. I have even less mobility for the future than I have for the present and the past. There is a kind of routine in me which does not allow me to envisage the future. The creative power in me is abolished. I see the future as a repetition of the past.
>
> *(277)*

What Minkowski's patient depicts in terms of a pervasive and unescapable feeling of motionlessness is rooted in an initial impairment in the protentional function of consciousness. As Fuchs (2007) has noted, in fact, the prodromal stages of the schizophrenic syndrome are marked by the emergence of "gaps" in the temporal flow, gaps that "leave the patients with the task of 'rational reconstruction' of meaningful thinking or speaking" (233). One of the first symptoms that arises, thus, is a lack in the sense of being 'projected' towards the future modes of appearance of the intentional objects. For example, a patient of Bin Kimura (1994) complained about the fact that

> [w]hile watching TV . . ., though I can see every scene, I don't understand the plot. Every scene jumps to the next, there is no connection. The course of time is strange, too. Time splits up and doesn't run forward anymore.
>
> *(194)*

When interviewed, many other patients reported different kinds of unusual experience of the dynamics of time (see Sass et al., 2017: 22–26), expressing an overall inability to anticipate even the most predictable outcomes in the unfolding of perceptual events and a correlated condition of uncertainty that often resulted in a sense of anxiety or in the feeling that anything – but especially bad things – could happen. This deficit in the anticipatory function of consciousness was also experimentally tested. For example, Frith (1992; Frith and Done, 1988) showed that, during the execution of an intentional movement correction task, schizophrenics perform like normal subjects when they are provided with a visual feedback, but, unlike normal subjects, fail to correct their mistakes when they are deprived of such a feedback. In line with these findings, a study conducted by Singh et al. (1992) evidenced abnormal pre-movement brain potentials in schizophrenia, which the authors addressed as the effect of a dysfunction in those brain areas that are "associated with physiological constructs such as readiness, preparation, initiation, planning, volition and intention to act" (39).

Consistent with the foregoing data and with the observations made by Merleau-Ponty about the interdependency between the temporal structure of consciousness and operative intentionality (see Section 2.2), once the protentional function is impaired "even bodily movements appear 'out of the blue' and interrupt the intentional arc" (Fuchs, 2007: 234). This happens because the protentional function of consciousness is a necessary (even though not sufficient) condition for the sense of agency (see Gallagher, 2000: 222), that is, the pre-reflective sense of being the source or the willful initiator of my intentional action:

> [W]ithout protention, whatever intention I may have, whatever sense I would have of what I will do or think, what I *will* to do or to think, is disrupted. My non-observational, pre-reflective sense of agency, which is tied to control over my own actions, and control over my own thoughts, and which I normally experience within a protentional framework, will be deferred by the lack of protention.
>
> *(223)*

(2) In one of the most important papers on the issue of disorders of attention and perception in schizophrenia, McGhie and Chapman (1961) explained that, in the early stages of the disease, patients struggle to keep their attention focused on just one element of their surroundings. According to one of their patients, trying to concentrate is like "trying to do two or three different things at the one time" (104). Moreover, some of the subjects who were interviewed by the authors talked about a desynchronization between visual and auditory stimuli, whilst some others reported they could never avoid getting distracted from what they were doing or thinking about (see also Oltmanns, 1978). These symptoms were often accompanied by a failure in distinguishing between salient and secondary aspects of the scene (figure/ground reversal) and by a heightened awareness of background auditory sensations (see Sass et al., 2017). In other words, with the onset of the pathology, schizophrenics' attention is directed "not by the individual's volition but by the diffuse pattern of stimuli existing in the total environment situation" (McGhie and Chapman, 1961: 105). This lack of selective attention has the immediate effect of depriving the patients of their implicit know-how, preventing them from having a tacit understanding of how to perform actions in a way that is appropriate to the circumstances (action gist). As Chapman (1966) puts it, the patients

> appear to have lost access to previous learning so that they are often unable to initiate an action simply by contemplating its goal. Instead, their attention seems to be taken up with the intermediate steps, which now require conscious co-ordination. . . . The schizophrenic's psychomotor performance is consequently slow and deliberate and readily interfered with.
>
> *(240)*

The psychopathological literature is full of reports on subjects who suffer from a complete absence of spontaneity when it comes to perform even the automatized and easiest motor tasks. This symptom can be accounted as a deficit in action gist, because the pre-reflective control that is usually associated with intentional actions and that manifests itself as an effortless parameterization of the movements is superseded, in schizophrenia, by an exasperated thematic attention towards every aspect of the bodily action, a hyper-reflexive attitude (Sass, 1992, 2000) that takes over operative intentionality. This is shown, for example, by the following excerpts:

> I can't do simple habits like walking or cleaning my teeth. I have to use all my mind to do these things and sometimes I find myself . . . having to use tremendous control to direct my feet and force myself round a corner as if I'm on a bicycle.
>
> *(Chapman, 1966: 231)*

> I am not sure of my own movements anymore. It's very hard to describe this but at times I am not sure about even simple actions like sitting down. It's not so much thinking out what to do, it's the doing of it that sticks me.
>
> *(McGhie and Chapman, 1961: 107)*

> At times, I could do nothing without thinking about it. I could not perform any movement without having to think how I would do it.
>
> *(Fuchs and Röhricht, 2017:132)*

> If I do something like going for a drink of water, I've to go over each detail – find cup, walk over, turn tap, fill cup, turn tap off, drink it.
>
> *(Chapman, 1966: 239)*

The fundamental indication coming from the foregoing passages is that the performative dimension, as one of the first cornerstones on which the experience of the lived body is grounded, is impaired. In short, in the prodromal phase of the illness, patients start to feel overwhelmed by the pattern of perceptual stimuli that surrounds them, reporting a lack of fluency in the unfolding of time and events. The breakdown in the fluency of perceptual experience results in the loss of the dynamicity intrinsic to every action, a disruption of the pre-reflective, implicit control over one's movements that the patient tries to gain back through a deliberate and thematic reconstruction of the single steps he has to follow in order to carry out the action. However, this hyper-reflexive tendency towards one's body and movements has a counterproductive effect and "can easily become a kind of self-propagating spiral. The person who attempts, for example, to reassert control and re-establish a sense of self by means of introspective scrutiny may end up exacerbating his self-alienation and fragmentation" (Sass, 2001: 261).

Hyper-reflexivity is linked to another typical symptom of schizophrenia, namely what Minkowski (1927) has called *morbid rationalism*. Morbid rationalism is "an attitude comprising an effort to submit some or all aspects of life under [a set of] schematic and often algorithmic rules, typically associated with focus on irrelevant details" (Parnas, 2019: 4). Defined as such, morbid rationalism may be thought of as something very similar to hyper-reflexivity; however, there are a few important differences. First of all, whereas hyper-reflexivity is considered a phenomenon that is "equiprimordial" (Sass, 2000: 152) with the alteration in the implicit sense of being a source of intentionality (that is to say, they arise together and fuel each other, according to the spiral structure described previously), morbid rationalism has "a secondary status in relation to the decline of the 'intimate dynamism of our life' and of vital contact with reality" (Sass, 2001: 256) caused by the joint effect of hyper-reflexivity and the lack of intentionality. Secondly, whereas hyper-reflexivity is the exaggerated way in which "an agent or self takes itself or some aspect of itself as its own object of awareness" (Sass, 2000: 152), i.e., focusing on the different parts of one's body during a motor act, morbid rationalism is an exaggerated form of awareness that affects many (if not all) aspects of the patient's life. Morbid rationalism, in fact, is the tendency to see not only oneself, but other people and even objects as guided by merely logical rules; in this sense, morbid rationalism may be conceived as the more evident manifestation of the patient's "loss of natural self-evidence" (Blankenburg, 1971), as the paradigmatic example of what happens when rationality is reduced to simply knowing-that. Consider an example mentioned by Parnas et al. (2002):

> A famous vignette of a schizoid father, who buys, as a Christmas present for his dying daughter, a coffin, illustrates this odd friction. The act is rational from a formal-logical point of view, because a coffin is something that the daughter eventually is going to need, yet nevertheless it is bizarre by any ordinary human standard.
>
> *(132)*

This example shows not only why "schizophrenic rationalism is not merely an *exaggerated* rationalism, but one that lacks both the vitality and the flexibility or *souplesse* that is characteristic of human rationality in its more normal forms" (Sass, 2001: 256), but also why it is important to highlight the differences between hyper-reflexivity and morbid rationalism. These phenomena, in fact, represent two different "stages" of the patient's detachment from the embodied aspects of life. On the one hand, the hyper-reflexive attitude is a sort of "compensatory mechanism" through which the patient tries to make sense out of a world that starts to fall to pieces due to perceptual disturbances (fragmentation of the intentional arc, loss of selective attention); however, this mechanism has the immediate effect of further distancing the patient from the embodied and performative dimension of the self, i.e., preventing him from relying on the 'know-how' that manifests itself in action gist and leading him to parameterize the action in a deliberate way, in the form of "I need to think how to move my body to carry out even the most banal actions". On the other hand, morbid rationalism is a form of detachment from the social and intersubjective dimension of our being in the world (i.e., loss of common sense) that might be rooted in the hypertrophy of the tendency to objectify one's own bodily experience; therefore, morbid rationalism shows how fundamental it is for the subject to follow a rationality that is not only the application of logical or language-based rules, but rather is based in those embodied and pre-reflective processes that allow us to optimize our cognitive and bodily responses to the environment.

This last consideration is corroborated by the data on another symptom of schizophrenia, which is typically observed in patients with persecutory delusions: hyper-intentionality, namely the tendency to attribute an excessive amount of intentions to others and even to inanimate objects (Peyroux et al., 2014; Bara et al., 2011; Ciaramidaro et al., 2014; Backasch et al., 2013). Hyper-intentionality is an interesting phenomenon for two reasons: first of all, because it shows that the ability to understand other people's intentions is deeply interconnected to the concept of operative intentionality. As Fuchs (2005) puts it, in fact, "we use the operative intentionality of our body as an instrument for understanding the other's intentions" (99); therefore, if the patient's intentional arc and body-schematic process are impaired due to perceptual disturbances and hyper-reflexivity, it follows that even others' actions will be perceived as fragmented and will call forth an explicit, pseudo-logical explanation. Secondly, our ability to understand other people's intentions is another example of 'embodied rationality', because it is the product of the activity of the kind of bodily attunement associated with primary intersubjectivity (Trevarthen, 1979; Gallagher, 2020b) and of our practical attunement to the world and to others that comes with experience. Traditionally, however, it has been explained as a form of 'linguistic' or 'intellectual' competence (Theory of Mind), which ignores embodied rationality. Here again, well-known problems with social cognition in schizophrenia[5] suggest that hyper-intentionality can be accounted for as one of the effects of the breakdown in the embodied processes of operative intentionality and the social forms of understanding that are deeply rooted in the embodied and performative aspects of intentional behaviour.

4 Conclusion

In this chapter, we showed how the phenomenology of perception and the study of skilled performance can challenge the principles of the intellectualist picture of rationality, first by delineating the intrinsic temporal-normative patterns that characterize perception and its embodied mechanisms, and second, by arguing that such mechanisms are foundational to the peculiar kind of intelligence we called 'embodied rationality'. We argued that embodied rationality does not downgrade the importance of our higher order cognitive functions, but rather explains how the latter integrate with a complex system of implicit forms of non-conceptual know-how which include body-schematic processes, performative awareness, and such intrinsic aspects involving strategic control, selective attention, and action gist. We then considered how schizophrenia involves a breakdown in the processes of interaction between tacit and explicit knowledge such that the embodied aspects of rational behaviour are distorted by hyper-reflexivity, hyper-intentionality, and morbid rationalism. We suggested that such disruptions lead to a form of inflexible *disembodied rationality* that prevents schizophrenic patients from optimizing their bodily and cognitive engagements with their environment. As evidenced in clinical reports, symptoms of this kind of disembodied rationality include a breakdown in operative intentionality, and specifically in body-schematic processes, and the disruption of the protentional function of time consciousness.

Notes

1 This point about following a rule is more generally, of course, a famous point also made by Wittgenstein. See, e.g., Gallagher (2020c).

2 The harshest critic of intellectualism is Hubert Dreyfus, who is well known for claiming that what distinguishes the novice, the advanced beginner, and the competent person from the expert is the fact that, whereas the former three need to think while they act, the latter does not rely on any kind of mindful process and "acts arationally" (Dreyfus and Dreyfus, 2000: 36). Following this line of thought, Dreyfus defines expert performers as "absorbed copers" (see Dreyfus, 2002, 2007) whose skilfulness lies precisely in their capacity to "ignore" the rules they know and to let themselves go to the automatisms acquired during the many hours of practice. We do not have enough room to provide a critical account of Dreyfus' position (see Gallagher, 2018b; Montero, 2010; Sutton et al., 2011); however, we want to highlight that some authors (Noë, 2015; Fridland, 2014; Sutton et al., 2011) have noticed that intellectualism and the anti-intellectualist view of Dreyfus, rather than being opposite poles, can be considered as the two sides of the same coin, for they both misrepresent the role played by cognition in the carrying out of skillful performances.

3 In a series of interviews conducted by Høffding (2018) with the Danish String Quartet, some of the musicians reported that in certain occasions "you [just] let the body function on its own. . . . You're surprised about how much the fingers remember themselves. Let the fingers play. Just use the activity of the brain not on what you're playing. Let go and think about something else" (198–199). As Høffding explains, however, this is just one of the several modalities of experiencing one's engagement with the performance that an expert musician may undergo; many others, conversely, require mindfulness and situation awareness.

4 In order to avoid such a controversial position, Stanley and Krakauer claim that skills also require "motor acuity" (Shmuelof et al., 2012), namely those "practice-related reductions in movement variability and increases in movement smoothness" (Stanley and Krakauer, 2013: 7) that are involuntary, mechanistic, and independent of the agent's attention. However, as Fridland (2014) argues, adding motor acuity to the equation does not make the intellectualist account of skillful performance more accurate. To prove this point, Fridland uses the following example: "Carrie wants to improve her basketball playing skills. Carrie has played basketball before . . . [Therefore] she knows that in order to play basketball, she needs a basketball and a basket and she needs to pick up the basketball in order to start playing (that is, she knows how to initiate her basketball playing actions), and she also knows how to hold the basketball and shoot and dribble. . . . Now, if all there is to developing her expertise at basketball is knowing these things plus improving her low-level motor acuity, say, reducing the variability in the trajectory of her finger, wrist, and elbow movements, then Carrie is as skilled before she practices as after. This is because reducing the variability in her movements is just basic, non-epistemic, non-intelligent procedural stuff and skill is not this sort of stuff but knowledge – it is knowledge how. If this is right, however, then the intelligence of skilled action and the intelligence of unpracticed intentional actions are exactly the same" (2743).

5 As Parnas et al. (2002) indicate, "the dimension of intersubjectivity is also fundamentally impaired (disorders of social and interpersonal functioning, inappropriate behavior). These three dimensions are inseparable: I, we, and the world belong together – and they are all afflicted in the schizophrenic autism" (132).

References

Ansuini, C., Giosa, L., Turella, L., Altoè, G., and Castiello, U. (2008). An object for an action, the same object for other actions: Effects on hand shaping. *Experimental Brain Research*, 185(1), 111–119.

Ansuini, C., Santello, M., Massaccesi, S., and Castiello, U. (2006). Effects of end-goal on hand shaping. *Journal of Neurophysiology*, 95, 2456–2465.

Babinski, J. (1899). De l'asynergie cérébelleuse. *Revue de Neurologie*, 7, 806–816.

Backasch, B., Straube, B., Pyka, M., Klöhn-Saghatolislam, F., Müller, M. J., Kircher, T. T., and Leube, D. T. (2013). Hyperintentionality during automatic perception of naturalistic cooperative behavior in patients with schizophrenia. *Social Neuroscience*, 8(5), 489–504.

Bara, B. G., Ciaramidaro, A., Walter, H., and Adenzato, M. (2011). Intentional minds: A philosophical analysis of intention tested through fMRI experiments involving people with schizophrenia, people with autism, and healthy individuals. *Frontiers in Human Neuroscience*, 5, 7.

Berthoz, A. (2000). *The brain's sense of movement*. Cambridge, MA: Harvard University Press.

Blaiklock, J. (2017). Husserl, protention, and the phenomenology of the unexpected. *International Journal of Philosophical Studies*, 25(4), 467–483.

Blankenburg, W. (1971). *Der Verlust der natürlichen selbstverständlichkeit: ein Beitrag zur Psychopathologie symptomarmer Schizophrenien*. Stuttgart: Enke.

Butterworth, G., and Hopkins, B. (1988). Hand-mouth coordination in the newborn baby. *British Journal of Developmental Psychology*, 6, 303–314.

Chapman, J. (1966). The early symptoms of schizophrenia. *The British Journal of Psychiatry*, 112(484), 225–251.

Christensen, W., Sutton, J., and McIlwain, D. J. (2016). Cognition in skilled action: Meshed control and the varieties of skill experience. *Mind and Language*, 31(1), 37–66.

Ciaramidaro, A., Bölte, S., Schlitt, S., Hainz, D., Poustka, F., Weber, B., . . . and Walter, H. (2015). Schizophrenia and autism as contrasting minds: Neural evidence for the hypo-hyper-intentionality hypothesis. *Schizophrenia Bulletin*, 41(1), 171–179.

Crowell, S. G. (2013). *Normativity and phenomenology in Husserl and Heidegger*. Cambridge: Cambridge University Press.

De Sousa, R. (2007). *Why think? Evolution and the rational mind*. Oxford: Oxford University Press.

Doyon, M. (2015a). Perception and normative self-consciousness. In M. Doyon and T. Breyer (Eds.), *Normativity in perception* (pp. 38–55). London: Palgrave Macmillan.

Doyon, M. (2015b). Intentionality and normativity. *International Journal of Philosophical Studies*, 23(2), 279–295.

Dreyfus, H. L. (2002). Intelligence without representation: Merleau-Ponty's critique of mental representation The relevance of phenomenology to scientific explanation. *Phenomenology and the Cognitive Sciences*, 1(4), 367–383.

Dreyfus, H. L. (2007). The return of the myth of the mental. *Inquiry*, 50(4), 352–365.

Dreyfus, H. L., and Dreyfus, S. E. (2000). *Mind over machine: The power of human intuition and expertise in the era of the computer*. New York: Free Press.

Fourkas, A. D., Bonavolontà, V., Avenanti, A., and Aglioti, S. M. (2008). Kinesthetic imagery and tool-specific modulation of corticospinal representations in expert tennis players. *Cerebral Cortex*, 18(10), 2382–2390.

Fridland, E. (2014). They've lost control: Reflections on skill. *Synthese*, 191(12), 2729–2750.

Frith, C. D. (1992). *The cognitive neuropsychology of schizophrenia*. Hove: LEA.

Frith, C. D., and Done, D. J. (1988). Towards a neuropsychology of schizophrenia. *The British Journal of Psychiatry*, 153(4), 437–443.

Fuchs, T. (2005). Corporealized and disembodied minds: A phenomenological view of the body in melancholia and schizophrenia. *Philosophy, Psychiatry, and Psychology*, 12(2), 95–107.

Fuchs, T. (2007). The temporal structure of intentionality and its disturbance in schizophrenia. *Psychopathology*, 40(4), 229–235.

Fuchs, T., and Röhricht, F. (2017). Schizophrenia and intersubjectivity: An embodied and enactive approach to psychopathology and psychotherapy. *Philosophy, Psychiatry, and Psychology*, 24(2), 127–142.

Fuchs, T., and Schlimme, J. E. (2009). Embodiment and psychopathology: A phenomenological perspective. *Current Opinion in Psychiatry*, 22(6), 570–575.

Gallagher, S. (1986). Body image and body schema: A conceptual clarification. *The Journal of Mind and Behavior*, 541–554.

Gallagher, S. (2000). Self reference and schizophrenia. *Exploring the Self*, 203–239.

Gallagher, S. (2005a). *How the body shapes the mind*. Oxford: Oxford Scholarship Online.

Gallagher, S. (2005b). Dynamic models of body schematic processes. In H. De Preester and V. Knockaert (Eds.), *Body image and body schema*. Amsterdam: John Benjamins Publishers.

Gallagher, S. (2012). Multiple aspects of agency. *New Ideas in Psychology*, 30, 15–31.

Gallagher, S. (2017). Theory, practice and performance. *Connection Science*, 29(1), 106–118.

Gallagher, S. (2018a). Embodied rationality. In G. Bronner and F. Di Iorio (Eds.), *The mystery of rationality: Mind, beliefs and the social sciences*. Cham: Springer.

Gallagher, S. (2018b). Mindfulness and mindlessness in performance. *Reti, saperi, linguaggi*, (1), 5–18.

Gallagher, S. (2020a). Mindful performance. In A. Pennisi and A. Falzone (Eds.), *The extended theory of cognitive creativity: Interdisciplinary approaches to performativity*. Cham: Springer.

Gallagher, S. (2020b). *Action and interaction*. Oxford: Oxford University Press.

Gallagher, S. (2020c). To follow a rule: Lessons from baby logic. In D. Weinstock and J. Levy (Eds.), *Interpreting modernity: Essays in honor of Charles Taylor*. Montreal: McGill-Queen's University Press.

Gallagher, S., and Aguda, B. (2020). Anchoring know-how: Action, affordance and anticipation. *Journal of Consciousness Studies*, 27(3–4), 3–37.

Gallagher, S., and Meltzoff, A. N. (1996). The earliest sense of self and others: Merleau-Ponty and recent developmental studies. *Philosophical Psychology*, 9(2), 211–233.

Gallagher, S., and Varga, S. (2020). The meshed architecture of performance as a model of situated cognition. *Frontiers in Psychology* 11: 2140. doi: 10.3389/fpsyg.2020.02140

Gallagher, S., and Zahavi, D. (2021). *The phenomenological mind* (3rd Edition). London: Routledge.

Georgieff, N., and Jeannerod, M. (1998). Beyond consciousness of external reality: A 'who' system for consciousness of action and self-consciousness. *Consciousness and Cognition*, 7(3), 465–477.

Gray, R. (2004). Attending to the execution of a complex sensorimotor skill: Expertise differences, choking, and slumps. *Journal of Experimental Psychology: Applied*, 10(1), 42–54.

Hagendoorn, I. (2003). Cognitive dance improvisation: How study of the motor system can inspire dance (and vice versa). *Leonardo*, 36(3), 221–228.

Haith, M. M. (1993). Future-oriented processes in infancy: The case of visual expectations. In C. Granrud (Ed.), *Carnegie-Mellon symposium on visual perception and cognition in infancy*. Hillsdale, NJ: Lawrence Erlbaum Associates.

Head, H. (1920). *Studies in neurology*, Vol. 2. London: Oxford University Press.

Høffding, S. (2018). *A phenomenology of musical absorption*. Cham: Springer International Publishing.

Husserl, E. (1991). *On the phenomenology of the consciousness of internal time (1893–1917).* Dordrecht: Kluwer Academic.

Husserl, E. (2001). *Analyses concerning passive and active synthesis: Lectures on transcendental logic.* Dordrecht: Kluwer Academic Publishers.

Jeannerod, M. (2001). Neural simulation of action: A unifying mechanism for motor cognition. *Neuroimage*, 14, S103–S109.

Kimura, B. (1994). Psychopathologie der Zufaelligkeit oder Verlust des Aufenthaltsortes beim Schizophrenen. *Daseinsanalyse*, 11, 192–204.

Legrand, D. (2007). Pre-reflective self-consciousness: On being bodily in the world. *Janus Head*, 9(2), 493–519.

Lew, A., and Butterworth, G. E. (1995). Hand-mouth contact in newborn babies before and after feeding. *Developmental Psychology*, 31, 456–463.

MacKay, D. (1966). Cerebral organization and the conscious control of action. In J. C. Eccles (Ed.), *Brain and conscious experience.* New York: Springer.

Maravita, A., and Iriki, A. (2004). Tools for the body (schema). *Trends in Cognitive Sciences*, 8(2), 79–86.

McDowell, J. (1994). *Mind and world.* Cambridge, MA: Harvard University Press.

McGhie, A., and Chapman, J. (1961). Disorders of attention and perception in early schizophrenia. *British Journal of Medical Psychology*, 34(2), 103–116.

Merleau-Ponty, M. (2002). *Phenomenology of perception.* London: Routledge Classics.

Milton, J., Solodkin, A., Hluštík, P., and Small, S. L. (2007). The mind of expert motor performance is cool and focused. *Neuroimage*, 35(2), 804–813.

Minkowski, E. (1927). *La schizophrénie: Psychopathologie des schizoides et des schizophrènes.* Paris.

Minkowski, E. (1970). *Lived time: Phenomenological and psychopathological studies.* Evanston, IL: Northwestern University Press.

Montero, B. (2010). Does bodily awareness interfere with highly skilled movement? *Inquiry*, 53(2), 105–122.

Montero, B. G. (2015). Thinking in the zone: The expert mind in action. *The Southern Journal of Philosophy*, 53, 126–140.

Noë, A. (2005). Against intellectualism. *Analysis*, 65(4), 278–290.

Noë, A. (2009). *Out of our heads: Why you are not your brain, and other lessons from the biology of consciousness.* New York: Hill and Wang.

Noë, A. (2015). Concept pluralism, direct perception, and the fragility of presence. In T. Metzinger and J. M. Windt (Eds.), *Open MIND.* Frankfurt am Main: MIND Group.

Oltmanns, T. F. (1978). Selective attention in schizophrenic and manic psychoses: The effect of distraction on information processing. *Journal of Abnormal Psychology*, 87(2), 212–225.

Pacherie, E. (2006). Towards a dynamic theory of intentions. In S. Pockett, W. P. Banks, and S. Gallagher (Eds.), *Does consciousness cause behavior? An investigation of the nature of volition.* Cambridge, MA: MIT Press.

Parnas, A. F. U. (2019). Eugéne Minkowski. In G. Stanghellini, M. R. Broome, A. V. Fernandez, P. Fusar-Poli, A. Raballo, and R. Rosfort (Eds.), *Oxford handbook of phenomenological psychopatology.* Oxford: Oxford University Press.

Parnas, J., Bovet, P., and Zahavi, D. (2002). Schizophrenic autism: Clinical phenomenology and pathogenetic implications. *World Psychiatry*, 1(3), 131.

Peyroux, E., Strickland, B., Tapiero, I., and Franck, N. (2014). The intentionality bias in schizophrenia. *Psychiatry Research*, 219(3), 426–430.

Sass, L. A. (1992). *Madness and modernism: Insanity in the light of modern art, literature, and thought.* New York: Basic Books.

Sass, L. A. (2000). Schizophrenia, self-experience, and the so-called negative symptoms. In D. Zahavi (Ed.), *Exploring the self: Philosophical and psychopathological perspectives on self-experience*. Amsterdam: Benjamins.

Sass, L. A. (2001). Self and world in schizophrenia: Three classic approaches. *Philosophy, Psychiatry, and Psychology*, 8(4), 251–270.

Sass, L., Pienkos, E., Skodlar, B., Stanghellini, G., Fuchs, T., Parnas, J., and Jones, N. (2017). EAWE: Examination of anomalous world experience. *Psychopathology*, 50(1), 10–54.

Shmuelof, L., Krakauer, J. W., and Mazzoni, P. (2012). How is a motor skill learned? Change and invariance at the levels of task success and trajectory control. *Journal of Neurophysiology*, 108(2), 578–594.

Shusterman, R. (2008). *Body consciousness: A philosophy of mindfulness and somaesthetics*. Cambridge: Cambridge University Press.

Siewert, C. (2013). Intellectualism, experience, and motor understanding. In J. K. Schear (Ed.), *Mind, reason, and being-in-the-world: The McDowell-Dreyfus debate*. Abingdon, OX: Routledge.

Singh, J., Knight, R. T., Rosenlicht, N., Kotun, J. M., Beckley, D. J., and Woods, D. L. (1992). Abnormal premovement brain potentials in schizophrenia. *Schizophrenia Research*, 8(1), 31–41.

Stanghellini, G., Ballerini, M., Presenza, S., Mancini, M., Raballo, A., Blasi, S., and Cutting, J. (2016). Psychopathology of lived time: Abnormal time experience in persons with schizophrenia. *Schizophrenia Bulletin*, 42(1), 45–55.

Stanley, J. (2011). *Know how*. Oxford: Oxford University Press.

Stanley, J., and Krakauer, J. W. (2013). Motor skill depends on knowledge of facts. *Frontiers in Human Neuroscience*, 7(503), 1–11.

Stanovich, K. E. (2011). *Rationality and the reflective mind*. Oxford: Oxford University Press.

Sutton, J., McIlwain, D., Christensen, W., and Geeves, A. (2011). Applying intelligence to the reflexes: Embodied skills and habits between Dreyfus and Descartes. *Journal of the British Society for Phenomenology*, 42(1), 78–103.

Trevarthen, C. (1979). Communication and cooperation in early infancy: A description of primary intersubjectivity. In M. Bullowa (Ed.), *Before speech: The beginning of interpersonal communication*. Cambridge: Cambridge University Press.

Williamson, T., and Stanley, J. (2001). Knowing how. *The Journal of Philosophy*, 98(8), 1–40.

Wu, W. (2014). *Attention*. London: Routledge.

INDEX

Note: Page numbers in *italics* indicate a figure and page numbers in **bold** indicate a table on the corresponding page.

For Product Safety Concerns and Information please contact our EU
representative GPSR@taylorandfrancis.com
Taylor & Francis Verlag GmbH, Kaufingerstraße 24, 80331 München, Germany

www.ingramcontent.com/pod-product-compliance
Lightning Source LLC
LaVergne TN
LVHW021120300926
849160LV00010B/794

* 9 7 8 0 3 6 7 4 4 4 5 8 7 *